Quick

Reference Guide

for Using

Essential Oils

Connie and Al

This book has been designed to provide information to help educate the reader in regard to the subject matter covered. It is sold with the understanding that the publisher and the authors are not liable for the misconception or misuse of the information provided. It is not provided in order to diagnose, prescribe, or treat any disease, illness, or injured condition of the body. The authors and publisher shall have neither liability nor responsibility to any person or entity with respect to any loss, damage, or injury caused or alleged to be caused directly or indirectly by the information contained in this book. The information presented herein is in no way intended as a substitute for medical counseling. Anyone suffering from any disease, illness, or injury should consult a qualified health care professional.

Library of Congress Cataloging-in-Publication Data.

Higley, Connie.
       Quick reference guide for using essential oils / Connie and Alan Higley.
           p. cm.
       Includes bibliographical references and index.
       1. Essences and essential oils–Therapeutic use–Handbooks, manuals, etc.
       2. Aromatherapy–Handbooks, manuals, etc. I. Title.

       RM666.A68 H543 1998
       615/.321–dc21

                                  99-191655

Published and distributed by Abundant Health
P.O. Box 281 Spanish Fork, UT 84660
Phone: 1-888-718-3068 / 801-705-4831
Fax: 1-877-568-1988 / 801-705-4830
Internet: www.abundant-health4u.com
E-Mail: orders@abundant-health4u.com

Printed and bound in the United States of America

International Standard Book Number: 0-9706583-1-1

Dedication

We, the authors (compilers) of this information, were introduced to Young Living Essential Oils in 1995. At that time, there was no compiled information on the use of these valuable oils, so together with Pat Leatham, we set out to find what we could. We gathered notes from lectures and seminars by D. Gary Young, N.D. and product information from Young Living Essential Oils. Extensive research into the works of other aromatherapy experts have shown us that Dr. Young, through his own research and clinical study, not only supports, but expands their solid foundation of knowledge and expertise. When this book was first made available in 1996, we made a conscious decision to keep the names of D. Gary Young and Young Living Essential Oils out of this book so as to remove all possibility of recrimination or harm to Dr. Young or his company. However, all past, present, and future readers of this work need to understand that all of us, author and reader alike, are deeply indebted to Dr. Young for his brilliant insight, extensive research, and incredible vision of the healing power of essential oils.

We, therefore, dedicate this book to D. Gary Young, N.D. as a tribute to his vision of health for all who will embrace the oils and use them to their fullest potential. Dr. Young is one of the foremost experts on the organic cultivation, distillation, and clinical use of essential oils in North America. His unwavering passion for maintaining the highest quality in his products have produced some astounding healing results. We applaud his heroic and often solitary effort to continue proving, by clinical study, the efficacy of essential oils as indispensable tools for combating disease.

Acknowledgments

To our 5 young children who demonstrate much patience and responsibility with the freedom they are given during the on-going compilation and updating of this book.

To the late Pat Leatham who provided the initial impetus for its creation.
Her many hours of research and meticulous note-taking will forever be appreciated.

And to all of you who are discovering, or re-discovering, for yourselves the healing powers of essential oils. May this book provide quick access to the information you need to help yourself, and those you love, progress on the road to better health.

A special thanks goes to our families and to all of our "Essential Oil" friends! Without your love, suggestions, support, and patience, we would have crumbled under the strain of compiling a book such as this while trying to raise a family and have a life.

Contents

The section tabs in the personal guide section, correspond to the alphabetical listing of health topics. By holding the spine of the book in the left hand and bending the right side back with the right hand, section markings become visible along the right edge. This should allow you quick and easy reference to any particular topic.

FACTS ABOUT ESSENTIAL OILS

How long have essential oils been around?

Essential oils were mankind's first medicine. From Egyptian hieroglyphics and Chinese manuscripts, we know that priests and physicians have been using essential oils for thousands of years. In Egypt, essential oils were used in the embalming process and well preserved oils were found in alabaster jars in King Tut's tomb. Egyptian temples were dedicated to the production and blending of the oils and recipes were recorded on the walls in hieroglyphics. There is even a sacred room in the temple of Isis on the island of Philae where a ritual called "Cleansing the Flesh and Blood of Evil Deities" was practiced. This form of emotional clearing required three days of cleansing using particular essential oils and oil baths.

There are 188 references to essential oils in the Bible. Oils such as frankincense, myrrh, rosemary, hyssop, and spikenard were used for anointing and healing the sick. In Exodus, the Lord gave the following recipe to Moses for "an holy anointing oil":

Myrrh ("five hundred shekels"— approximately 1 gallon)
Sweet Cinnamon
    ("two hundred and fifty shekels"— approximately ½ gallon)
Sweet Calamus ("two hundred and fifty shekels")
Cassia ("five hundred shekels")
Olive Oil ("an hin"— approximately 1⅓ gallons)

The three wise men presented the Christ child with essential oils of frankincense and myrrh. There are also accounts in the New Testament of the Bible where Jesus was anointed with spikenard oil; "And being in Bethany in the house of Simon the leper, as he sat at meat, there came a woman having an alabaster box of ointment of spikenard very precious; and she brake the box, and poured [it] on his head" (Mark 14:3). "Then took Mary a pound of ointment of spikenard, very costly, and anointed the feet of Jesus, and wiped his feet with her hair: and the house was filled with the odour of the ointment" (John 12:3).

What are *PURE, THERAPEUTIC-GRADE* essential oils?

Essential oils are the volatile liquids that are distilled from plants (including their respective parts such as seeds, bark, leaves, stems, roots, flowers, fruit, etc.). One of the factors that determine the purity of an oil is its chemical constituents. These constituents can be affected by a vast number of variables including: the part(s) of the plant from which the oil was produced, soil condition, fertilizer (organic or chemical), geographical region, climate, altitude, harvest season and methods, and distillation process. For example, common thyme, or thyme vulgaris, produces several different chemotypes (biochemical specifics or simple species) depending on the conditions of its growth, climate, and altitude. One will produce high levels of thymol depending on the time of year it is distilled. If distilled during mid-summer or late fall, there can be higher levels of carvacrol which can cause the oil to be more caustic or irritating to the skin. Low pressure and low temperature are also keys to maintaining the purity, the ultimate fragrance, and the therapeutic value of the oil.

As we begin to understand the power of essential oils in the realm of personal, holistic healthcare, we comprehend the absolute necessity for obtaining the purest essential oils possible. No matter how costly pure essential oils may be, there can be no substitutes. Chemists have yet to successfully recreate essential oils in the laboratory.

The information in this book is based upon the use of pure, therapeutic-grade essential oils. Those who are beginning their journey into the realm of aromatherapy and essential oils, must actively seek for the purest quality and highest therapeutic-grade oils available. Anything less than pure, therapeutic-grade essential oil may not produce the desired results and can, in some cases, be extremely toxic.

Why is it so difficult to find *PURE, THERAPEUTIC-GRADE* essential oils?

Producing the purest of oils can be very costly because it may require several hundred pounds, or even several thousand pounds of plant material to extract one pound of pure essential oil. For example, one pound of pure melissa oil sells for $9,000 - $15,000. Although this sounds quite expensive, one must realize that three tons of plant material are required to produce that single pound of oil. Because the vast majority of all the oils produced in the world today are used by the perfume industry, the oils are being purchased for their aromatic qualities only. High pressure, high temperatures, rapid processing and the use of chemical solvents are often employed during the distillation process so that a greater *quantity* of oil can be produced at a faster rate. These oils may smell just as good and cost much less, but will lack most, if not all, of the chemical constituents necessary to produce the expected therapeutic results.

What benefits do *PURE, THERAPEUTIC-GRADE* essential oils provide?

1. Essential oils are the regenerating, oxygenating, and immune defense properties of plants.
2. Essential oils are so small in molecular size that they can quickly penetrate the tissues of the skin.
3. Essential oils are lipid soluble and are capable of penetrating cell walls, even if they have hardened because of an oxygen deficiency. In fact, essential oils can affect every cell of the body within 20 minutes and are then metabolized like other nutrients.
4. Essential oils contain oxygen molecules which help to transport nutrients to the starving human cells. Because a nutritional deficiency is an oxygen deficiency, disease begins when the cells lack the oxygen for proper nutrient assimilation. By providing the needed oxygen, essential oils also work to stimulate the immune system.
5. Essential oils are very powerful antioxidants. Antioxidants create an unfriendly environment for free radicals. They prevent all mutations, work as free radical scavengers, prevent fungus, and prevent oxidation in the cells.
6. Essential oils are anti-bacterial, anti-cancerous, anti-fungal, anti-infectious, anti-microbial, anti-tumoral, anti-parasitic, anti-viral, and antiseptic. Essential oils have been shown to destroy all tested bacteria and viruses while simultaneously restoring balance to the body.
7. Essential oils may detoxify the cells and blood in the body.
8. Essential oils containing sesquiterpenes have the ability to pass the blood brain barrier, enabling them to be effective in the treatment of Alzheimer's disease, Lou Gehrig's disease, Parkinson's disease, and multiple sclerosis.
9. Essential oils are aromatic. When diffused, they provide air purification by:
   A. Removing metallic particles and toxins from the air;
   B. Increasing atmospheric oxygen;
   C. Increasing ozone and negative ions in the area, which inhibits bacterial growth;
   D. Destroying odors from mold, cigarettes, and animals; and
   E. Filling the air with a fresh, aromatic scent.
10. Essential oils help promote emotional, physical, and spiritual healing.
11. Essential oils have a bio-electrical frequency that is several times greater than the frequency of herbs, food, and even the human body. Clinical research has shown that essential oils can quickly raise the frequency of the human body, restoring it to its normal, healthy level.

What is frequency and how does it pertain to essential oils?

Frequency is a measurable rate of electrical energy that is constant between any two points. Everything has an electrical frequency. Bruce Tainio of Tainio Technology in Cheny, Washington, developed new equipment to measure the bio-frequency of humans and foods.

Bruce Tainio and D. Gary Young, a North American expert on essential oils, used this bio-frequency monitor to determine the relationship between frequency and disease. Some of the results of their studies are as follows:

Human Brain	72-90 MHz	Processed/canned food	0 MHz
Human Body (day)	62-68 MHz	Fresh Produce	up to 15 MHz
Cold Symptoms	58 MHz	Dry Herbs	12-22 MHz
Flu Symptoms	57 MHz	Fresh Herbs	20-27 MHz
Candida	55 MHz	Essential Oils	52-320 MHz
Epstein Barr	52 MHz	**Note:** Due to the sensitivity of the instruments, these results are not easily duplicatable. What is important is the relativity of the numbers and the fact that the higher frequency of the essential oils can help raise the frequency of the human body to a more normal level.	
Cancer	42 MHz		
Death Begins	25 MHz		

Another part of this same study measured the frequency fluctuations within the human body as different substances were introduced. The chart shown below illustrates the frequency reaction of the human body to the introduction of coffee. The subsequent time necessary for the frequency to return to its original measurement was shown to be substantially reduced with the use of essential oils.

Frequency Reaction to Substance

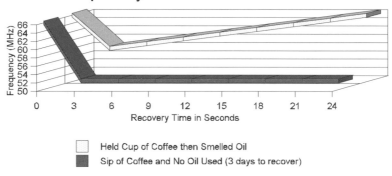

Held Cup of Coffee then Smelled Oil
Sip of Coffee and No Oil Used (3 days to recover)

Initially, the frequency of each of two different individuals—the first a 26 yr. old male and the second a 24 yr. old male—was measured at 66 MHz for both. The first individual held a cup of coffee (without drinking any) and his frequency dropped to 58 MHz in 3 seconds. He then removed the coffee and inhaled an aroma of essential oils. Within 21 seconds, his frequency had returned to 66 MHz. The second individual took a sip of coffee and his frequency dropped to 52 MHz in the same 3 seconds. However, no essential oils were used during the recovery time and it took 3 days for his frequency to return to the initial 66 MHz.

Another very interesting result of this study was the influence that thoughts have on our frequency as well. Negative thoughts lowered the measured frequency by 12 MHz and positive thoughts raised the measured frequency by 10 MHz. It was also found that prayer and meditation increased the measured frequency levels by 15 MHz.

What effect do *PURE, THERAPEUTIC-GRADE* essential oils have on the brain?

The blood-brain barrier is the barrier membrane between the circulating blood and the brain that prevents certain damaging substances from reaching brain tissue and cerebrospinal fluid. The American Medical Association (AMA) determined that if they could find an agent that would pass the blood-brain barrier, they would be able to cure Alzheimer's disease, Lou Gehrig's disease, multiple sclerosis, and Parkinson's disease. In June of 1994, it was documented by the Medical University of Berlin, Germany and Vienna, Austria that sesquiterpenes have the ability to go beyond the blood-brain barrier.

High levels of sesquiterpenes, found in the essential oils of Frankincense and Sandalwood, help increase the amount oxygen in the limbic system of the brain, particularly around the pineal and pituitary glands. This leads to an increase in secretions of antibodies, endorphins, and neurotransmitters.

Also present in the limbic system of the brain, is a gland called the amygdala. In 1989, it was discovered that the amygdala plays a major role in the storing and releasing of emotional trauma. The only way to stimulate this gland is with fragrance or the sense of smell. Therefore, with Aromatherapy and essential oils, we are now able to release emotional trauma.

What enables *PURE, THERAPEUTIC-GRADE* essential oils to provide such incredible benefits?

Essential oils are chemically very heterogenetic; meaning they are very diverse in their effects and can perform several different functions. Synthetic chemicals are completely opposite in that they have basically one action. This gives essential oils a paradoxical nature which can be difficult to understand. However, they can be compared to another paradoxical group—human beings. For example, a man can play many roles: father, husband, friend, coworker, accountant, school teacher, church volunteer, scout master, minister. etc. and so it is with essential oils. Lavender can be used for burns, headaches, PMS, insomnia, stress, etc.

APPLICATION OF ESSENTIAL OILS

1. **Direct Application.** Apply the oils directly on the area of concern using 1-6 drops of oil. More is not necessarily better since a large amount of oil can trigger a detoxification of the surrounding tissue and blood. Hot, moist compresses can be applied over top of the application area. The moist heat will force the oils deeper into the tissues.
2. **Baths.** Add three to six drops of your favorite essential oil to the bath water as the tub is filling. Adding the oils to a bath and shower gel base first allows one to obtain the greatest benefit from the oils as they are more evenly dispersed throughout the water and not allowed to immediately seperate.
3. **Diffuse.** A diffuser will disperse the essential oils into a micro-mist that will stay suspended for several hours to reduce bacteria, fungus, mold and freshen the air with natural fragrances. Diffusing releases oxygenating molecules, anti-viral, anti-bacterial and antiseptic properties, as well as negative ions, which kill bacteria. When diffused, essential oils have been found to reduce airborne chemicals, bacteria and metallics in the air as well as help to create greater spiritual, physical and emotional harmony. It is usually best to diffuse an oil 15 to 30 minutes at a time as you become accustomed to them. You may mix the single oils, but do not mix the blends together.
4. **Feet Massage.** Your feet are the second fastest area of your body to absorb oils because of the large pores. Three to six drops per foot are adequate to experience a feeling of peace, relaxation or energy.
5. **Body Massage.** If massaging a large area of the body, always dilute the oils by 15 to 30 percent with the V-6 Mixing Oil.
6. **Vita Flex Technique.** One to three drops of oil may be applied to the Vita Flex points (contact points) of the foot. Refer to the VITA FLEX FEET CHART.
7. **Auricular Therapy.** Apply oils to the rim of the ear using auricular therapy. Try using this therapy for emotional clearing. Refer to the Auricular Emotional Therapy chart in the Basic Information section of this book.
8. **Raindrop Technique.** A technique of dropping oils onto the spine that helps bring the body into balance, align the energy centers of the body, and release them if blocked. The oils used in this technique will continue to work in the body for about 5 to 7 days after the treatment with continued realignment taking place during this time. The following oils are used: ***Thyme, Oregano, Cypress, Birch/Wintergreen, Basil, Peppermint, Marjoram, Aroma Siez, Valor, Ortho Ease Massage Oil, and V-6 Mixing Oil.*** For more information on this technique, see the Science and Application section of the Reference Guide for Essential Oils. The video entitled Raindrop Technique by D. Gary Young (*available from Abundant Health*) provides step-by-step instructions for this technique.

KEY PRINCIPLES OF VITA FLEX THERAPY

1. **Fingernails should be cut and filed as short as possible, to reduce any discomfort.**
2. Remove all jewelry and watches to prevent an interference of energy.
3. Always **DROP** the oils in the palm of your hand and use the dominant hand to stir the oils clockwise three times before applying them on location. This method will increase the electrical frequency of the oils and significantly improve the results. **To prevent contamination of your oils, do not touch the top of the bottle.**
4. Put a drop of White Angelica on each shoulder to protect yourself from any possible negative energies of the person you are working on.
5. Always start on the bottom of the feet. Put 3-6 drops of <u>Valor</u> on the bottom of each foot. Some may be applied to the brain stem. Hold the bottoms of the feet with your hands. Right hand to right foot and left hand to left foot. Continue holding the feet until you feel the body's energy balance, which may feel like an energy pulse beating in both feet. Another way to balance, which may be preferable to some, is to put 1 drop of <u>Valor</u> on the wrists and hold the wrists crossed together for a few minutes. You may feel an energy pulse in your finger tips (thumb and index finger) when the energy balances.
6. Use the Vita Flex charts to determine where the oils should be placed during the therapy. The Vita Flex chart combines the work of Stanley Burroughs (Vita Flex Charting) and D. Gary Young (Electrical Frequency Tracing). Apply 1-3 drops of oil(s) to the specific Vita Flex points on the feet.
7. Apply the Vita Flex technique as follows: Starting with the fingers on their pads, curl the fingers up and over onto the nails (see photo examples below). Increasing pressure is applied until the fingers are curled almost completely over on the nails. Pressure is then immediately released to create the spark of energy and send it on its way. The curling should be one continuous motion, not jerky, with medium to heavy pressure being placed on the contact point. Never press and hold while performing this technique. This may be done several times on the same spot to obtain the desired results. Some leverage can be achieved by placing the thumb of the same hand around to the other side of the foot or hand on which the Vita Flex is being performed. This allows the hand to operate in a fashion similar to a pipe wrench, which increases pressure on the pipe as it is twisted.

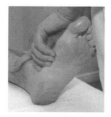
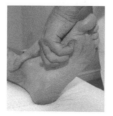
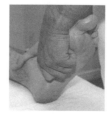

Comments: For a detailed explanation of the entire Vita Flex system, refer to Stanley Burroughs' book, <u>Healing for the Age of Enlightenment</u>.

For step-by-step instructions of the full Vita Flex treatment, refer to the video, <u>Vita Flex Instruction</u> with Tom Woloshyn. This video teaches the proper Vita Flex technique as developed by Stanley Burroughs, including the Atlas Adjustment (a non-chiropractic technique used to quickly and efficiently re-align the spine or any other misalignment in the body). Another excellent tool for use with this technique is the Vita Flex Roller or "Relax-a-Roller". This unique massage roller was specifically designed by Stanley Burroughs to provide the same stimulating effect as the fingers of the hand. It is excellent for personal use. (*Both of these products are available from Abundant Health*)

VITA FLEX HAND CHART

Vita Flex points in this hand chart correspond to those in the feet. Occasionally the feet can be too sensitive for typical Vita Flex Therapy. Working with the hands will not only affect the specific body points, but may also help to provide some pain relief to the corresponding points on the feet. (Refer to Stanley Burroughs' book, <u>Healing for the Age of Enlightenment</u>, pg. 78 for a more detailed explanation.)

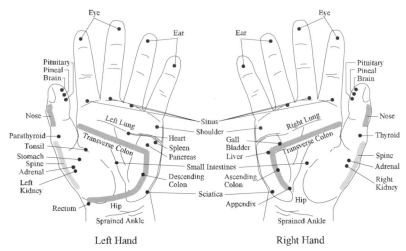

Left Hand   Right Hand

VITA FLEX FEET CHART

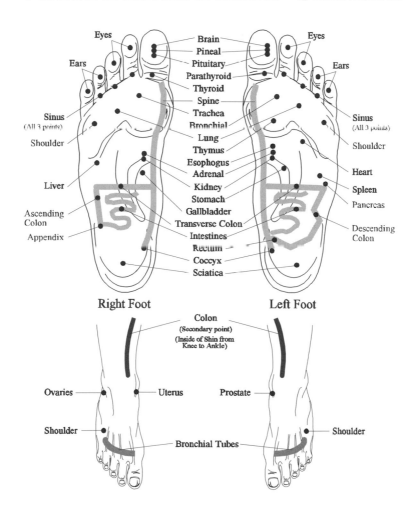

Eyes
Brain
Pineal
Pituitary
Parathyroid
Thyroid
Spine
Trachea
Bronchial
Lung
Thymus
Esophogus
Adrenal
Kidney
Stomach
Gallbladder
Transverse Colon
Intestines
Rectum
Coccyx
Sciatica

Ears

Sinus
(All 3 points)

Shoulder

Liver

Ascending
Colon

Appendix

Eyes

Ears

Sinus
(All 3 points)

Shoulder

Heart

Spleen

Pancreas

Descending
Colon

Right Foot   **Left Foot**

Colon
(Secondary point)
(Inside of Shin from
Knee to Ankle)

Ovaries   Uterus   Prostate

Shoulder   Shoulder

Bronchial Tubes

AURICULAR EMOTIONAL THERAPY

MOTHER: Geranium

Sexual Abuse: Geranium, Ylang Ylang
Abandonment: Geranium, Forgiveness, Acceptance

FATHER: Lavender

Sexual Abuse: Lavender, Ylang Ylang, Release
Male Abuse: Helichrysum, Lavender

DEPRESSION

Any of the following: Valor, Joy, Hope, White Angelica, Peace & Calming, Citrus Fresh, Christmas Spirit, Gentle Baby. Use whichever blend(s) work best for you.

OVERWHELMED

Use Hope and Acceptance

BEARING BURDENS OF THE WORLD

Use Release and Valor

ANGER & HATE

Use Joy to stimulate the pituitary. Use Valor and Release to release the anger.

SELF EXPRESSION

Use Valor and Motivation. Take deep breaths to express oneself.

FEAR

Apply Valor, Release, Joy.

OPEN THE MIND

Apply 3 Wise Men.

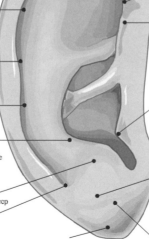

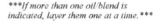

****If more than one oil/blend is indicated, layer them one at a time.* ***

*** *When working on the ear, apply Harmony and Forgiveness to the entire ear and apply Valor on the feet.* ***

SYMPATHY & GUILT

Use Joy and Inspiration.

SELF PITY

Use Acceptance.

REJECTION

Use Forgiveness and Acceptance. Work the rejection points on both ears. For rejection from Mother, use Geranium. For rejection from Father, use Lavender. While applying the oils, say "I choose to accept my Mother/Father for what they have done or not done. It is their life and not mine."

EYES and VISION

To improve eyesight, use 10 Lemongrass, 5 Cypress, 3 Eucalyptus, in ½ oz. of V-6 Mixing Oil.
For Vision of goals, use Dream Catcher, Acceptance, and 3 Wise Men.

HEART

To strengthen the heart and lower blood pressure, use Aroma Life.
For self acceptance, apply Joy, Forgiveness, and Acceptance.

RAINDROP TECHNIQUE

This application technique was developed by Dr. Don Gary Young, N.D. Aromatologist, and one of North America's leading experts on the art and science of aromatherapy. This technique involves dropping the oils directly onto the spine from about six inches above the body. The oils are then worked into the spine using light strokes with the fingers which stimulate energy impulses and disperse the oils along the nervous system throughout the entire body. In this way, the body can be brought into balance and the energy centers can be cleared and re-aligned. It will also help to reduce spinal inflammations and kill viruses that hibernate along the spinal column, as well as help to straighten any spinal curvatures. Although a session lasts for about 45 minutes to an hour, the oils will continue to work in the body for a week or more following the treatment. The Raindrop Technique that is explained below is an abbreviated form. The video entitled <u>Raindrop Technique</u> by D. Gary Young (*available from Abundant Health*) provides step-by-step instructions for this technique.

<u>Oils used in the Raindrop Technique</u>

VALOR—is the first and most important oil used in this technique because it helps balance the electrical energies within the body. It also helps create an environment where structural alignment can occur.

THYME—is used for its ability to support the immune system by attacking any bacteria, fungus, infection, or virus that may be present. It may also help one overcome fatigue and physical weakness after an illness.

OREGANO—works in conjunction with thyme to strengthen the immune system and to attack bacteria and viruses. It may also act as an antiseptic for the respiratory system, help balance metabolism, and strengthen the vital centers of the body.

CYPRESS—is used for its anti-bacterial, anti-infectious, antimicrobial, and diuretic properties. In addition, it may function as a decongestant for the circulatory and lymphatic systems.

BIRCH/WINTERGREEN—is great for removing discomfort associated with the inflammation of bones, muscles, and joints. It may also help cleanse the lymphatic system.

BASIL—is relaxing to spastic muscles and is stimulating to the nerves and the adrenal cortex.

PEPPERMINT—is used to calm and strengthen the nerves, reduce inflammation, and is highly effective when dealing with conditions related to the respiratory system. It also has a synergistic and enhancing effect on all other oils.

MARJORAM — is used to relax spastic muscles, soothe the nerves, relieve cramps, aches, and pains, and to help calm the respiratory system.

AROMA SIEZ — may help to relax, calm, and relieve the tension of spastic muscles resulting from sports injury, fatigue, or stress.

ORTHO EASE — is the crowning oil to this application. It is used to help relax all the muscles of the back and legs and to help reduce any stress, arthritic pain, or tension that may exist.

V-6 MIXING OIL — is used to help dilute any of the oils that may be somewhat caustic to the skin. It should always be used with oregano and thyme and can be used with any of the other oils based upon the person's skin sensitivity.

Note: The oils used in this technique have many more benefits than those listed above. *For more specific information, please refer to the sections in this book on Singles and Blends.*

Raindrop Technique

1. Remove all jewelry or metal to allow the energy to flow freely. Put a drop of **White Angelica** on each of your shoulders to protect you against any negative energies coming from the person receiving the treatment.

2. Have the person lie face up on a table with their body as straight as possible on the table. The person receiving the treatment should be as comfortable as possible, so the arms can be resting along side the body or resting on the top of their hips, whichever they prefer (don't let their hands touch each other as this will tend to short circuit the flow of energy through their body). By covering the person with a sheet, their modesty can be protected as you roll them over and they can be kept warm as you alternate between working on the back and working on the legs and feet.

3. Apply **three** drops of **Valor** on each shoulder as well as six drops on each foot. Hold right foot/shoulder with right hand and left foot/shoulder with left hand (crossing hands if necessary – see the following photo illustration entitled, "Valor Balance on Feet") for five to ten minutes or until you can feel an energy pulse in the person's feet. For this part of the

application, it works best if there is another person assisting in the treatment. If you are working by yourself, do the feet only. **Valor** is used to balance and it works well on the energy alignment of the body. **This is the most important oil that is used in this application.**

Valor Balance on Feet

4. First apply 2 drops of **thyme** to the Vita Flex spine points along the inside edge of each foot, working it in three times with the Vita Flex technique (*refer to Vita Flex Technique in this same section, Key Principle #7 and photo illustrations for an explanation of this technique*). Repeat this procedure with each of the following oils, one at a time: **Oregano**, **cypress**, **birch/wintergreen**, **basil**, and **peppermint**. Then, have the person roll over onto their stomach and perform steps 5 through 14 on their spine.

5. Hold the bottle of **thyme** about six inches from the spine and evenly space **four to five** drops from the sacrum (tailbone) to the neck. Work it in evenly along the curvature of the spine with gentle upward strokes. Apply **five** drops of **oregano** and work it in the same way. Then, apply **ten to fifteen** drops of **V-6 Mixing Oil** to prevent any discomfort since both these oils can be quite caustic.

6. Using the very tips of the fingers, alternate between left hand and right hand as you very lightly work up the spine from the sacrum to the base of the neck with short, brush-like strokes. Follow the curvature of the spine and repeat two more times.

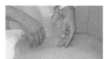 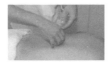 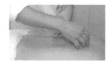

7. Using your finger tips again, softly brush up a few inches from the sacrum then out to either side of the body; right hand to the right and left hand to the left.

 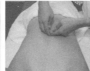 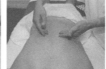 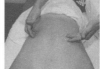

Repeat this step from the sacrum but go a few more inches up the spine then out to the sides. Then again from the sacrum, going up a few more inches then out. Then again, each time going further up the spine until you reach the base of the neck and flare out along the shoulders. This entire step should then be repeated two more times.

8. Using your finger tips again, start at the sacrum and in full-length strokes, lightly brush all the way up the spine to the base of the neck and then out over the shoulders. Repeat two more times.

9. Evenly space **four to five** drops of **cypress** from the sacrum to the neck. Work it in evenly along the curvature of the spine with gentle upward strokes. Then apply the oils of **birch/wintergreen, basil, and peppermint** in the same manner.

10. Place both hands side by side (parallel to the spine) and using the tips of the fingers, massage in a circular, clock-wise motion, just off to one side of the spine, from the sacrum up to the neck. **Remember to never work directly on the spine**. Apply moderate pressure and move a finger's width at a time. This will help to loosen the muscles and allow the spine to straighten itself. After doing one side of the spine, 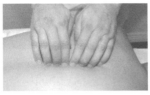 move around the person and work the other side of the spine from the sacrum to the neck in the same manner. Repeat two more times on either side.

11. Using whichever hand is most comfortable to you, place the index and middle finger on either side of the spine at the sacrum. Place the other hand on top of the first, part way down the two fingers. Apply moderate pressure and with a quick, forward and back continued sawing motion of the hand on top, slide the fingers a little at a time up the spine to the skull. Move the fingers upward slowly during the sawing motion. Once the skull is reached, apply gentle but firm pressure to push the skull forward, stretching the spine. Return to the sacrum and repeat two more times.

 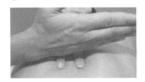 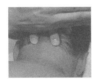

12. Place the thumbs of each hand on either side of the spine at the sacrum and point them towards each other. Next, using the Vita Flex technique, roll the thumbs up and over onto the thumbnails, applying some pressure straight down during the roll (refer to the photo illustrations at the top of the following page). Then release and slide the thumbs up an inch or so and repeat the roll with pressure. Continue up to the base of the neck, then return to the sacrum and repeat two more times. This will become easier with practice.

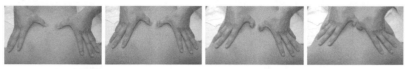

13. Apply five to six drops of **marjoram** up the spine and work it in. Then apply five to six drops of **Aroma Siez** to each side and away from the spine. Gently massage these oils into the muscle tissue all over the back to soothe and relax the patient. After the oils have been massaged in well, you may cover the person with the sheet and rest for approximately five minutes. Apply **Ortho Ease** over the entire area of the back and gently massage it in. Then cover the person to keep them warm and massage **Ortho Ease** into the legs. This will help to relax the muscles that may be pulling on the spine.

14. Fold a hand towel, soak it in hot water, wring it out and lay it along the entire length of the spine. Take a dry towel and fold it in half lengthwise and place it over the hot wet towel. Be extremely sensitive to the feelings of the person as the heat will build along the spine. Areas of the spine where more inflammation, virus, or bacteria exist will be the hottest. The heat will gradually build for five to eight minutes then cool right down to normal. If the heat becomes too uncomfortable, remove the towels and apply V-6 Mixing Oil. Then replace the towels and continue until the wet towel becomes cold. If the person's back is still hot, cover with a dry towel and allow the back to cool down slowly.

15. After the person's back begins to cool down, gently stretch the spine by crossing hands and straddle the spine with your hands, one pointing towards the top of the spine and the other towards the bottom as shown in the adjacent photo. Starting in the middle, gently press the hands downwards and apart towards opposite ends of the spine. Then move the hands apart more and repeat the stretch. Continue moving the hands and stretching until the ends of the spine are reached.

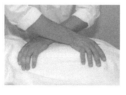

16. Remove the wet towels and have the person roll over onto their back. Apply two to three drops of **birch/wintergreen** along the inside of each leg from the knee to the heel and up the inside of the foot to the big toe. Layer it in and apply the oils of **cypress, basil, and peppermint** in the same fashion. Then work the same area using the Vita Flex technique. The inside of the shin corresponds to the colon. By working this area, you are opening the colon and allowing it to expel any toxins released during the Raindrop Technique.

17. The final step is to perform another gentle stretching of the spine. If you are working alone, put your right hand behind the base of the head and your left hand under the chin. Very gently pull to create a slight tension and release. Do three times then move to the

feet. Hold above the ankles and gently pull and release three times. If you have an assistant, one person can hold the head and the other hold the feet. Then together, apply a gentle tension and hold for a few minutes. This is then completed by the person at the head doing a very slight pull and release three times.

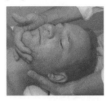 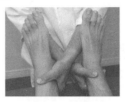

By stimulating the Central Nervous System, you have just given someone a total treatment, affecting every system in the body, including emotional release and support. Even though the oils continue to work in the body for a week or more, one application may last months or it may be necessary to repeat the application every week until the body begins to respond. And in cases of more severe health conditions, this treatment can be done every day or two. The object is to develop a new memory in the tissues of the body and train it to hold itself in place.

Note: There have been a couple of excellent videos created to help demonstrate this very effective technique for oils application. They are great tools for providing instruction and should be studied by those individuals who are interested in performing this technique appropriately. See the *Video Listing* in the Bibliography section for more information.

Personal Guide

NOTES AND EXPLANATIONS

1. *Aromatic* means diffuse, breathe, or inhale.
2. A superscripted "F" (i.e. ^FClary sage) means the oil has been used medicinally in France.
3. *Neat* means to apply the oil without diluting it with a pure vegetable oil.
4. If essential oils get into your eyes by accident or they burn a little, do not try to remove the oils with water. This will only drive the oils deeper into the tissue. It is best to dilute the essential oils with a pure vegetable oil.
5. The FDA has not approved essential oils for internal use and given them the following designations: GRAS (Generally Regarded As Safe for internal consumption), FA (Food Additive), or FL (FLavoring agent). These designations are listen in the Single Oil Summary Information chart in the Appendix of this book under Safety Data.
6. Using Citrus oils such as lemon, orange, grapefruit, mandarin, bergamot, angelica, etc. during exposure to direct sunlight may cause a rash or pigmentation. It is best to dilute the oil first with a pure vegetable oil, then apply a little to determine how the skin responds.
7. Caution should be used with oils such as Clary sage, sage, and fennel during pregnancy. These oils contain active constituents with hormone-like activity and could possibly stimulate adverse reactions in the mother, though there are no recorded cases in humans.
8. Particular care should be taken when using cinnamon, lemongrass, oregano, and thyme as they are some of the strongest and most caustic oils. Dilute them with a pure vegetable oil.
9. Essential oils are not listed in a specific order (an attempt was made to list them alphabetically) so you will have to be intuitive on which one(s) to use. It is not necessary to use all of the oils listed. Try one oil at a time. If you do not see a change soon, try a different one. What one person needs may be different than another person. (Hint: Use Kinesiology to test yourself on the oils that are right for you.)
10. In this document, several homemade blends are suggested. However, it is done with great hesitancy. Some of the blends listed come from individuals who may not be experts in the field of essential oils and aromatherapy. Rather than mix the oils together, it may be better to layer the oils; that is, apply a drop or two of one oil, rub it in, and then apply another oil. If dilution is necessary, a pure vegetable oil can be applied on top.
11. When someone is out of electrical balance, try the following:
    A. Place a drop or two of <u>Harmony</u> into one hand, then rub the palms of both hands together in a clockwise motion.
    B. Place one hand over the thymus (heart chakra) and the other hand over the navel.

C.   Take three deep breaths and switch hands, then take three more deep breaths.

12. Less is often better; use one to three drops of oil and no more than six drops at a time. Stir and rub on in a clockwise direction.

13. When applying oils to infants and small children, dilute one to two drops pure essential oil with ½-1 teaspoon (tsp.) of a pure vegetable oil (V-6 Mixing Oil). If the oils are used in the bath, always use a bath gel base as a dispersing agent for the oils. See BABIES for more information about the recommended list of oils for babies and children.

14. The body absorbs oils the fastest through inhalation (breathing) and second fastest through application to the feet or ears. Testing on the thyroid, heart, and pancreas showed that the oils reached these organs in three seconds. Layering the oils can increase the rate of absorption.

15. When an oil causes discomfort it is because it is pulling toxins, heavy metals, chemicals, poisons, parasites, and mucus from the system. Either stop applying the oils for a short time, to make sure your body isn't eliminating (detoxifying) too fast, or dilute the oils until the body catches up with the releasing. These toxins go back into the system if they cannot be released.

16. When the cell wall thickens, oxygen cannot get in. The life expectancy of the cell is 120 days (4 months). Cells divide, making two duplicate cells. If the cell is diseased, two new diseased cells will be made. When we stop the mutation of the cells (create healthy cells), we stop the disease. Essential oils have the ability to penetrate and carry nutrients through the cell wall to the nucleus and improve the health of the cell.

17. Each oil has a frequency, and each of our organs and body parts have a frequency. The frequency of an oil is attracted by a like frequency within the body. Lower oil frequencies become a sponge for negative energy. The frequency is what stays in the body to maintain the longer-lasting effects of the oil.

 Low frequencies can make **physical** changes in the body.

 Middle frequencies can make **emotional** changes in the body.

 High frequencies can make **spiritual** changes in the body.

A.   Average frequency of the human body during the day time is between 62 and 68 Megahertz (MHz).

 1)   Bone frequency is 38 to 43 MHz.

 2)   Frequencies from the neck down vary between 62 and 68 MHz.

B.   Spiritual frequencies range from 92 to 360 MHz.

18. *Use extreme caution when diffusing cinnamon bark* because it may burn the nostrils if you put your nose directly next to the nebulizer of the diffuser.

19. When traveling by air, you should always have your oils hand-checked. X-ray machines may interfere with the frequency of the oils.

20. Keep oils away from the light and heat, although they seem to do fine in temperatures up to 90 degrees. If stored properly, they can maintain their maximum potency for many years.

21. The following information will be useful to those who are familiar with the art and technique of blending. (*See the Science and Application section of Reference Guide for Essential Oils for more information.*)

1ˢᵗ—The **Personifier** (1-5% of blend) oils have very sharp, strong and long-lasting fragrances. They also have dominant properties with strong therapeutic action.
Oils in this classification may include: Angelica, birch, cardamom, German chamomile, cinnamon, cistus, Clary sage, clove, coriander, ginger, helichrysum, mandarin, neroli, nutmeg, orange, patchouly, peppermint, petitgrain, rose, spearmint, tangerine, tarragon, wintergreen, ylang, ylang

2ⁿᵈ—The **Enhancer** (50-80% of blend) oil should be the predominant oil as it serves to enhance the properties of the other oils in the blend. Its fragrance is not as sharp as the personifiers and is usually of a shorter duration.
Oils in this classification may include: Basil, bergamot, birch, Roman chamomile, Black cumin, cajeput, cedarwood, dill, eucalyptus, frankincense, galbanum, geranium, grapefruit, hyssop, jasmine, lavender, lemon, lemongrass, lime, marjoram, melaleuca (Tea Tree), melissa, myrtle, orange, oregano, palmarosa, patchouly, petitgrain, ravensara, rose, rosemary, sage, spruce, thyme, wintergreen

3ʳᵈ—The **Equalizer** (10-15% of blend) oils create balance and synergy among the oils contained in the blend. Their fragrance is also not as sharp as the personifier and is of a shorter duration.
Oils in this classification may include: Basil, bergamot, cedarwood, Roman chamomile, cypress, fennel, fir, frankincense, geranium, ginger, hyssop, jasmine, juniper, lavender, lemongrass, lime, marjoram, melaleuca (Tea Tree), melissa, myrrh, myrtle, neroli, oregano, pine, rose, rosewood, sandalwood, spruce, tarragon, thyme.

4ᵗʰ—The **Modifier** (5-8% of blend) oils have a mild and short fragrance. These oils add harmony to the blend.
Oils in this classification may include: Angelica, bergamot, cardamom, coriander, eucalyptus, fennel, grapefruit, hyssop, jasmine, lavender, lemon, mandarin, melissa, myrrh, neroli, petitgrain, rose, rosewood, sandalwood, tangerine, ylang ylang.

Depending upon the topical application of your blend, you will want to add some carrier/base oil. When creating a **therapeutic essential oil blend**, you may want to use about **28 drops of essential oil to ½ oz. of V-6 Mixing Oil**. When creating a **body massage blend**, you will want to use a total of about **50 drops of essential oils to 4 oz. of V-6 Mixing Oil**. Remember to store your fragrant creation in dark-colored glass bottles.

Learn to trust your nose as it can help you decide which classification an oil should be in. For additional information on blending, we highly recommend Marcel Lavabre's Aromatherapy Workbook.

ABANDONED: See EMOTIONS. Acceptance, Forgiveness, Valor.

ABSCESS: See ANTI-FUNGAL, ANTI-BACTERIAL, FUNGUS: FUNGAL INFECTION
     or INFECTION. Bergamot, birch, elemi, frankincense, galbanum, lavender,
     melaleuca (Tea Tree), Melrose, myrrh, Purification, Roman chamomile, Thieves,
     thyme, wintergreen. To reduce swelling, pain, inflammation, and to draw out
     toxins, it may help to apply the oil(s) with a hot compress.
     BLEND—Roman chamomile, lavender, and melaleuca (Tea Tree).
     SUPPLEMENTS—ImmuGel, Royaldophilus, Super B. Put ImmuGel and Thieves on
         a rolled-up gauze and place over abscess to pull out the infection.
     DENTAL—Helichrysum, Purification, Roman chamomile. Apply using a hot compress
         on face. It may also help to apply one drop of oil to a cotton ball and apply
         directly to the abscess. Put ImmuGel and Thieves on a rolled-up gauze and place
         over abscess to pull out the infection.
     BLEND #1—Use clove, birch/wintergreen, and helichrysum to help with infection.
     MOUTH—ʳLavender.
     ****COMMENTS—Some sources recommend a non-toxic diet and an increase in liquid
         intake.*

ABSENT MINDED: See MEMORY. Basil, Brain Power, cardamom, Clarity, frankincense,
     lemongrass, M-Grain, peppermint, rosemary, sandalwood.
     SUPPLEMENTS—Mineral Essence, Power Meal, Sulfurzyme, Ultra Young,
         VitaGreen.

ABUNDANCE: Abundance, Acceptance, bergamot, cinnamon bark, cypress, Harmony,
     Gathering.
     ATTRACTS—Abundance, cinnamon bark.
     MONEY—Ginger, patchouly.
     ****COMMENTS—One waitress demonstrated her luck when she wore Abundance and
         Harmony together; she received a whopping $120.00 tip! Who knows, it may
         work for you too!*

ABUSE: Acceptance, Brain Power, Citrus Fresh, Christmas Spirit, geranium, Forgiveness,
     Grounding, Harmony, Hope, Humility, Inner Child, Joy, lavender, melissa, Peace
     & Calming, Release, 3 Wise Men, sandalwood, SARA (releases memory and
     trauma of sexual or ritual abuse), Surrender, Trauma Life, Valor, ylang ylang.
     Apply l drop of the oils desired on each Chakra to allow blocked emotions to
     come out.
     SUPPLEMENTS—Power Meal, Super B, Super C.
     BY FATHER—Forgiveness, lavender, Sacred Mountain (empowers self).
     BY MOTHER—Forgiveness, geranium, lavender.

***COMMENTS—*Refer to the page on Auricular Emotional Therapy in the Basic Information section of this book for points where oils can be applied.*

FEELINGS OF REVENGE—<u>Forgiveness</u> (around navel), <u>Present Time</u> (on thymus), <u>Surrender</u> (on sternum over heart).

PROTECTION or BALANCE—<u>Harmony</u> (over thymus; on energy centers/chakras), <u>White Angelica</u> (on shoulders).

SEXUAL/RITUAL—<u>Forgiveness</u> (around navel), <u>Harmony</u>, <u>Joy</u>, <u>Present Time</u>, <u>Release</u> (liver Vita Flex point on feet; under nose), sage, <u>SARA</u> (over area of abuse), <u>3 Wise Men</u>, <u>Trauma Life</u>, <u>Valor</u>, and <u>White Angelica</u>.

ESPOUSAL—<u>Acceptance</u>, <u>Envision</u>, <u>Forgiveness</u>, <u>Joy</u>, <u>Release</u>, <u>Trauma Life</u>, <u>Valor</u>.

SUICIDAL—<u>Brain Power</u>, <u>Hope</u> (on rim of ears), melissa, <u>Present Time</u>.

ACCIDENTS: See EMOTIONS. <u>Trauma Life</u>.

ACHES/PAINS: Blue cypress, Idaho balsam fir, <u>PanAway</u>, <u>Relieve It</u>.

   MASSAGE OILS—Ortho Ease or Ortho Sport (stronger). *These massage oils help seal in and enhance the effectiveness of following the single oils or oil blends.*

   SUPPLEMENTS—Sulfurzyme contains MSM which has been shown to be very effective in controlling pain, especially in the joints and tissues.

BONE—All the tree oils–**Birch**, cedarwood, cypress, fir, helichrysum, juniper, <u>PanAway</u>, peppermint, sandalwood, spruce, **wintergreen**.

   SUPPLEMENTS—Coral Sea (highly bio-available calcium, contains 58 trace minerals), Super Cal, ArthroTune (1 capsule twice a day).

CHRONIC—Basil, birch, clove, cypress, cedarwood, elemi, fir, helichrysum, Idaho tansy, ginger, juniper, <u>PanAway</u> (add 1-2 drops birch for extra strength), peppermint, rosemary cineol, <u>Relieve It</u>, sandalwood, spruce, valerian, wintergreen.

   BLEND—Equal parts of birch/wintergreen, elemi, and Idaho tansy.

   MASSAGE OILS—Ortho Ease or Ortho Sport (stronger).

   SUPPLEMENTS—Coral Sea (highly bio-available calcium, contains 58 trace minerals), Super Cal, ArthroTune (1 capsule twice a day).

GENERAL—<u>Aroma Siez</u>, birch, Blue cypress, frankincense, ginger, helichrysum, Idaho balsam fir, lavender, marjoram, <u>PanAway</u>, <u>Relieve It</u>, Roman chamomile, rosemary, **White fir** (pain from inflammation), wintergreen.

GROWING—Massage with birch/wintergreen, cypress, peppermint, wait 5 minutes and apply <u>PanAway</u>, then seal with Ortho Ease.

   MASSAGE OILS—Ortho Ease.

   SUPPLEMENTS—Coral Sea (highly bio-available calcium, contains 58 trace minerals). Sulfurzyme, Super Cal, 1 ArthroTune twice a day.

JOINTS—Birch (discomfort), Idaho balsam fir, nutmeg, Roman chamomile (inflamed), spruce, wintergreen.

MUSCLE—<u>Aroma Siez</u>, ᶠbirch, basil, ᶠclove, ginger, helichrysum, Idaho balsam fir, lavender, lemongrass (especially good for ligaments), marjoram, nutmeg, oregano,

PanAway, peppermint, <u>Relieve It</u>, Roman chamomile, rosemary verbenon,
spearmint, spruce (torn muscles), thyme, vetiver, **White fir** (pain from
inflammation), wintergreen.
TISSUE—Helichrysum, <u>PanAway</u>, <u>Relieve It</u> (good for deep tissue pain).

ACIDOSIS: See ALKALINE and
pH BALANCE.
Lemon, peppermint.
ACID-FORMING FOODS—
Avoid meat, dairy
products, whole wheat
or rye bread, coffee,
tea, wine, beer, root
beer, cider, yeast
products, soy sauce,
cold cereals, potato
chips, etc.
SUPPLEMENTS—
AlkaLime (acid-
neutralizing mineral),
Body Balance, Exodus
(may increase oxygen),
Mineral Essence,
Power Meal,
Royaldophilus,
VitaGreen (for
alkaline/acid balance).
***COMMENTS*—*Cancer and
candida need an acid*
condition in order to thrive and spread. In acidic conditions, the oils will take
longer to work and won't last as long. When a person does not like the smell of
an oil it is usually because of an acidic condition. THE BODY CAN ONLY
HEAL IN AN ALKALINE STATE.

> *Acidosis is a condition of over-acidity in the blood and
> body tissues. When the body loses its alkaline reserve,
> pleomorphic virus, bacteria, yeast, and fungus take over
> and cause degenerative diseases such as, diabetes,
> cancer, aids, arteriosclerosis, arthritis, osteoporosis,
> chronic fatigue, etc.*
>
> *Symptoms of acidosis may include: frequent sighing,
> insomnia, water retention, recessed eyes, rheumatoid
> arthritis, migraine headaches, abnormally low blood
> pressure, and alternating constipation and diarrhea.*
>
> *Causes of acidosis may include: improper diet, kidney,
> liver, and adrenal disorders, emotional disturbances,
> fever, and an excess of niacin, vitamin C, and aspirin.*
>
> *Oxygen reduces the acidity of the blood. All essential
> oils contain oxygen. We like to flavor our water with 1-2
> drops of lemon or peppermint oil. Lemon has the ability
> to counteract acidity in the body. The citric acid found
> in lemons is neutralized during digestion, giving off
> carbonates and bicarbonates of potassium and calcium,
> which helps maintain the alkalinity of the system.*

ACNE: See HORMONAL IMBALANCE, SCARRING, SKIN, and STRESS. Bergamot,
cedarwood, <u>Clarity</u> (on temples), Clary sage, clove, eucalyptus, *Eucalyptus
radiata*, frankincense, <u>Gentle Baby</u>, geranium, FGerman chamomile, Fjuniper,
Flavender, lemon, lemongrass, marjoram, melaleuca (Tea Tree), <u>Melrose</u>, myrtle,
patchouly, petitgrain, <u>Purification</u>, <u>Raven</u>, ravensara, <u>RC</u>, rosemary, Frosewood,
sage, sandalwood, <u>Sensation</u>, spearmint, thyme, vetiver, yarrow. Apply one of the
above oils on location or try putting about 10 drops of an oil into a small spray
bottle and mist your face several times a day.

PERSONAL CARE—
Prenolone/Prenolone+,
Rose Ointment,
Sensation Massage Oil.
SUPPLEMENTS—
ComforTone, ICP,
Megazyme, JuvaTone,
and Sulfurzyme.
Cleansing the colon
may help (see
CLEANSING).
ADULT ONSET—
Prenolone/Prenolone+
if the acne stems from a
hormonal imbalance.
CELLULAR
REGENERATIVE—
Palmarosa, rosewood.
HEALING—Use anti-bacterial
and anti-inflammatory

> *Acne is often a result of seborrhea (an overproduction of fat from the sebaceous glands), which can oftentimes be traced back to a hormonal imbalance. Stress is another reason for increased sebum production. Consequently, it may be of help to use oils that balance the hormones and reduce stress.*
>
> *Essential oil treatments combined with a good diet (lots of vegetables and lots of water), exercise, and increased lymphatic and circulatory flow, will allow the toxic wastes to leave the body as the oxygen and nutrients reach the skin in greater proportions.*
>
> *One of the best ways to release toxins through the skin is to sweat. Chamomile, hyssop, juniper, lavender, rosemary, and thyme contain sudorific properties and may facilitate the sweating process. The anti-bacterial and anti-inflammatory oils may assist in the healing process.*

oils like geranium, melaleuca (Tea Tree), Melrose, and rosewood.
INFECTIOUS—Clove.
MENSTRUAL—Premenstrual or mid-menstrual cycle acne may be helped by balancing
the hormones.
PERSONAL CARE—Prenolone/Prenolone+.
SUPPLEMENTS—CortiStop (Women's), FemiGen, ProMist, Super B.
TINCTURES—Femalin.
TOXIN RELEASE—Use sudorific oils like chamomile, hyssop, juniper, lavender,
rosemary, and thyme to help promote sweating.

ACNE ROSACEA: See ROSACEA.

ADD: See ATTENTION DEFICIT DISORDER.

ADENITIS: See LYMPHATIC
SYSTEM. Garlic,
onion, pine, rosemary,
sage.

> *Adenitis is an acute or chronic inflammation of the lymph glands or nodes. Drink a lot of water to help remove the toxins from the body.*

ADDICTIONS: Acceptance,
bergamot (helps with over indulgences), calamus (tobacco), JuvaFlex, Peace &
Calming, Purification.

SUPPLEMENTS—JuvaTone, Mineral Essence, Super C.

The following recipe has worked for individuals who are trying to break addictions:

RECIPE #1—Use JuvaTone, ComforTone, JuvaFlex and Acceptance together.

ALCOHOL—(to stop drinking) Purification, Peace & Calming. Do not use Clary sage and alcohol together; it may result in nightmares. *For professional assistance, contact the local chapter of Alcoholics Anonymous.*

COFFEE/TOBACCO—Bergamot, calamus. Apply to stomach, abdomen, liver area, and bottom of feet.

DRUGS—Basil, bergamot, birch, eucalyptus, fennel, grapefruit (withdrawal), lavender, marjoram, nutmeg, orange, Peace & Calming, Purification, Roman chamomile, sandalwood, wintergreen. Apply to Vita Flex points on feet.

SUPPLEMENTS—Super C (at least 250 mg per day).

SMOKING—Use the above recipe. Applying either clove or Thieves to the tongue before lighting up helps remove the desire to smoke. Calamus may also help.

****COMMENTS—One individual used JuvaTone to break a habit of smoking 2 ½ packs of cigarettes a day for 20 years. It only took him three to five days!*

SUGAR—Dill, Purification, Peace & Calming. Apply to Vita Flex points on feet. Place dill on wrists to help remove addiction to sweets.

SUPPLEMENTS–Allerzyme (aids the digestion of sugars, starches, fats, and proteins), Cleansing Trio (ComforTone, Megazyme, and ICP).

WITHDRAWAL—Dill, grapefruit, lavender, marjoram, nutmeg, orange, sandalwood. Apply to temples and diffuse. Applying dill to the wrists helps reduce the sweating that often accompanies withdrawal.

ADDISON'S DISEASE: See ADRENAL GLANDS. En-R-Gee, EndoFlex, Joy, nutmeg (increases energy; supports adrenal glands),sage (combine with nutmeg).

> *Addison's Disease is an autoimmune disease where the body's own immune cells attack the adrenal glands and either severely limit or completely shut down the production of the adrenal cortex hormones. Extreme fluid and mineral loss are the life-threatening results.*

SUPPLEMENTS—ImmuPro, Master Formula His/Hers, Mineral Essence (help supplement mineral loss), **Sulfurzyme** (shown to slow or reverse autoimmune diseases), Super B, VitaGreen.

TINCTURES—Royal Essence (for energy).

ADRENAL GLANDS: See ENDOCRINE SYSTEM, LUPUS, THYROID. EndoFlex, nutmeg (increases energy; supports adrenal glands).

BLEND—Add 3 drops clove, 4 nutmeg, and 6 rosemary to 1 tsp. V-6 Mixing Oil. Apply 4-5 drops of this mixture to kidney areas and cover with hot compress.

Also apply 1-2 drops of mixture to Vita Flex kidney points on the feet and work in with fingers using Vita Flex technique.

STIMULANT—ᶠBasil, geranium, pine, rosemary, ᶠsage.

STRENGTHEN—Spruce (Black), peppermint.

UNDERACTIVE ADRENALS— See ADDISON'S DISEASE.

PERSONAL CARE— EndoBalance.

SUPPLEMENTS—

> *The **adrenal glands** are made up of an inner part (medulla) and an outer part (cortex). The outer portion (or cortex) produces critical steroid hormones, including glucocorticoids and aldosterone. These hormones directly affect blood pressure and mineral content. They also help regulate the conversion of carbohydrates into energy. Nutmeg displays similar properties and is contained in EndoFlex.*
>
> *When the adrenal glands are working properly, it is easier to correct low thyroid function.*

Thyromin (1-4 tablets daily. *See Suggested Use under Thyromin in the Supplements section of the Reference Guide for Essential Oils.*)

AFTERSHAVE: see SKIN. Valor. Awaken can be used instead of aftershave lotion. Try adding Awaken to Sandalwood Moisture Creme, Satin Body Lotion, Sensation Hand & Body Lotion, or Genesis Hand & Body Lotion as an aftershave.
PERSONAL CARE–Genesis Hand & Body Lotion, KidScents Lotion (soothes and rehydrates the skin- smells great too), Prenolone/Prenolone+, Rose Ointment, Sandalwood Moisture Creme, Satin Body Lotion, Sensation Hand & Body Lotion.

AGENT ORANGE POISONING:

JuvaFlex (over liver with hot compress), EndoFlex (over adrenal glands/kidneys).

> *Agent Orange is a toxic herbicide that was used to defoliate areas of the forest during the Vietnam War.*

BATH—in 1 cup Epsom salts and 4 oz. of food grade hydrogen peroxide.
SUPPLEMENTS—ComforTone, ICP, ImmuneTune, ImmuPro, Megazyme, Radex, Thyromin.
RECIPE #1— 3 drops EndoFlex on throat, feet (under big toes and kidney Vita Flex point). Also across the back over the kidneys. After 90 days, start the Cleansing Trio (ComforTone, Megazyme, and ICP) and continue for one year.
RECIPE #2— 2 Radex three times a day, 3 ImmuneTune four times a day, 2 Thyromin at bedtime. After 90 days, start on Cleansing Trio (ComforTone, Megazyme, and ICP) and continue for one year.

AGING: See WRINKLES. Carrot, frankincense, Longevity (take as a dietary supplement to help prevent premature aging), rosehip, rosewood, sandalwood.

SUPPLEMENTS—Berry Young Juice (a delicious blend of highly antioxidant fruit juices - measures higher on the ORAC (oxygen radical absorbent capacity) scale than even Tahitian Noni Juice), Berry Young Delights (a pack of six cookies packed full of antioxidant ingredients), Longevity Capsules.

MOISTURIZERS—

PERSONAL CARE—Boswellia Wrinkle Creme, Satin Facial Scrub - Mint or Juniper, Prenolone/Prenolone+, Rose Ointment, Sandalwood Moisture Creme, Sensation Hand & Body Lotion, Wolfberry Eye Creme.

SUPPLEMENTS— Megazyme, Mineral Essence (antioxidant), Wolfberry Bar *(Refer to the Wolfberry Bar in the Supplements section of the Reference Guide for Essential Oils for more information on the benefits of the Chinese Wolfberry).*

AGITATION: ᶠBergamot, cedarwood, Clary sage, <u>Forgiveness</u>, frankincense, geranium, <u>Harmony</u>, <u>Joy</u>, juniper, lavender, marjoram, myrrh, <u>Peace & Calming</u>, rose, rosewood, sandalwood, <u>Trauma Life</u> (calms), <u>Valor</u>, ylang ylang.

AIDS: <u>Brain Power</u>, cistus, cumin (supports immune system; inhibits HIV virus), <u>Exodus II</u>, helichrysum, <u>ImmuPower</u>, lemon, nutmeg, <u>Thieves</u>, <u>Valor</u>. Apply to Thymus and bottom of feet.

SUPPLEMENTS—Cleansing Trio (ComforTone, Megazyme, and ICP), Exodus, ImmuGel, ImmuneTune, ImmuPro, Mineral Essence, Power Meal (contains wolfberry which is an immune stimulator), Super B, Super C, Thyromin, Ultra Young, VitaGreen.

****COMMENTS—Refer to the chapter entitled "How to Use - The Personal Usage Reference" in the Essential Oils Desk Reference under "AIDS" for specific oil blend and supplement recommendations.*

AIRBORNE BACTERIA:
Cinnamon bark, fir, Idaho balsam fir, Mountain savory, oregano, <u>Purification</u>, and <u>Thieves</u>.

AIR POLLUTION: <u>Abundance</u>, <u>Christmas Spirit</u>, cypress, eucalyptus, fir, grapefruit, <u>ImmuPower</u>, lavender, lemon (sterilize air), lime, <u>Purification</u>, rosemary, <u>Thieves</u>.

> *Diffusing essential oils in the home or work place is one of the best ways to purify our environment. The anti-viral, anti-bacterial, and antiseptic properties of the oils, along with the negative ions and oxygenating molecules that are released when essential oils are diffused, all help to reduce chemicals, bacteria, and metallics in the air.*
>
> *Cinnamon bark, Mountain savory, oregano, and Thieves. were all tested by Weber State University and were shown to kill 100% of the airborne bacteria present. This was all done by diffusing the oils into the atmosphere.*
> *(KID-Radio with Lance Richardson and Dr. Gary Young, N.D., Aromatologist, March 5, 1996)*

DISINFECTANTS—Birch, citronella, clove, eucalyptus, grapefruit, ᶠlemon, peppermint, Purification, sage, spruce, wintergreen.
  SUPPLEMENTS—Radex helps prevent the build-up of free radicals within the body due to air pollution.

ALCOHOLISM: See ADDICTIONS. Fennel, juniper, and rosemary (Alternative Medicine—A Definitive Guide, p. 492). Can also use Acceptance, elemi, Forgiveness, helichrysum, Joy, JuvaFlex, lavender, Motivation, orange, Roman chamomile, rosemary verbenon, Surrender.
  SUPPLEMENTS—Cleansing Trio (ComforTone, ICP, Megazyme), JuvaTone, Mineral Essence, Power Meal, Thyromin. Work on cleaning out the colon and liver with the Cleansing Trio and JuvaTone or the Master Cleanser (see CLEANSING).

ALERTNESS: Basil, Citrus Fresh, Clarity, lemon, peppermint, rosemary. Apply to temples and bottom of feet.

ALKALINE: See ACIDOSIS, pH BALANCE.
  ALKALI-FORMING FOODS—Dark green and yellow vegetables, sprouted grains, legumes, seeds, nuts, essential fats (omega 3 and 6), and low sugar fruits like avocados and lemons.
  PERSONAL CARE—Genesis Hand & Body Lotion balances pH on the skin.

> *Alkaline refers to a substance or solution that has a pH of 7.0 or above. The optimum pH for our blood and body tissues is about 7.2 (The use of saliva and urine test strips will show a much lower pH level due to the protein present in the solution. Saliva and urine tests from a healthy body should be about 6.6 to 6.8).*
>
> *The body heals best when it is slightly alkaline. To keep the blood and body tissue at an optimum pH, avoid acid-forming food. See ACIDOSIS. Make sure your food intake is 80 percent alkaline and drink plenty of water.*

  SUPPLEMENTS—AlkaLime, Mineral Essence, Power Meal (pre-digested protein), Royaldophilus (replaces intestinal flora), Stevia Select (with FOS to help rebuild and protect friendly intestinal flora), VitaGreen (helps normalize blood pH levels).

ALKALOSIS: See pH BALANCE. Anise, Di-Tone, ginger, tarragon.
  SUPPLEMENTS—Body Balance, Megazyme, Mineral Essence, Power

> *Alkalosis refers to a condition where the blood and intestinal tract becomes excessively alkaline. Slight alkalinity is important for a healthy body but excessive alkalinity can cause depression, fatigue, and sickness.*

Meal (pre-digested protein), Royaldophilus (replaces intestinal flora), Sulfurzyme, VitaGreen (helps normalize blood pH levels).

ALONE (Feeling): See EMOTIONS. <u>Acceptance</u>, <u>Valor</u>.

ALLERGIES: Elemi (rashes), eucalyptus, <u>Harmony</u>, ᶠlavender, ledum, *Melaleuca ericifolia*, *Melaleuca quinquenervia*, melissa (skin and respiratory), ᶠpatchouly, peppermint, <u>ImmuPower</u>, <u>Raven</u>, <u>RC</u>, Roman chamomile, spikenard. Apply to sinuses, bottom of feet, and diffuse.

  ****COMMENTS—According to the <u>Essential Oils Desk Reference</u>, ". . . rub three drops [<u>Harmony</u>] on sternum, breathing deeply." (EDR-June 2002; Ch. 8; Harmony; Application)*

  SUPPLEMENTS—AlkaLime, ComforTone, Coral Sea (highly bio-available calcium, contains 58 trace minerals), ICP fiber beverage (beneficial when there is an allergy to psyllium), ImmuneTune, ImmuPro, Mineral Essence, Super C, Super Cal.

COUGHING—<u>Purification</u> (diffuse).

FOOD ALLERGIES—Cleanse the body!

HAY FEVER—See HAY FEVER.

PHYSICAL ALLERGIES—Need to detoxify the body.

> *If you have a reaction to the oils, it is only a reaction to all of the chemicals you have been dumping into your body throughout the years. The oils are merely reacting with the toxins in the sub-dermal tissues and beginning their removal.* **Cleanse the body!**

PSYCHOLOGICAL ALLERGIES (in the mind)—Put <u>Harmony</u> on feet, neck, navel, or in your shoes for one to five days.

TO OILS—Put one drop of the oil, to which there is an allergy reaction, on a cotton ball and place it in a shoe. Add a drop each day until the allergy to that particular oil is gone. Since allergies often indicate an electrical imbalance, try the following:

  A. Place a drop or two of <u>Harmony</u> into one hand, then rub the palms of both hands together in a clockwise motion.

  B. Place one hand over the thymus (heart chakra) and the other hand over the navel.

  C. Take three deep breaths and switch hands, then take three more deep breaths. Harmony helps open the energy meridians and balance the bio-electrical field of the body.

The following recipes have been used for allergies:

  RECIPE #1—Apply 1 drop of peppermint on the base of the neck two times a day. Tap the thymus (located just below the notch in the neck) with pointer and index fingers (energy fingers). Diffuse peppermint. For some individuals, the use of peppermint oil has resulted in no more allergy shots!

RECIPE #2—Apply 1 drop of <u>RC</u> and <u>Raven</u> on the base of the neck two times a day. Tap on thymus, massage chest and back with 5 <u>Raven</u>, 5 <u>RC</u>, and 2 tsp. V-6 Mixing Oil. Diffuse <u>RC</u> and <u>Raven</u>.

RECIPE #3—For allergy rashes and skin sensitivity, Dr. Gary Young applies 3 lavender, 6 Roman chamomile, 2 myrrh, and 1 peppermint on location.

ALOPECIA AREATA: (Inflammatory hair-loss disease) See HAIR: LOSS.

ALUMINUM TOXICITY: See
ATTENTION
DEFICIT DISORDER.
SUPPLEMENTS—Chelex
helps remove
aluminum from the
body.

> *Aluminum toxicity may contribute to the cause of rickets, colic, digestion, kidney and liver dysfunction, speech and memory problems, osteoporosis, and Alzheimer's disease.*

ALZHEIMER'S DISEASE: See
BRAIN, MEMORY,
PINEAL GLAND,
PITUITARY GLAND.
SUPPLEMENTS—Chelex,
Cleansing Trio
(ComforTone,
Megazyme, and ICP),
JuvaTone, Power Meal,
Sulfurzyme.
    COMMENTS—*The
gingko biloba that is
found in Power Meal
has been shown to help*

> *Autopsies have revealed that victims of **Alzheimer's disease** have four times the normal amount of aluminum in the nerve cells of their brain.*
>
> ***Prevention:*** *Use glass, iron, or stainless steel cookware. Avoid products containing aluminum, bentonite, or dihydroxyaluminum. Some of these products are: aluminum cookware, foil, antacids, baking powders, buffered aspirin, most city water, antiperspirants, deodorants, beer, bleached flour, table salt, tobacco smoke, cream of tartar, Parmesan and grated cheeses, aluminum salts, douches, and canned goods.*

improve memory loss, brain function, depression, cerebral and peripheral circulation, oxygenation, and blood flow.

BLOOD-BRAIN BARRIER—Frankincense and sandalwood contain sesquiterpenes, which enable these oils to pass the blood-brain barrier. Blends containing both of these oils include: <u>3 Wise Men</u>, <u>Acceptance</u>, <u>Forgiveness</u>, <u>Gathering</u>, <u>Harmony</u>, <u>Inspiration</u>, <u>Into the Future</u>, and <u>Trauma Life</u>. Apply to temples, bottom of feet, and diffuse.

    COMMENTS—*Oils that pass through the blood-brain barrier cannot carry unwanted substances with them.*

BRAIN FUNCTION—<u>Clarity</u>.

EMOTIONS—<u>Acceptance</u>, cypress, <u>Peace & Calming</u>, <u>3 Wise Men</u> (crown).

AMINO ACIDS: Lavender.

> *Amino acids* have the ability to neutralize and help eliminate free radicals in the system.

    SUPPLEMENTS—Body Balance, Cleansing Trio (ComforTone, Megazyme, and ICP), Exodus, FemiGen, JuvaTone, ImmuGel, Master Formula His/Hers, Mighty Mist/Vites, Mineral Essence, Power Meal, Radex, Thyromin.

    TINCTURES—Royal Essence.

AMNESIA: See MEMORY. Basil, clove, rosemary.

ANALGESIC: Bergamot, birch, clove, eucalyptus, geranium, helichrysum, lavender, lemongrass, marjoram, melaleuca, oregano, PanAway, peppermint, Roman chamomile, rosemary, wintergreen.

    ***COMMENT—See the "single oil property chart" in the APPENDIX of this book for additional analgesic oils and their strengths.*

ANEMIA: Carrot, ImmuPower, lavender, ᶠlemon. Apply to bottom of feet and stomach.

    FOOD—Flavor water with a drop of lemon. Can also use an H2Oils packet of lemon to infuse the drinking water with lemon oil.

    SUPPLEMENTS—Rehemogen tincture (10 drops twice a day) and JuvaTone together help raise blood cell count.

ANESTHESIA: Helichrysum, PanAway.

    ***COMMENTS—One individual applied helichrysum every 15 minutes during gum surgery and there was no bleeding and no pain. No other anesthetic was used.*

ANEURYSM: See BLOOD. Aroma Life (chelates plaque), cypress (strengthens the capillary walls and increases circulation), frankincense, helichrysum, Idaho tansy. Apply to temples, heart, Vita Flex heart points, and diffuse.

    BLEND—5 frankincense, 1 helichrysum, and 1 cypress. DIFFUSE.

    HERBS—Cayenne pepper, Garlic, Hawthorn Berry.

    MASSAGE OIL—Cel-Lite Magic dilates blood vessels for better circulation.

    SUPPLEMENTS—Cleansing Trio (ComforTone, Megazyme, and ICP), Sulfurzyme, Super C.

    TINCTURES—HRT.

ANGER: See LIVER. Bergamot, cedarwood, cypress, Forgiveness, frankincense, geranium, German chamomile, Grounding, Joy, Harmony, helichrysum, Hope, Humility, Inspiration, lavender, lemon, mandarin, marjoram, melissa, myrrh (soothes), myrtle, orange, Peace & Calming, petitgrain, Present Time, Release, Roman chamomile, rose, <u>Sacred Mountain</u>, sandalwood, <u>Trauma Life</u>, <u>Valor</u>, ylang ylang.

***COMMENTS—*Refer to the Emotional Release part of the Science and Application section of the <u>Reference Guide for Essential Oils</u>.*

CALMS ANGER—<u>Inspiration</u>, <u>Peace & Calming</u>, spruce, <u>Trauma Life</u>.

CLEANSING AFTER ARGUMENT and PHYSICAL FIGHTING—Eucalyptus.

CLEANSE THE LIVER—(Anger is stored in the liver) <u>JuvaFlex</u>, ᶠgeranium (cleanses and detoxifies the liver), grapefruit (liver disorders).

DISPELS ANGER—Ylang ylang.

FOR COMMUNICATION WITHOUT ANGER—Roman chamomile.

LESSENS ANGER—Myrrh.

OVERCOME—Bergamot, ᶠcedarwood, <u>Release</u>, Roman chamomile.

RELEASES LOCKED UP ANGER and FRUSTRATION—Roman or German chamomile, <u>Release</u> (together with <u>JuvaFlex</u>), <u>Sacred Mountain</u>, sandalwood, <u>Valor</u>.

> *BLEND*—4 drops lavender, 3 geranium, 3 rosewood, 3 rosemary, 2 tangerine, 1 spearmint, 2 Idaho tansy, 1 German chamomile, and 1 oz. V-6 Mixing Oil. Apply to back of neck, wrist, and heart.
> *SUPPLEMENTS*—JuvaTone, Thyromin, Super B.
> *TINCTURES*—Royal Essence.

ANGINA: <u>Aroma Life</u>, ᶠginger, laurel, ᶠorange (for false angina). Apply to heart and Vita Flex heart point.

Angina pectoris is a severe spasmodic pain in the chest that is due to an insufficient supply of blood to the heart.

TINCTURES—HRT.

ANIMALS: Only a 1-2 drops of oil is all that is necessary on animals as they respond much more quickly to the oils than do humans. V-6 Mixing Oil can be added to extend oil over larger areas and to heavily dilute the essential oil for use on smaller animals, especially cats.

PERSONAL CARE—Alkaline shampoos without chemicals are good for animals.
SUPPLEMENTS—Power Meal and Sulfurzyme.

BLEEDING—Geranium, helichrysum.

BONES (Pain)—Birch/wintergreen, lemongrass, <u>PanAway</u>, spruce.

> *MASSAGE OILS*—Ortho Ease or Ortho Sport.

CALM—<u>Citrus Fresh</u>, lavender, <u>Peace & Calming</u>, Roman chamomile (for horses, add to feed), <u>Trauma Life</u>. Dilute well for cats.

CANCER—

SKIN—Frankincense and cumin.

CATS—Valerie Worwood says that you can treat a cat like you would a child (see
    BABIES). Dilute oils heavily with V-6 Mixing Oil. Avoid melaleuca.
    ***COMMENTS—Cat physiology is so different from other animals and from
    humans that oils should be used with extreme caution on cats. In fact,
    melaleuca (or Tea Tree oil) should never be used on a cat as death can result.
    Some cases exist where a blend of oils containing melaleuca have killed cats.***
COLDS and COUGHS—Eucalyptus, melaleuca (not for cats). Apply on fur or stomach.
COWS—For scours, use 5 drops <u>Di-Tone</u> on stomach (can mix with V-6 Mixing Oil to
    cover larger area) and repeat 2 hours later.
CUTS and SORES—<u>Melrose</u> (not on cats). 1 drop on location. Work in with finger.
DOGS—There was a dog that walked with its head down and its tail between its legs.
    <u>Valor</u> was put on its feet and <u>3 Wise Men</u> and <u>Joy</u> on its crown. The next day its
    head was up and it was happy.
    ANXIETY/NERVOUSNESS—Lavender, <u>Peace & Calming</u>, valerian, <u>Valor</u>. Rub 1-
        2 drops between hands and apply to muzzle, between toes, on top of feet to smell
        when nose is down, and on edge of ears.
    ARTHRITIS—A blend of rosemary, lavender, and ginger diluted with V-6 Mixing
        Oil. Ortho Ease Massage Oil can also be applied to arthritic areas. Add
        Sulfurzyme (powder) or Vitamin C to their food.
    BONE INJURY—Birch/wintergreen and Ortho Ease Massage Oil on injury.
        Sulfurzyme in food.
    CHEWING ON FURNITURE—Mineral Essence (helps satisfy mineral deficiency).
    DIGESTION—Megazyme.
    HEART PROBLEMS—Myrtle, ravensara, and <u>Thieves</u> on back using Raindrop
        Technique with warm wet pack. Peppermint on paws. HRT Tincture can also be
        added to food.
    LIMPING—4 ArthroTune per day for two weeks, then 3 per day until healed. Use 2
        per day for maintenance.
    PAIN and STRESS—Do Raindrop Technique (*the video "Essential Tips for Happy,*
        Healthy Pets" demonstrates this technique on a dog and a horse). This
        technique helps relieve stress on the back, shoulders, and legs as well as raise
        immune function and protect against illness.
    SLEEP—Lavender (on paws), <u>Peace & Calming</u> (on stomach).
    STROKE—<u>Brain Power</u> (on head), frankincense (on brain stem/back of neck), <u>Valor</u>
        (on each paw).
    TICKS and BUG BITES—<u>Purification</u>. 1 drop directly on live tick. Can also be
        applied to untreated tick wound and worked in with finger.
    TRAVEL SICKNESS—Peppermint. Dilute with V-6 Mixing Oil and rub on
        stomach. Also helps calm stomachaches.
    TRAUMATIZED—<u>Trauma Life</u>. Rub 1-2 drops between hands and cup over nose
        and mouth for dog to inhale.

EARACHE—1 drop <u>Melrose</u> or a blend of 1 drop melaleuca (Tea Tree), 1 lavender, and 1 Roman chamomile diluted in V-6 Mixing oil. Put in ear and rub around the ear.

EAR INFECTIONS—<u>ImmuPower</u>, <u>Purification</u> (helps ward off insects too). Dip cotton swab in oil and apply to inside and front of ear.

FLEAS—Citronella, eucalyptus, lemongrass, <u>Melrose</u>, pine. Add 1-2 drops of oil to shampoo.

    BLEND—Combine eucalyptus, orange, citronella, and cedarwood. Add blend to distilled water in a spray bottle, shake well, and mist over entire animal.

HORSES—

    ANXIETY/NERVOUSNESS—<u>Peace & Calming</u>. Rub 1-2 drops between hands and apply to nose, on front of chest, knees, and tongue.

    FLIES—Idaho Tansy Floral Water. Spray over animal to keep flies and other insects away.

    HOOF ROT—Blend of Roman chamomile, thyme, and melissa diluted in V-6 Mixing Oil.

    INFECTION—<u>Melrose</u>, <u>Thieves</u>.

        ****COMMENTS—One couple had a horse that got kicked in the flank, creating a large wound. The Vet treated the wound and gave her some medication. Unfortunately, the wound became reinfected and worsened to the point that the horse almost died. The Vet came over and reopened the wound and flushed out nearly two gallons of blood clots. However, the Vet had no medication with him and would not be able to deliver any more for a couple of days. So, the wife put 15 drops of <u>Thieves</u> in about 1/4 cup of olive oil and while the husband held open the horse's mouth, she poured the oil down its throat. This was repeated three or four times and within just a few days, the horse was fully recovered.*

    INJURIES—Do Raindrop Technique (*the video "Essential Tips for Happy, Healthy Pets" demonstrates this technique on a dog and a horse*). When a frisky race horse took a fall and was unable to walk, application of the oils using the Raindrop Technique brought the horse out of it in a matter of days.

    LEG FRACTURES—Ginger and V-6 Mixing Oil. Wrap the leg with a hot compress. Massage leg after the fracture is healed with a blend of rosemary and thyme with V-6 Mixing Oil. This may strengthen the ligaments and prevent calcification.

    MUSCLE TISSUE/LIGAMENTS—Equal parts lemongrass and lavender on location and wrap to help regenerate torn muscle tissue.

    WOUNDS—Helichrysum, <u>Melrose</u>, and Rose Ointment.

    SADDLE SORES—<u>Melrose</u> and Rose Ointment.

INFECTION—<u>Di-Tone</u> and <u>ImmuPower</u> on the paws.

PARASITES—Cedarwood, lavender, <u>Di-Tone</u>. Rub on paws to release parasites.

    SUPPLEMENTS—ParaFree.

SNAKE BITES (Venomous Wounds)—Do Raindrop Technique (*the video "Essential Tips for Happy, Healthy Pets" demonstrates this technique on a dog and a horse*).

ANOREXIA: Angelica, Christmas Spirt, Citrus Fresh, coriander, grapefruit, Purification, Melrose, ᶠtarragon, Valor. Apply to stomach and bottom of feet. It may also help to diffuse anti-depressant oils.
>   ****COMMENTS—Some studies have shown that people suffering from anorexia have a tendency to have lower levels of zinc.*
>   *SUPPLEMENTS*—Mineral Essence.
>   ANTI-DEPRESSANTS— Acceptance, basil, bergamot, Clary sage, lavender, neroli, Roman chamomile, ylang ylang.

ANTHRAX: ᶠThyme.

> *Anthrax is an infectious, fatal animal disease found in cows and sheep. It can be transmitted to human beings through contact with contaminated animal substances, such as hair, feces, or hides. It may also be used in biological warfare and is transmitted as spores through the air. It is characterized by ulcerative skin lesions.*

ANTI-BACTERIAL: ᶠBasil, bergamot, cassia, Canadian Red cedar, cedarwood, citronella, Christmas Spirit, Citrus Fresh, ᶠcinnamon bark, Clary sage, ᶠclove, ᶠcypress, eucalyptus, Evergreen Essence, fir, geranium, grapefruit, Idaho tansy, juniper, lavender, lemon, marjoram, melaleuca, *Melaleuca ericifolia*, Mountain savory, neroli, ᶠoregano, palmarosa, petitgrain, pine, Purification, ravensara, RC, Roman chamomile, ᶠrosemary, ᶠrosewood, Sacred Mountain, ᶠspearmint, tarragon, Thieves (annihilates bacteria), ᶠthyme, valerian, Western Red cedar
>   ****COMMENTS—All oils are anti-bacterial; see the "single oil property chart" in the APPENDIX of this book for additional anti-bacterial oils and their strengths.*

> *Research at Weber State University has shown that out of 67 oils tested, 66 of them were powerful anti-bacterial agents. Oregano, cinnamon bark, Mountain savory, ravensara, and peppermint were all more powerful as anti-bacterial agents than Penicillin or Ampicillin. Thieves was shown to be 60 percent higher in activity against bacteria, germs, and anti-microbial action than either Ampicillin or Penicillin!*
> *(KID-Radio with Lance Richardson and Dr. Gary Young, N.D., Aromatologist, March 5, 1996)*

>   *ESSENTIAL WATERS (HYDROSOLS)*—Mountain Essence. Spray into air directly on area of concern, or diffuse using the Essential Mist Diffuser.
>   AIRBORNE—See AIRBORNE BACTERIA. Cinnamon bark, fir, Mountain savory, oregano, Purification, Thieves.

CLEANSING—Purification.
INFECTION—Nutmeg (fights).
PREVENTS GROWTH OF—Melrose.

ANTI-CANCEROUS: Clove, frankincense, ImmuPower, ledum (may be more powerful than
frankincense).
SUPPLEMENTS—Exodus, Power Meal, Sulfurzyme.

ANTI-CATARRHAL: Black pepper, ᶠcypress, elemi, eucalyptus, ᶠfir, frankincense, ginger,
ᶠhelichrysum (discharges mucus), hyssop (opens respiratory system and discharges
toxins and mucous), jasmine, onycha (benzoin), RC, Raven, ravensara, and
rosemary. Apply on lung area, feet, around nose, Vita Flex lung points, and
diffuse.
***COMMENTS*—*See the "single oil property chart" in the APPENDIX of this book
for additional anti-catarrhal oils and their strengths.*

ANTI-COAGULANT: Angelica, cassia, ᶠhelichrysum, lavender, tangerine, tarragon. Apply
on location, bottom of feet, and diffuse.

ANTI-DEPRESSANT: See DEPRESSION. Elemi, ᶠfrankincense, lavender, onycha
(combine with rose for massage). Apply to bottom of feet, heart, and diffuse.
SUPPLEMENTS—Essential Omegas
***COMMENTS*—*See the "single oil property chart" in the APPENDIX of this book
for additional anti-depressant oils and their strengths.*
RECOVERY FROM COMMERCIAL ANTI-DEPRESSANTS LIKE PROZAC—

Brain Power, Clarity, Joy, and Valor all help repair brain damage from the
commercial drugs that inhibit serotonin metabolism. They also stimulate the
pineal gland which normally metabolizes 50% of the serotonin in the body.
SUPPLEMENTS—Carbozyme (to help control blood sugar levels), Essential Omegas

ANTI-FUNGAL: Abundance, ᶠcinnamon bark, ᶠclove, geranium, ImmuPower, juniper,
lavender, lemon, lemongrass, mandarin, ᶠmelaleuca, *Melaleuca ericifolia*,
Mountain savory, ᶠoregano, palmarosa, ᶠrosewood, sage, ᶠspearmint, ᶠthyme.
Apply to bottom of feet, on location, and diffuse.
***COMMENTS*—*See the "single oil property chart" in the APPENDIX of this book
for additional anti-fungal oils and their strengths.*
BLEND—2 myrrh and 2 lavender. Rub on location.
SUPPLEMENTS—AlkaLime, ICP, Megazyme, ImmuGel.

ANTI-HEMORRHAGING: See HEMORRHAGING. Helichrysum, rose.

ANTI-INFECTIOUS: ᶠBasil, cassia, ᶠcinnamon bark, clove, ᶠcypress, davana, elemi, eucalyptus, hyssop, Idaho tansy, ᶠlavender, marjoram, melaleuca, *Melaleuca ericifolia*, myrrh, ᶠpatchouly, petitgrain, ᶠpine, ᶠravensara, rose, ᶠrosemary, ᶠrosewood, <u>Purification</u>, Roman chamomile, spearmint, spikenard, ᶠspruce, tarragon, ᶠthyme. Apply on location and bottom of feet.
   ***COMMENTS—*See the "single oil property chart" in the APPENDIX of this book for additional anti-infectious oils and their strengths.*
   *SUPPLEMENTS—*ImmuGel, Radex, Super C.

ANTI-INFLAMMATORY: ᶠBirch, Black pepper, Blue cypress, calamus (gastrointestinal), citronella, coriander, cypress, eucalyptus, ᶠGerman chamomile, helichrysum, hyssop (of the pulmonary), ᶠlavender, lemongrass, melaleuca, ᶠmyrrh, onycha (benzoin), ᶠpatchouly, peppermint, petitgrain, ravensara, ᶠRoman chamomile, spearmint, spikenard, ᶠspruce, tangerine, ᶠtarragon, wintergreen. Apply on location.
   ***COMMENTS—*See the "single oil property chart" in the APPENDIX of this book for additional anti-inflammatory oils and their strengths.*

ANTI-PARASITIC: ᶠCinnamon bark, clove, <u>Di-Tone</u>, fennel, ginger, hyssop, lemon, lemongrass, melaleuca, Mountain savory, oregano, ᶠRoman chamomile, rosemary, rosewood, spearmint, spikenard, tarragon. Apply to stomach, liver, intestines, and Vita Flex points on feet.
   ***COMMENTS—*See the "single oil property chart" in the APPENDIX of this book for additional anti-parasitic oils and their strengths.*
   *SUPPLEMENTS—*Cleansing Trio (ComforTone, Megazyme, and ICP), ImmuneTune, ParaFree.

ANTI-RHEUMATIC: Birch, eucalyptus, juniper, onycha (benzoin), oregano, rosemary, thyme, wintergreen.
   ***COMMENTS—*See the "single oil property chart" in the APPENDIX of this book for additional anti-rheumatic oils and their strengths.*

ANTI-SEXUAL: ᶠMarjoram (helps balance sexual desires).

ANTI-TUMORAL: Clove, ᶠfrankincense, <u>ImmuPower</u>, ledum (may be more powerful than frankincense).

ANTI-VIRAL: <u>Abundance</u>, bergamot, ᶠcinnamon bark, Clary sage, ᶠclove, <u>Cumincense</u> (available through Creer Labs 801-465-5423), *Eucalyptus radiata*, galbanum, geranium, hyssop, Idaho tansy, <u>ImmuPower</u>, juniper, lavender, lemon, ᶠmelaleuca, melissa, Mountain savory, myrrh, ᶠoregano, palmarosa, pine, <u>RC</u>, ᶠravensara, ᶠrosewood, sandalwood, tarragon, <u>Thieves</u>, ᶠthyme.

***COMMENTS**—See the "single oil property chart" in the APPENDIX of this book
for additional anti-viral oils and their strengths. Dr. J. C. Lapraz found that
viruses cannot live in the presence of cinnamon oil. However, because of its
high phenol content, it must be diluted before applied on the skin.
SUPPLEMENTS—ParaFree.

ANTIBIOTIC: Bergamot, cinnamon bark, clove, eucalyptus, hyssop, lavender, lemon,
melaleuca, <u>Melrose</u>, myrtle, nutmeg, oregano, patchouly, <u>Purification</u>, ravensara,
Roman chamomile, <u>Thieves</u>, thyme. Apply on location, liver area, bottom of feet,
and diffuse.

ANTIHISTAMINE: Lavender, Roman chamomile. Apply to sinuses, Vita Flex points, and
diffuse.

ANTIMICROBIAL: <u>Abundance</u>, cinnamon bark, cypress, helichrysum, jasmine, lavender,
lemongrass, *Melaleuca ericifolia* (powerful), melissa (shown in lab tests to be
effective against *Streptococcus haemolytica*), myrrh, palmarosa, pine, rosemary,
rosewood, sage, thyme.
***COMMENTS**—See the "single oil property chart" in the APPENDIX of this book
for additional antimicrobial oils and their strengths.
ESSENTIAL WATERS (HYDROSOLS)—Idaho Tansy, Melissa. Spray into air directly
on area of concern, or diffuse using the Essential Mist Diffuser.
SUPPLEMENTS—ImmuGel.

ANTIOXIDANTS: Cinnamon
bark, <u>Di-Tone</u>, <u>Exodus II</u>, frankincense,
helichrysum, hyssop,
<u>ImmuPower</u>, <u>JuvaFlex</u>,
melaleuca, <u>Longevity</u>

> ***Antioxidants*** *create an unfriendly environment for free radicals. They prevent all mutations, work as free radical scavengers, prevent fungus, prevent oxidation in the cells, and help to oxygenate the cells.*

(take as a dietary supplement to promote longevity), melaleuca, <u>Melrose</u>, onycha
(benzoin), oregano, <u>PanAway</u>, <u>Purification</u>, ravensara, <u>RC</u>, <u>Relieve It</u>, Roman
chamomile, <u>Thieves</u>, thyme.
SUPPLEMENTS—ArthroTune, Berry Young Juice {a delicious blend of highly
antioxidant fruit juices - measures higher on the ORAC (oxygen radical absorbent
capacity) scale than even Tahitian Noni Juice}, Berry Young Delights (a pack of
six cookies packed full of antioxidant ingredients), Exodus, ImmuGel,
ImmuneTune, JuvaTone, CardiaCare (with *Rhododendron caucasicum*),
Longevity Capsules (highest known ORAC score), Master Formula His/Hers,
Megazyme. Mineral Essence, Radex, Super C, Super B, VitaGreen, Wolfberry
Bar (*Refer to the Wolfberry Bar in the Supplements section of the <u>Reference</u>*

> *Guide for Essential Oils for more information on the benefits of the Chinese Wolfberry).*
> *TINCTURES*—AD&E

ANTISEPTIC: Bergamot, Canadian Red cedar, ᶠcedarwood, cinnamon bark, citronella, clove, cumin, <u>Di-Tone</u> (all oils in this blend are antiseptic), elemi, eucalyptus, <u>Evergreen Essence</u>, fennel, ᶠfir, frankincense, Idaho balsam fir, lavender, lemon, mandarin, marjoram, melaleuca, <u>Melrose</u>, Mountain savory, mugwort, ᶠmyrtle (skin), ᶠnutmeg (intestinal), orange, onycha (benzoin), ᶠoregano, ᶠpatchouly, ᶠpeppermint, ᶠpine (pulmonary, urinary, hepatic), <u>Purification</u>, ravensara, Roman chamomile, rosemary cineol, rosemary verbenon, ᶠsage, ᶠsandalwood, ᶠspearmint, ᶠthyme, thyme linalol, Western Red cedar, ylang ylang. Apply on location.

> *ESSENTIAL WATERS (HYDROSOLS)*—Eucalyptus, Western Red Cedar, Thyme. Spray directly onto area of concern.

> ***COMMENTS**—Most oils can be used as antiseptics. See the "single oil property chart" in the APPENDIX of this book for additional antiseptic oils and their strengths.*

> *PERSONAL CARE*—Rose Ointment (apply over oils to increase antiseptic properties and extend effectiveness).
> *SUPPLEMENTS*—ImmuGel, Super C.
> *TINCTURES*—AD&E.

ANTISPASMODIC: Anise, ᶠ**basil**, calamus, citronella, cumin, fennel, ᶠGerman chamomile, helichrysum, ᶠlavender, mandarin, ᶠmarjoram, mugwort ᶠpeppermint, petitgrain, ᶠRoman chamomile (relaxes spastic muscles of the colon wall), ᶠrosemary, ᶠsage, spearmint, spikenard, ᶠspruce, tarragon, valerian, ylang ylang.

> ***COMMENTS**—See the "single oil property chart" in the APPENDIX of this book for additional antispasmodic oils.*

ANXIETY: Basil, bergamot, cedarwood, Clary sage, cypress, <u>Evergreen Essence</u>, frankincense, geranium, hyssop, jasmine, juniper, lavender, lemon, lime, marjoram, melissa, onycha (combine with rose for massage), patchouly, pine, <u>Release</u>, Roman chamomile, rose, sandalwood, <u>Surrender</u>, tangerine, tsuga (grounding), ᶠylang ylang.

APATHY: Frankincense, geranium, <u>Harmony</u>, <u>Hope</u>, jasmine, <u>Joy</u>, marjoram, orange, peppermint, rose, rosemary, rosewood, sandalwood, <u>3 Wise Men</u>, thyme, <u>Valor</u>, <u>White Angelica</u>, ylang ylang.

APHRODISIAC: Cinnamon bark, Clary sage, ginger, jasmine, patchouly, rose, ᶠsandalwood, Sensation, neroli, ylang ylang.

> *Many books of aromatherapy tout the **aphrodisiac** qualities of a number of oils. Perhaps an aphrodisiac to one individual may not be to another. The most important factor is to find an oil that brings balance to the mind and body. A balanced individual is more likely to extend love.*

    BATH & SHOWER GELS— Sensation Bath & Shower Gel.
    *MASSAGE OILS—*Sensation Massage Oil.
    *PERSONAL CARE—*Sensation Hand & Body Lotion.

APNEA: Brain Power, Clarity (diffuse), Raven, RC, Valor (on feet).

> **Apnea** is the cessation of breathing. During sleep, periods of apnea can occur for a few seconds before breathing resumes. May be due to irregular heartbeats, high blood pressure, obesity, or damage to the area of the brain responsible for controlling respiration.

    *SUPPLEMENTS—*Super B, Thyromin, VitaGreen.
    *TINCTURES—*Royal Essence.
    *RECIPE #1—*Try 3 droppers of Royal Essence four times per day, 3 VitaGreen twice per day, 1 Super B three times per day with meals, and 1 Thyromin before bed.

APPETITE-LOSS OF: ᶠBergamot, calamus, cardamom, ginger, hyssop, lemon, myrrh, ᶠnutmeg, orange, spearmint. Apply to stomach, bottom of feet, and diffuse.
    *SUPPLEMENTS—*ComforTone, Megazyme, Mint Condition.

APPETITE SUPPRESSANT:
    *SUPPLEMENTS—*ThermaBurn (tablets), ThermaMist (oral spray).

ARGUMENTATIVE: Acceptance, cedarwood, eucalyptus, frankincense, Harmony, Hope, Humility, jasmine, joy, orange, Peace & Calming, Roman chamomile, thyme, Trauma Life, Valor, ylang ylang.

ARMS-FLABBY: Cypress, fennel, juniper, lavender.

ARTERIAL VASODILATOR: Aroma Life, ᶠmarjoram. Apply to carotid arteries in neck, over heart, Vita Flex points on feet.

ARTERIAL WALLS: Aroma Life (strengthens).

ARTERIES: (blocked after surgery), Aroma Life, lavender, Melrose.

MASSAGE OIL (body)—Cel-Lite Magic and drink Chamomile Tea.
SUPPLEMENTS—Cleansing Trio (ComforTone, Megazyme, and ICP).

ARTERIOSCLEROSIS: See BLOOD. <u>Aroma Life</u>, birch, [F]cedarwood, ginger, juniper, lemon (increase white and red blood cells), rosemary, thyme, wintergreen. Apply to heart and Vita Flex points on feet.

BLOOD CLOTS—Grapefruit, helichrysum.
SUPPLEMENTS—In addition to Vitamins E and C, all supplements containing essential oils should help increase the supply of oxygen in the blood stream. Rehemogen (tincture) together with JuvaTone may help build blood and hemoglobin platelets (raise cell count). ImmuneTune is good for building white blood cells.

ARTHRITIS: See ACIDOSIS. <u>Aroma Life</u>, <u>Aroma Siez</u>, basil, birch (drains toxins that cause pain), cedarwood, clove, [F]cypress, eucalyptus, fir (has cortisone-like action), ginger, <u>Harmony</u> (with <u>Valor</u>), helichrysum, hyssop, Idaho balsam fir, Idaho tansy, <u>ImmuPower</u>, lavender, [F]marjoram, <u>Melrose</u>, nutmeg, onycha (benzoin), <u>PanAway</u>, <u>Peace & Calming</u>, peppermint, pine, <u>Purification</u>, Roman chamomile, [F]rosemary, [F]spruce, <u>Valor</u>, white fir (has cortisone-like action), wintergreen (drains toxins that cause pain). Apply oils on location and diffuse.

BLEND #1—Combine 1 oz. Ortho Ease with 25 drops birch/wintergreen, 12 cypress, 9 Roman chamomile, and 3 juniper. Massage on location.
BLEND #2—Combine Ortho Ease with birch/wintergreen alone and apply on location.
BLEND #3—Birch/wintergreen with <u>PanAway</u>.
MASSAGE OILS—Ortho Ease.
PERSONAL CARE—Prenolone/Prenolone+, Regenolone.
SUPPLEMENTS—AlkaLime, ArthroTune, CardiaCare (with *Rhododendron caucasicum* which inhibits the enzyme hyaluronidase), Coral Sea (highly bio-available calcium, contains 58 trace minerals), Mineral Essence, Power Meal (contains wolfberry), Sulfurzyme (contains wolfberry), Super C, Super Cal, Thyromin (improves thyroid function and energy levels), VitaGreen.
TINCTURES—Arthro Plus.

ARTHRITIC PAIN—Birch, ginger, <u>PanAway</u>, spruce, wintergreen.

OSTEOARTHRITIS—Basil, birch, eucalyptus, lavender, lemon, marjoram, thyme, wintergreen.

RHEUMATOID—Angelica, [F]birch, [F]bergamot, Black pepper, cajeput, cinnamon bark, coriander, [F]cypress, eucalyptus, fennel, fir,

Detoxify with cypress, fennel, and lemon. Massage affected joints with rosemary, chamomile, juniper and lavender (Alternative Medicine—A Definitive Guide, p. 537).

galbanum, geranium, ᶠginger, hyssop, Idaho balsam fir, juniper, lavender, ᶠlemon, ᶠmarjoram, ᶠnutmeg, oregano (chronic), <u>PanAway</u>, <u>Peace & Calming</u>, peppermint, ᶠpine, Roman chamomile, rosemary, ᶠspruce, tarragon, thyme, wintergreen.
PERSONAL CARE—Prenolone/Prenolone+, Regenolone.
BLEND #4—Combine 2 oz. of Ortho Ease with 7 drops birch/wintergreen, 6 ginger, 19 eucalyptus, 6 juniper, 8 marjoram, and 3 peppermint. Rub on location.

ASHAMED: See EMOTIONS. <u>Acceptance</u>, <u>Forgiveness</u>, <u>Valor</u>.

ASSAULT: See EMOTIONS. <u>Trauma Life</u>.

ASSIMILATING FOOD:
SUPPLEMENTS—Enzyme products. Allerzyme (aids the digestion of sugars, starches, fats, and proteins), Carbozyme (aids in the digestion of carbohydrates), Detoxzyme (helps maintain and support a healthy intestinal environment), Fiberzyme (aids the digestion of fiber and enhances the absorption of nutrients), Lipozyme (aids the digestion of fats) and Polyzyme (aids the digestion of protein and helps reduce swelling and discomfort). Megazyme, Power Meal (pre-digested protein), Super B.

ASTHMA: See RESPIRATORY SYSTEM. Cajeput, calamus, Clary sage, cypress, ᶠeucalyptus, <u>Evergreen Essence</u>, fir, ᶠfrankincense (on crown), hyssop, laurel, lavender, ᶠlemon, ᶠmarjoram, myrrh, myrtle, onycha (benzoin), ᶠoregano, ᶠpeppermint, ᶠpine, <u>Raven</u> (diffuse), ravensara, <u>RC</u> (some people use <u>RC</u> or <u>Raven</u> instead of inhaler), rose, rosemary, ᶠsage, ᶠthyme, tsuga (opens respiratory tract). Avoid steam inhalation. Apply topically over lungs and throat. Drop on pillow or diffuse. May insert <u>RC</u> and <u>Raven</u> with 1 tsp. V-6 Mixing Oil in rectum, OR <u>Raven</u> rectally with <u>RC</u> on chest and back; reverse each night.
BLEND #1—Combine 10 drops cedarwood, 10 eucalyptus, 2 Roman chamomile, and 2 oz. water. Put on hanky and inhale. Can also be used to gargle.
BLEND #2—Combine 10 drops <u>Raven</u>, 5 hyssop, and 2 tsp. V-6 Mixing Oil. Massage on spine and chest.
PERSONAL CARE—Prenolone/Prenolone+.
SUPPLEMENTS—ImmuneTune (for drainage), Super C, Thyromin.
***COMMENTS*—*Do a colon and liver cleanse with either the MASTER CLEANSER (see CLEANSING) or the Cleansing Trio supplements (ComforTone, ICP, Megazyme) and JuvaTone.*
ATTACK—<u>RC</u> or <u>Raven</u>. Just smelling from bottle has stopped attacks.
RECIPE #1—<u>3 Wise Men</u> on crown, <u>Raven</u> on throat, <u>RC</u> on lungs, <u>Thieves</u> on feet, <u>ImmuPower</u> on spine. May insert <u>RC</u> and <u>Raven</u> with V-6 Mixing Oil in rectum, OR <u>Raven</u> rectally with <u>RC</u> on chest and back; reverse each night.

RECIPE #2—Inhale or diffuse bergamot, eucalyptus, hyssop, lavender, or marjoram. Try frankincense for calming. (<u>Alternative Medicine—The Definitive Guide</u>, p. 824).

RECIPE #3—Apply frankincense to the crown, <u>RC</u> on the throat and chest and <u>Raven</u> on the back. Then, inhale the aroma of the oils from your hands.

ASTRINGENT: Lemon, onycha (benzoin).

ATHLETES FOOT: Cajeput, cypress, *Eucalyptus citriodora*, geranium, lavender, ᶠmelaleuca, myrrh, thyme.

BLEND—Combine 2 oz. of Genesis Hand & Body Lotion with 10 drops thyme, 10 lavender, and 10 melaleuca. Rub on feet.

ATTENTION DEFICIT DISORDER (ADD): See HYPERACTIVITY. Ledum.

BLEND—Lavender with basil (on crown), <u>Harmony</u>, or <u>Peace & Calming</u>; Basil with <u>Clarity</u>; Frankincense with <u>Valor</u>. Apply 1-3 drops of any of these blends on the bottom of the feet and on the spine; diffuse.

MASSAGE, BATH, DIFFUSE—<u>Citrus Fresh</u>, lavender.

SUPPLEMENTS—Allerzyme (aids the digestion of sugars, starches, fats, and protiens), Chelex, Essential Omegas (absolutely necessary), Mineral Essence.

CHELATING AGENT—Helichrysum.

SLEEPING—Diffuse either <u>Peace & Calming</u> or <u>Gentle Baby</u>.

****COMMENTS—Avoid sweeteners such as sugar and corn syrup. Eliminate caffeine and food additives from diet. Individuals who have ADD often have high aluminum toxicity. Chelex may help remove aluminum from the body.*

AURA: <u>Awaken</u>, <u>Joy</u>, <u>Sacred Mountain</u>, <u>White Angelica</u>.

INCREASE AURA AROUND BODY—<u>White Angelica</u> (use with <u>Awaken</u> and <u>Sacred Mountain</u>).

PROTECTION OF—<u>White Angelica</u>.

STRENGTHEN—<u>White Angelica</u>.

AUTISM:

REDUCE ANXIETY/FEAR—Bergamot, geranium, and Clary sage. Layer or dilute in V-6 Mixing Oil for a massage.

STIMULATE THE SENSES—Basil, lemon, peppermint, and rosemary. Layer or dilute in V-6 Mixing Oil for a massage.

****COMMENTS—Make sure that no negativity exists when the oils are used because the autistic child will make those associations when the oil is used again.*

AUTO-IMMUNE SYSTEM: For diseases, see GRAVES DISEASE, HASHIMOTO'S DISEASE, and LUPUS. Cistus, <u>ImmuPower</u>.

SUPPLEMENTS—ImmuPro, Sulfurzyme (helps mitigate effects of autoimmune
    diseases), Thyromin, VitaGreen.

AVOIDANCE: See EMOTIONS. Magnify Your Calling, Motivation.

AWAKE:
    JET LAG—Eucalyptus, geranium, grapefruit, lavender, lemongrass, peppermint.
    STAYING AWAKE WHILE DRIVING—Clarity and En-R-Gee together.

AWAKEN THE MIND, SPIRIT: Awaken, myrrh.

AWAKEN THE PAST: Cypress.

AWARENESS:
    GREATER AWARENESS OF ONES POTENTIAL—Believe, Into the Future, White
        Angelica.
    INCREASES SENSORY SYSTEM—Awaken, birch, wintergreen.
    OPENS SENSORY SYSTEM—Birch, peppermint, wintergreen.
    REVITALIZES—Lemongrass.
    SELF—Acceptance, Believe.
    SPIRITUAL—Believe, Frankincense, Inspiration (enhances spiritual mood), myrrh, 3
        Wise Men.

BABIES/CHILDREN:
        FORMULA—Body Balance. Mix 1/3 scoop in 10 oz. distilled water or Rice Dream.
        PERSONAL CARE— KidScents Bath Gel, KidScents Detangler, KidScents Lotion,
            KidScents Shampoo, KidScents Tender Tush, KidScents Toothpaste, Rose
            Ointment.
        SUPPLEMENTS—Mighty Mist (vitamin spray), Mighty Vites (chewable tablets).
    BONDING—Gentle Baby (one drop gently rubbed on baby's feet and another drop or two
        brushed over mom's hair and aura–open palms skimming body surface, head to
        foot).
    COLIC—ᶠBergamot, ginger, mandarin, ᶠmarjoram, Roman chamomile, rosemary, or ylang
        ylang.
        BLEND #1—Combine 2 Tbs. Almond oil with 1 drop Roman chamomile, 1 drop
            lavender, and 1 drop geranium. Mix and apply to stomach and back.
        ***COMMENTS—*Burping the baby, and keeping the abdomen warm with a warm
            water bottle will often bring relief.*
    COMMON COLD—Cedarwood, lemon, *Melaleuca ericifolia*, rosemary, rose,
        sandalwood, or thyme.

BLEND #2—Combine 2 Tbs. V-6 Mixing Oil with 2 drops melaleuca (Tea Tree), 1 lemon, and 1 rose otto. Massage a little of the blend on neck and chest.

CONSTIPATION—Ginger, mandarin, orange, or rosemary. Dilute one of the oils and massage stomach and feet.

CRADLE CAP REMEDY—
BLEND #3—Combine 2 Tbs. Almond oil with 1 drop lemon and 1 geranium or with 1 drop cedarwood and 1 sandalwood. Mix and apply a small amount on head.

CROUP—Marjoram, ravensara, rosewood, sandalwood, or thyme. Dilute for massage; diffuse. Bundle the baby up and take outside to breathe cold air.

CRYING—Cypress, frankincense, geranium, lavender, Roman chamomile, rose otto, or ylang ylang. Dilute for massage or diffuse.

DIAPER RASH—Lavender (dilute and apply).
BLEND #4—Combine 1 drop Roman

When using essential oils on babies and children, it is always best to dilute 1-2 drops of pure essential oil with ½-1 tsp. V-6 Mixing Oil. If the oils are used in the bath, always use a bath gel base as a dispersing agent for the oils.

Keep the oils out of children's reach. If an oil is ever ingested, give the child an oil-soluble liquid such as milk, cream, or half & half. Then call your local poison control center or seek emergency medical attention. A few drops of pure essential oil shouldn't be life-threatening, but for your protection, it is best to take these precautions.

In Shirley Price's book, Aromatherapy for Babies and Children, she mentions twenty oils that are safe for children. Nineteen of them are oils with the same botanical names as those mentioned in this book. These oils are:

Bergamot (Citrus bergamia)*
Cedarwood (Cedrus atlantica)**
Chamomile, Roman (Chamaemelum nobile),
Cypress (Cupressus sempervirens)
Frankincense (Boswellia carteri)
Geranium (Pelargonium graveolens)
Ginger (Zingiber officinale)
Lavender (Lavandula angustifolia)
Lemon (Citrus limon)*
Mandarin (Citrus reticulata)*
Marjoram (Origanum majorana)
Melaleuca-Tea Tree (Melaleuca alternifolia)
Orange (Citrus aurantium)*
Rose Otto (Rosa damascena)
Rosemary (Rosmarinus officinalis)**
Rosewood (Aniba rosaeodora)
Sandalwood (Santalum album)
Thyme (Thymus vulgaris CT linalol)
Ylang Ylang (Cananga odorata)

*These oils are photosensitive; always dilute. To prevent a rash or pigmentation of the skin, do not use citrus oils when exposed to direct sunlight.

B

chamomile and 1 lavender with V-6 Mixing Oil or Genesis Hand & Body Lotion. Apply.

> *PERSONAL CARE*—KidScents Tender Tush (formulated specifically for diaper rash), Rose Ointment.

DIGESTION (sluggish)—Lemon or orange. Dilute and massage feet and stomach.

DRY SKIN—Rosewood or sandalwood. Dilute and apply.

EARACHE—Lavender, melaleuca (Tea Tree), *Melaleuca ericifolia*, Roman chamomile, or thyme (sweet). Put a diluted drop of oil on a cotton ball and place in the ear; rub a little bit of diluted oil behind the ear.

> *BLEND #5*—Combine 2 Tbs. V-6 Mixing Oil with 2 drops lavender, 1 Roman chamomile, and 1 melaleuca (Tea Tree). Put a drop on a cotton ball and put in ear, rub behind the ear and on the ear Vita Flex feet points.

> *OTHER*—Garlic oil works great too, but it is stinky!

FEVER—Lavender. Dilute in V-6 Mixing Oil and massage baby (back of neck, feet, behind ears, etc.). Peppermint (diffuse only).

FLU—Cypress, lemon, *Melaleuca ericifolia*. Dilute 1 drop of each in 1 Tbs. Bath Gel Base for a bath; diffuse.

HICCOUGHS—Mandarin. Diffuse.

JAUNDICE—Geranium, lemon, lime, mandarin, or rosemary. Dilute and apply on the liver area and on the liver Vita Flex feet points.

PREMATURE—Since premature babies have very thin and sensitive skin, it is best to avoid the use of essential oils.

RASHES—Lavender, Roman chamomile, rose otto, or sandalwood. Dilute and apply.

TEETH GRINDING—Lavender (rub on feet), <u>Peace & Calming</u> (on feet or diffuse).

TEETHING—German chamomile, ginger, lavender, marjoram, or melaleuca (Tea Tree). Dilute and apply.

TONSILLITIS—Ginger, lavender, lemon, or melaleuca (Tea Tree), Roman chamomile. Dilute and apply.

THRUSH—Geranium, lavender, lemon, melaleuca (Tea Tree), *Melaleuca ericifolia*, rosewood, or thyme. Dilute and apply.

> *BLEND*—2 Tbsp. garlic oil, 8 drops lavender, 8 drops *Melaleuca ericifolia*, 1 ml. (1 softgel) Vitamin E oil. Apply to nipples just before nursing, or with a clean finger into baby's mouth.

****COMMENTS—Besides <u>Gentle Baby</u> listed under bonding, no other commercial blends are listed in this section because many of them contain oils that are not recommended for babies. The author's admit, however, that they have used many of the commercial blends mentioned in this book on their babies and children with great success and no side effects. We are careful, however, to use only a couple drops at a time, diluted in V-6 Mixing Oil, and only for external application. Also, we do not continue applications for any extended period of time.*

BACK: Basil, birch, Black pepper, cypress, <u>EndoFlex</u>, eucalyptus, geranium, ginger, juniper, lavender, oregano, peppermint, <u>PanAway</u>, <u>Relieve It</u>, Roman chamomile, rosemary, sage, tangerine, thyme (for virus in spine), <u>Valor</u> (aligns; a chiropractor in a bottle), wintergreen.

    CALCIFIED (spine)—Geranium, <u>PanAway</u>, rosemary.

    MASSAGE OILS—Ortho Ease and <u>PanAway</u> (on spine).

    DETERIORATING DISCS—Do RAINDROP THERAPY with just the application of the oils, none of the working along the spine.

    HERNIATED DISCS—Cypress (strengthens blood capillary walls, improves circulation, powerful anti-inflammatory), <u>PanAway</u>, <u>Relieve It</u>, (massage up disc area three times to help with pain), pepper, peppermint (a compress is good too). <u>Valor</u> (3 drops) on location may help relieve pressure. Do RAINDROP THERAPY with just the application of the oils, none of the working along the spine.

    MASSAGE OILS—Ortho Ease.

    SUPPLEMENTS—Super C.

    LOW BACK PAINS—

        RECIPE #1—Rub <u>Valor</u> on top and bottom of feet, <u>Di-Tone</u> on colon, Ortho Ease up the back. Massage cypress up the disc area three times. Cypress strengthens blood capillary walls, improves circulation, and is a powerful anti-inflammatory. Use helichrysum to increase circulation, decongest, and to reduce inflammation and pain. Use peppermint to stimulate the nerves (may need to dilute with Ortho Ease). Layer basil, <u>Aroma Siez</u>, <u>Relieve It</u>, and spruce.

    MUSCULAR FATIGUE—Clary sage, lavender, marjoram, rosemary.

    PAIN—

        BLEND #1—5 to 10 drops each rosemary, marjoram, sage **OR**

        BLEND #2—5 to 10 drops each of lavender, eucalyptus, ginger **OR**

        BLEND #3—5 to 10 drops each of peppermint, rosemary, basil.

        RECIPE #2—Apply <u>PanAway</u> and <u>Valor</u> on the shoulders. If the individual being worked on is laying on their stomach, the person applying the oils to the shoulders should cross their arms so the electrical frequency is not broken (right to right etc.). Apply the following oils **up** the spine, one at a time, using a probe on each vertebra if possible, stroke with fingers, feathering gently in 4" strokes three times for each oil: Peppermint (excites the back), cypress (anti-inflammatory), <u>Aroma Siez</u>, <u>Relieve It</u>, and spruce. Follow the procedure with a hot compress. The blends above have also been used with success. Follow the same stroking procedure and dilute the blends with a little V-6 Mixing Oil for a massage.

    SUPPLEMENTS—ArthroTune.

    TINCTURE—Arthro Plus.

BACTERIA: See ANTI-BACTERIAL.

B

BALANCE: <u>Acceptance</u>, <u>Aroma Siez,</u> <u>Awaken</u>, cedarwood, frankincense (balances electrical field), <u>Harmony</u>, <u>Mister</u>, Roman chamomile, <u>Valor</u>, ylang ylang.

    BALANCE MALE/FEMALE ENERGIES—<u>Acceptance</u>, ylang ylang.

    CHAKRAS—<u>Harmony</u>, <u>Valor</u>.

    EMOTIONAL—<u>Envision</u>.

    ELECTRICAL ENERGIES—Frankincense, <u>Harmony</u>, <u>Valor</u>. Start by applying 3-6 drops <u>Valor</u> on the bottom of each foot. Some may be applied to the neck and shoulders if desired. When working on someone else, place the palms of the hands on the bottom of each foot (left hand to left foot and right hand to right foot) and hold for 5 to 15 minutes. If working on yourself, perform the Cook's Hookup by lifting the right foot and placing the right ankle on top of the left knee in cross-legged fashion. Next place the left hand on the right ankle and cup the front of the ankle with the fingers. Then cross the right hand over the left and with the right hand grasp the heel of the right foot (with thumb around the back and fingers cupping the bottom of the heel). Hold this for 5 to 15 minutes. The balancing of the electrical energies can be felt by either a pulse in the hands and feet or a warming sensation.

    FEELING OF—<u>Envision</u>, spruce.

    HARMONIC BALANCE TO ENERGY CENTER—<u>Acceptance</u>, <u>Harmony</u>.

    SUPPLEMENTS—Body Balance, Master Formula His/Hers.

BALDNESS: See HAIR. Cedarwood, lavender, rosemary, sage. Apply 2-3 drops of each oil on location and on bottom of feet before bedtime and/or in the morning after washing with Lavender Volume products shown below.

    PERSONAL CARE—Lavender Volume Hair & Scalp Wash and Lavender Volume Nourishing Rinse together.

    SUPPLEMENTS—Sulfurzyme may help if the hair is falling due to a sulfur deficiency.

BATH: While tub is filling, add oils to the water; oils will be drawn to your skin quickly from the top of the water, so use gentle oils like: Lavender, Roman chamomile, rosewood, sage, ylang ylang, etc. For the most benefit, add 5-10 drops of your favorite essential oil to one-half ounce Bath and Shower Gel Base.

    BATH & SHOWER GELS—Evening Peace, Relaxation, and Sensation Bath and Shower Gels as well as Lavender Rosewood, Sacred Mountain, and Peppermint Cedarwood Moisturizing Soaps are all wonderfully soothing in the evening. Morning Start Bath and Shower Gel as well as Lemon Sandalwood and Thieves Cleansing Soaps are all terrific ways to jump-start your day.

    AQUA ESSENCE BATH PACKS—Finally, some of the most popular essential oil blends have been combined with the latest hydro-diffusion technology to create the perfect solution for adding oils to your bath water. Just place a packet in the tub while hot water is being added and the oils are perfectly dispersed into the water.

The packets contain 10 ml of oil and are reusable. Packets can be ordered with either Joy, Valor, Peace & Calming, or Sacred Mountain.

BED WETTING: See BLADDER. Before bedtime, rub the abdomen with a couple drops of cypress mixed with V-6 Mixing Oil.

BELCHING: Di-Tone. Apply to stomach and on Vita Flex points.

BEREAVEMENT: Basil, cypress.

BETRAYED (Feeling): See EMOTIONS. Acceptance, Forgiveness, Valor.

BIRTHING: See PREGNANCY.

BITES: See also INSECT. Basil, cinnamon bark, garlic, lavender, lemon, sage, thyme (all have antitoxic and anti-venomous properties).
ALLERGIC—Purification.
BEES AND HORNETS—Remove the stinger, apply a cold compress of Roman chamomile to area for several hours or as long as possible. Then, apply 1 drop of Roman chamomile three times a day for two days. Idaho tansy may also work.
GNATS AND MIDGES—Lavender, or 3 drops thyme in 1 tsp. cider vinegar or lemon juice. Apply to bites to stop irritation.
INSECT—Cajeput, patchouly.
MOSQUITO—Helichrysum, lavender.
SNAKE—Basil, patchouly.
SPIDERS, BROWN RECLUSE, BEE STINGS, ANTS, FIRE ANTS—Basil, cinnamon bark, lavender, lemon, lemongrass, peppermint, Purification, thyme.
SPIDERS—3 drops lavender and 2 drops Roman chamomile in 1 tsp. alcohol. Mix well in clockwise motion and apply to area three times a day.
TICKS—After getting the tick out, apply 1 drop lavender every 5 minutes for 30 minutes. How to remove:
• Do not apply mineral oil, Vaseline, or anything else to remove the tick as this may cause it to inject the spirochetes into the wound.
• Be sure to remove the entire tick. Get as close to the mouth as possible and firmly tug on the tick until it releases its grip. Don't twist. If available, use a magnifying glass to make sure that you have removed the entire tick.
• Save the tick in a jar and label it with the date, where you were bitten on your body, and the location or address where you were bitten for proper identification by your doctor, especially if you develop any symptoms.
• Do not handle the tick.
• Wash hands immediately.

        • Check the site of the bite occasionally to see if any rash develops. If it does, seek medical advice promptly.

WASPS (are alkaline)—1 drop basil, 2 Roman chamomile, 2 lavender, and 1 tsp. cider vinegar. Mix in clockwise motion and put on area three times a day.

BITTERNESS: See EMOTIONS. <u>Acceptance</u>, <u>Forgiveness</u>, Roman chamomile, <u>Valor</u>.

BLADDER: Apply <u>EndoFlex</u> over kidneys as a hot compress.

    BED WETTING AND INCONTINENCE—Before bed rub cypress on abdomen.
        TINCTURES—Take K&B morning, noon, and night.
    INFECTION—See CYSTITIS. Cedarwood, <u>Inspiration</u>, onycha (benzoin), and sandalwood (for 1st stages of bladder infection), ᶠlemongrass, or 1 drop <u>Thieves</u> in 8 oz. juice or water and drink three times a day.
        SUPPLEMENTS—ImmuGel, K&B.
    ***COMMENTS—*One individual who had bladder infection took 1 tsp. ImmuGel every two hours. They were over the infection in two days.*
    HANGING DOWN—<u>Valor</u> on feet, 3 drops ravensara and 1 drop lavender on calves, (bladder should pull up).

BLAME: See EMOTIONS. <u>Acceptance</u>, <u>Forgiveness</u>, <u>Valor</u>.

BLISTER:

    (on lips from sun): Lavender (Apply as often as needed. It should take fever out and return lip to normal).

BLOATING: <u>Di-Tone</u>. Apply to stomach, Vita Flex points, and diffuse.
    SUPPLEMENTS—ComforTone, Mint Condition.

BLOCKED (Emotionally): See EMOTIONS.

BLOOD: Red blood cells carry oxygen throughout the body.

    BLOOD TYPES—Different blood types have different dominating glands.
        <u>TYPE A</u>: more prone to be alkaline pH balanced. Natural vegetarians. Type A child living in a home of type O

> *Quoting from the book, <u>4 Blood Types, 4 Diets—Eat Right 4 your Type</u>, Dr. Peter J. D'Adamo states, "Your blood type is the key that unlocks the door to the mysteries of health, disease, longevity, physical vitality, and emotional strength. Your blood type determines your susceptibility to illness, which foods you should eat, and how you should exercise. It is a factor in your energy levels, in the efficiency with which you 'burn' calories, in your emotional response to stress, and perhaps even in your personality." Please refer to the "Blood Type" chart in the APPENDIX of this book.*

parent is affected by parents' programing or conditioning or visa versa. They have problems with their thyroid, may have tendency to gain weight, and need exercise.

TYPE AB: may want to be a vegetarian some days, but not on others. Can go either way like A or O types. They may be affected by either the A or O parent. AB types haven't decided whether to be an A or B type. They may even need more protein than O types.

TYPE B: down the middle more balanced. Takes them about 3 years to convert to being a vegetarian.

TYPE O: more prone to acidic condition in blood. AlkaLime is an acid-neutralizing mineral formulation and may help preserve the body's proper pH balance. Big eaters and may need to take more supplements because they are not assimilating the nutrients. If they are not assimilating their food, they eat and get full quick and one hour later they are hungry again. They get more gas because they lack enzyme secretion. They may need MEGAZYME for the enzymes. They eat more, digest less, but don't gain weight. May take 8 years to totally convert to vegetarian diet. Need more protein; BODY BALANCE, VITAGREEN and POWER MEAL are mainstays for O types as they are high protein and high energy formulas; nuts and seeds are good too. Nutrients in purest form reduces the need to eat. They have a harder time structuring their diet and they get cold because of poor circulation. If an O type is slender, has high energy, is compulsive in behavior, and/or is a hard worker, they may need as many as 16 VitaGreen and 10 Master Formula His/Hers per day.

BLOOD PRESSURE—

HIGH (hypertension)—<u>Aroma Life</u>, ᶠbirch, Clary sage, clove, goldenrod, ᶠlavender, lemon, ᶠmarjoram (regulates), nutmeg, ᶠspearmint, wintergreen, ᶠylang ylang (arterial; put in hand, rub palms together, cup over nose, and breathe deeply for 5 minutes and/or put on feet). Place oils on heart points on left arm, hand, foot, and over heart. Can also smell from palms of hands, diffuse, or place a few drops on a cotton ball and put in a vent.

***COMMENTS—Refer to the chapter entitled "How to Use - The Personal Usage Reference" in the <u>Essential Oils Desk Reference</u> under "Blood Pressure, High" for specific product recommendations.

> ### OILS TO AVOID IF HYPERTENSIVE
>
> **Single oils:** *Hyssop, rosemary, sage, thyme, and possibly peppermint.*
>
> *This list is a compilation of the safety data contained in aromatherapy books written by the following authors: Ann Berwick, Julia Lawless, Shirley & Len Price, Jeanne Rose, Robert Tisserand, and Tony Balacs.*

BATH—3 ylang ylang and 3 marjoram in bath water. Bathe in the evening twice a week.

©2002 Abundant Health

B

BLEND #1—5 geranium, 8 lemongrass, 3 lavender, and 1 oz. V-6 Mixing Oil. Rub over heart and heart Vita Flex points on left foot and hand.

BLEND #2—10 ylang ylang, 5 marjoram, 5 cypress, and 1 oz. V-6 Mixing Oil. Rub over heart and heart Vita Flex points on left foot and hand.

TINCTURES—HRT (1-2 droppers two to three times per day).

LOW—<u>Aroma Life</u>, hyssop (raises), pine, ^Frosemary, ylang ylang.

SUPPLEMENTS—CardiaCare (with *Rhododendron caucasicum* which helps to normalize blood pressure).

BLOOD PROTEIN—Body Balance, VitaGreen.

BLEEDING (STOPS)—<u>Aroma Life</u>, cistus, geranium (will increase bleeding first to eliminate toxins, then stop it), helichrysum, onycha (benzoin), Cayenne pepper, rose.

BROKEN BLOOD VESSELS—Grapefruit, helichrysum.

***COMMENTS—One woman had some blood vessels break in her brain which effected her short-term memory, concentration, focus, and emotions. She used the oils of Clarity, basil, rosemary, peppermint, and cardamom. Not only did her blood vessels heal, but her concentration, awareness, focus, and self-esteem increased.*

BUILD—Rehemogen (tincture) together with JuvaTone may help build blood and hemoglobin platelets (raise cell count). ImmuneTune is good for building white blood cells.

CHOLESTEROL—Helichrysum (regulates).

CLEANSING—^FHelichrysum, Roman chamomile. Apply on bottom of feet.

SUPPLEMENTS—VitaGreen.

TINCTURES—Rehemogen (purifier).

CLOTS—Grapefruit, helichrysum (anti-coagulant).

HEMORRHAGING—See FEMALE PROBLEMS. Cistus, helichrysum, rose, Cayenne pepper.

LOW BLOOD SUGAR—Cinnamon bark, clove, <u>Thieves</u> (balances blood sugar), thyme.

SUPPLEMENTS—AlkaLime, VitaGreen (balances blood sugar), Mineral Essence.

TINCTURES—Sugar-Up (balances blood sugar; available through Creer Labs 801-465-5423).

STIMULATES—^FLemon (helps with the formation of red and white blood cells).

VESSELS—<u>Aroma Life</u>, cypress (strengthens the capillary walls, and increases circulation), lemongrass (vasodilator).

SUPPLEMENTS—Cel-Lite Magic dilates blood vessels for better circulation.

BODY SYSTEMS:

CARDIOVASCULAR SYSTEM: See CARDIOVASCULAR SYSTEM. <u>Aroma Life</u>, clove, cypress, goldenrod, helichrysum, marjoram, onycha (benzoin), rosemary, tsuga (opens and dilates for better oxygen exchange), ylang ylang.

SUPPLEMENTS—CardiaCare (contains ingredients that have been scientifically tested for their abilities to support and strengthen the cardiovascular system), Coral Sea (highly bio-available calcium, contains 58 trace minerals), ICP, Mineral Essence, Super B, Super Cal.

TINCTURE—HRT.

DIGESTIVE SYSTEM: See DIGESTIVE SYSTEM. Clove, <u>Di-Tone</u> (acid stomach; aids and secretes digestive enzymes), ^Ffennel (sluggish), ginger, laurel, myrtle, ^Fpeppermint, rosemary, spearmint, tarragon (nervous and sluggish). Add the oil(s) to your food, rub on stomach, or apply as a compress over abdomen.

SUPPLEMENTS—Essential Manna, Megazyme (digestive enzymes; take before meals for acid stomach), Mint Condition (take after meals; soothing to irritated stomach; reduces inflammation), ParaFree, Royaldophilus, Stevia Select.

EMOTIONAL BALANCE: See EMOTIONS. <u>Forgiveness</u>, frankincense, geranium, <u>Grounding</u>, <u>Harmony</u>, <u>Hope</u>, Idaho balsam fir, <u>Inner Child</u>, <u>Joy</u>, juniper, lavender, onycha (combine with rose for massage), orange, <u>Present Time</u>, <u>Release</u>, Roman chamomile, sandalwood, <u>SARA</u>, <u>3 Wise Men</u>, <u>Trauma Life</u>, <u>Valor</u>, vetiver, <u>White Angelica</u>.

SUPPLEMENTS—ProMist.

HORMONAL SYSTEM: See HORMONAL SYSTEM. Clary sage, <u>EndoFlex</u>, fennel, goldenrod, <u>Mister</u>, myrrh, myrtle, peppermint, sage, ylang ylang. The most common places to apply oils for hormonal balance are the Vita Flex points on ankles, lower back, thyroid, liver, kidneys, gland areas, the center of the body and along both sides of the spine, and the clavicle area. Diffusing them may also help.

MASSAGE OILS—Dragon Time.

PERSONAL CARE—Prenolone/Prenolone+.

SUPPLEMENTS—CortiStop (Men's and Women's), FemiGen (female), ProGen (male), ProMist, Thyromin, Ultra Young+.

TINCTURES—Estro, Femalin.

IMMUNE SYSTEM: See IMMUNE SYSTEM. Clove, <u>Exodus II</u>, frankincense, <u>ImmuPower</u>, ledum (supports), lemon, Mountain savory, rosemary (supports), <u>Thieves</u> (enhances; massage on feet and body), thyme (supports immunological functions).

SUPPLEMENTS—Essential Manna, Exodus, ImmuneTune, ImmuPro, Super B, Super C, Ultra Young (may help raise levels of cytokines, interleukin 1 & 2, and tumor necrosis factor).

MUSCLES and BONES: See individual listings for BONES and MUSCLES. <u>Aroma Siez</u>, basil, birch, cypress, Idaho balsam fir, lavender, lemongrass, marjoram, oregano, peppermint, thyme, <u>Valor</u>, wintergreen.

MASSAGE OILS—Ortho Ease or Ortho Sport Massage Oils.

SUPPLEMENTS—Be-Fit, Coral Sea (highly bio-available calcium, contains 58 trace minerals), Essential Manna, Mineral Essence, Power Meal, Sulfurzyme, Super Cal, WheyFit.

B

NERVOUS SYSTEM: See NERVOUS SYSTEM. <u>Brain Power</u>, cedarwood (nervous tension), ginger, Idaho balsam fir, lavender, <u>Peace & Calming</u>, **peppermint** (soothes and strengthens), rosemary, vetiver.

PERSONAL CARE—NeuroGen, Regenolone (nerve regeneration).

SUPPLEMENTS—Mineral Essence, Sulfurzyme, Super B.

RESPIRATORY SYSTEM: See RESPIRATORY SYSTEM. ^FEucalyptus (general stimulant and strengthens), *Eucalyptus radiata*, ledum (supports), melaleuca, ^Fmyrtle, ^Fpeppermint (aids), pine (dilates and opens bronchial tract), <u>RC</u>, <u>Raven</u> (all respiratory problems), ravensara, rosemary verbenon, tsuga (dilates and opens respiratory tract).

ESSENTIAL WATERS (HYDROSOLS)—Canadian Red Cedar (supportive), Eucalyptus (calming), Mountain Essence (enhances respiratory action). Spray into air, onto chest, or diffuse using the Essential Mist Diffuser.

SUPPLEMENTS—ImmuGel, Super C.

SKIN: See SKIN. Frankincense, <u>Gentle Baby</u> (youthful skin), geranium, German chamomile (inflamed skin), lavender, ledum (all types of problems), <u>Melrose</u>, myrrh (chapped and cracked), onycha (chapped and cracked), patchouly (chapped; tightens loose skin and prevents wrinkles), rosewood (elasticity and candida), <u>Valor</u>, vetiver, Western Red cedar.

BAR SOAPS—Lavender Moisturizing Soap, Lemon Sandalwood Cleansing Soap, Peppermint Cedarwood Moisturizing Soap, Sacred Mountain Moisturizing Soap for oily skin, Thieves Cleansing Soap.

PERSONAL CARE—Boswellia Wrinkle Creme, Genesis Hand & Body Lotion (hydrates, heals, and nurtures the skin), Satin Facial Scrub - Mint or Juniper (eliminates layers of dead skin cells and slows down premature aging of the skin), Orange Blossom Facial Wash combined with Sandalwood Toner and Sandalwood Moisture Creme (cleans, tones, and moisturizes dry or prematurely aging skin), Prenolone, Regenolone (helps moisturize and regenerate tissues), Rose Ointment (for skin conditions and chapped skin), Satin Body Lotion (moisturizes skin leaving it feeling soft, silky, and smooth).

SUPPLEMENTS FOR SKIN—Sulfurzyme.

TINCTURES—AD&E.

BALANCING—<u>Harmony</u>, <u>Joy</u>, lavender, spruce, <u>Valor</u>.

CHEMICALS—Radex (prevents build up in the body).

CONTROLLING—Cedarwood.

ODORS—<u>Purification</u> (obnoxious odors), sage.

RADIATION—Radex (prevents build up in the body).

STRENGTHEN VITAL CENTERS—Oregano.

SUPPORT—Fir, ledum, <u>Valor</u>.

BOILS: Bergamot, Clary sage, frankincense, galbanum, <u>Gentle Baby</u>, lavender, lemon, lemongrass, melaleuca, <u>Melrose</u>, <u>Purification</u>, <u>Raven</u>, ravensara, <u>RC</u>, Roman chamomile.

PERSONAL CARE—Rose Ointment.

****COMMENTS—One individual put lemon oil on a sore that looked like a boil. The next day it turned black, puss came out and it got smaller and finally disappeared.*

BONDING: See EMOTIONS. <u>Gentle Baby</u>.

****COMMENTS—Use <u>Release</u> or other oils listed under Emotional Release in the Science and Application section of the <u>Reference Guide for Essential Oils</u> to help release emotional connections to one who has passed on. Also, to help children create good bonds with others, tell them about the person when working with the oils.*

BONES: All the tree oils, **birch**, cedarwood, cypress, fir, juniper, lavender, lemongrass, marjoram, <u>PanAway</u> (bone pain), peppermint, <u>Relieve It</u>, sandalwood, spruce, wintergreen.

SUPPLEMENTS—Be-Fit, Coral Sea (highly bio-available calcium, contains 58 trace minerals), Essential Manna, Mineral Essence, Power Meal, ProMist, Sulfurzyme, Super Cal.

BONE SPURS—Birch/wintergreen, cypress, marjoram, <u>RC</u> (dissolves). Rub on location.

****COMMENTS—One lady had a heel spur flare up one evening, so she took a bath with birch and cypress before retiring. The next morning, the pain was a little better. She then put 6 drops birch, 6 drops cypress, and on top of that, 5 drops <u>RC</u> on a cotton pad and applied it to her heel. In 10 minutes all pain was gone and even after four days, the pain had not returned.*

BROKEN HEAL—Birch/wintergreen and cypress (before bed), helichrysum, oregano and <u>Valor</u> (in morning).

BLEND—9 drops birch/wintergreen, 8 drops each of spruce, White fir, and helichrysum, 7 drops clove (good when inflammation is causing the pain).

MASSAGE OILS—3 droppers full of Ortho Ease mixed with lavender, lemongrass, and <u>PanAway</u>. Ortho Sport with juniper, lemongrass, and marjoram (apply over broken bones).

SUPPLEMENTS—4 Super Cal and 14 ArthroTune for three weeks, then cut in half.

BRUISED—Helichrysum, <u>Relieve It</u>, and <u>PanAway</u>.

CARTILAGE—Sandalwood (regenerates), White fir (pain from inflammation).

DEGENERATION—Ortho Ease then peppermint.

SUPPLEMENTS—Super C.

DEVELOPMENT—

SUPPLEMENTS—Super C, Ultra Young (may help boost bone formation).

B

PAIN—**Birch**, <u>PanAway</u>, White fir, wintergreen.
ROTATOR CUFF (Sore)—See SHOULDER. **Birch/wintergreen** (bone), lemongrass
(torn or pulled ligaments), <u>PanAway</u>, peppermint (nerves), <u>Relieve It</u>, spruce,
White fir (inflammation).

BOREDOM: <u>Awaken</u>, <u>Believe</u>, cedarwood, cypress, <u>Dream Catcher</u>, fir, frankincense,
<u>Gathering</u>, juniper, lavender, <u>Motivation</u>, pepper, Roman chamomile, rosemary,
sandalwood, spruce, thyme, <u>Valor</u>, ylang ylang.

BOWEL:
IRRITABLE BOWEL SYNDROME—<u>Di-Tone</u> and peppermint. Take 2 drops of each in
distilled water 1-2 times per day. Idaho tansy may also help. Dilute 1-2 drops
with V-6 Mixing Oil and apply over abdomen with a hot compress.
SUPPLEMENTS—Mint Condition (works harmoniously with Megazyme and <u>Di-
Tone</u>). ComforTone, JuvaTone, ICP (fiber beverage), Royaldophilus, Stevia
Select (with FOS).
NORMAL FUNCTION OF—
SUPPLEMENTS—ComforTone, ICP (fiber beverage for normal function of bowels),
Mint Condition.
PARALYSIS—ComforTone.
****COMMENTS—One women was paralyzed by surgery and had to have 2
colonics a day. She took ComforTone and then she was able to have natural
bowel movements.*

BOXED IN (Feeling): <u>Peace &
Calming</u>, <u>Valor</u>.

BRAIN: <u>Aroma Life</u>, Blue cypress
(improves circulation),
Clary sage (opens
brain, euphoria),
cypress, geranium,
lemongrass, spearmint.
ACTIVATES RIGHT
BRAIN— Bergamot,
birch, geranium,
grapefruit,
helichrysum, Roman
chamomile,
wintergreen.

> *The **blood-brain barrier** is the barrier membrane
> between the circulating blood and the brain that
> prevents certain damaging substances from reaching
> brain tissue and cerebrospinal fluid. The American
> Medical Association (AMA) determined that if they could
> find an agent that would pass the blood-brain barrier,
> they would be able to heal **Alzheimer's, Lou Gehrig's,
> Multiple Sclerosis, and Parkinson's disease**. In June of
> 1994, it was documented by the Medical University of
> Berlin, Germany and Vienna, Austria that
> **sesquiterpenes have the ability to go beyond the blood-
> brain barrier**. High levels of sesquiterpenes are found in
> the essential oils of frankincense and sandalwood.
> Blends containing both of these oils include: 3 Wise
> Men, Acceptance, Forgiveness, Gathering, Harmony,
> Inspiration, Into the Future, and Trauma Life.*

BROKEN BLOOD VESSELS— See BLOOD.

CEREBRAL (BRAIN)—ᶠNutmeg.

INJURY—Frankincense, Valor. Massage on brain stem and diffuse.

INTEGRATION—Clary sage, cypress, geranium, helichrysum, lemongrass, spearmint, Valor.

NEUROLOGICAL INJURY (break down of Myelin sheath)—Peppermint, lemongrass, frankincense, Valor. Massage on brain stem and spine; diffuse.

> *FOOD*—Omega 3 fatty acids found in Flax Seed Oil and Sesame Oil (taken internally). Can also try Essential Omegas supplement.

OXYGENATE—3 drops each of helichrysum and sandalwood once or twice a day on the back of neck, temples, and behind ears down to jaw. Also Blue cypress.

TUMOR—See CANCER. Frankincense, Valor. Massage on brain stem and diffuse.

BREAST: Clary sage, cypress, elemi (inflammation), fennel, geranium, lemongrass, sage, spearmint, vetiver.

> *PERSONAL CARE*—Prenolone/Prenolone+ (for tenderness and swelling).

ENLARGE AND FIRM—Clary sage, fennel, sage.

> *BLEND*—Equal parts vetiver, geranium, ylang ylang.
> *PERSONAL CARE*—Sandalwood Toner (to tone and tighten skin)

LACTATION—See PREGNANCY.

MASTITIS (breast infection)—Citrus Fresh (with lavender), Exodus II, lavender, tangerine.

> *BLEND*—Equal amounts of lavender and tangerine. Dilute with some V-6 Mixing Oil and apply to breasts and under arms twice a day.
> *SUPPLEMENTS*—Exodus, ImmuGel.

MILK PRODUCTION—See PREGNANCY.

SORE NIPPLES—Roman chamomile.

STRETCH MARKS—Gentle Baby.

BREATH(ING): Cinnamon bark, Exodus II, frankincense, ginger, hyssop, juniper, marjoram, nutmeg, Roman chamomile, rosemary, thyme. Raven or RC may work instead of an inhaler.

HYPERPNEA (Abnormal rapid breathing)—ᶠYlang ylang.

OXYGEN—Frankincense, sandalwood, all Essential Oils.

> *PERSONAL CARE*—Satin Facial Scrub - Mint or Juniper (deep cleansing that dispenses nutrients and oxygen). Mix with Orange Blossom Facial Wash for a milder cleanse.
> *SUPPLEMENTS*—Exodus, Radex (increases oxygen).

SHORTNESS OF—Aroma Life.

> *BLEND #1*—For shortness of breath due to overexertion (lots of work, no sleep, etc.) add 10 drops each of eucalyptus and peppermint to a basin of lukewarm water. Soak some cloths in this water and wring them out leaving them fairly moist.

Then wrap the joints (ankles, knees, wrists, elbows, and neck) with the cloths. While relaxing and allowing the compresses to cool the joints, have another person do Vita Flex on the points for the Pineal Gland and Adrenal Glands on the feet.

BRONCHITIS: See RESPIRATORY SYSTEM. <u>Abundance</u>, basil, bergamot, birch, cajeput, ᶠcedarwood, ᶠClary sage, clove, ᶠcypress, elemi, *Eucalyptus radiata*, ᶠfir (obstructions of Bronchi), frankincense, ginger, <u>ImmuPower</u>, lavender, ledum, lemon, ᶠmarjoram, ᶠmelaleuca, *Melaleuca ericifolia*, ᶠmyrtle, myrrh, nutmeg, onycha (benzoin), ᶠpeppermint, ᶠpine, <u>RC</u>, <u>Raven</u>, ravensara, Roman chamomile, rose, ᶠrosemary, sandalwood, ᶠspearmint, <u>Thieves</u> (drops in drinking water, also put on chest & feet, may need to dilute with V-6 Mixing Oil), ᶠthyme, tsuga (opens respiratory tract), wintergreen. Diffuse the oils or rub on chest (dilute with V-6 Mixing Oil if necessary).

> *BLEND #1*—10 cedarwood, 10 eucalyptus, 2 Roman chamomile, and 2 oz. water. Put on hanky and inhale. Blend can also be added to water for gargle.

> *BLEND #2*—Clove, cinnamon bark, melissa, and lavender (<u>Alternative Medicine—The Definitive Guide</u>, p. 55).

> ***COMMENTS*—*Refer to the chapter entitled "How to Use - The Personal Usage Reference" in the* <u>Essential Oils Desk Reference</u> *under "Bronchitis" for specific oil blend and supplement recommendations.*

> CHRONIC—Elemi, eucalyptus, laurel, ᶠravensara, ᶠsage, ᶠsandalwood, ᶠoregano.

> CHILDREN—Eucalyptus, lavender, melaleuca, *Melaleuca ericifolia*, Roman chamomile, rosemary, thyme (CT linalol).

> *SUPPLEMENTS*—ImmuneTune, ImmuGel.

> CLEAR MUCUS—Bergamot, sandalwood, and thyme (<u>Alternative Medicine—The Definitive Guide</u>, p. 824). Onycha (benzoin) may also help.

> ***COMMENTS*—*Diffusing the oils is a great way to handle a respiratory problem.*

According to Dr. Daniel Pénoël, bronchitis can be broken down into three separate areas, each of which should be considered separately. Following are the three areas and specific blends recommended by Dr. Pénoël:

> *Inflamation*—Mix equal portions of *Eucalyptus citriodora* and lemongrass. Apply 3-6 drops per foot to the sinus and lung Vita Flex points. Add to V-6 Mixing Oil and apply over the chest.

> *Infection*—Mix 1 tsp. melaleuca, 25 drops palmarosa or geranium, 3 drops peppermint, 1 drop thyme. Apply 3-6 drops per foot to the sinus and lung Vita Flex points. Add to V-6 Mixing Oil and apply over the chest.

> *Accumulation of Fluids (mucus)*—Mix 25 drops each of *Eucalyptus dives*, peppermint, dill. Apply 3-6 drops per foot to the sinus and lung Vita Flex points.

BRUISES: Angelica, fennel, geranium, helichrysum, hyssop, lavender, <u>Melrose</u>, <u>PanAway</u>, <u>Thieves</u>. Apply on location.

> ***COMMENTS—*Refer to the chapter entitled "How to Use - The Personal Usage
> Reference" in the* <u>Essential Oils Desk Reference</u> *under "Bruising" for some
> excellent blend recipes and supplement recommendations.*

BUGGED (Feeling): See EMOTIONS. <u>Acceptance</u>, <u>Forgiveness</u>, <u>Peace & Calming</u>, <u>Valor</u>.

BUGS (Repel): See BITES and INSECT. Lemon (kills bugs), <u>Purification</u>. Diffuse.
    BITES (All spiders, Brown Recluse, bee stings, ants, fire ants)—Basil, cinnamon bark,
        lavender, lemon, lemongrass, peppermint, <u>Purification</u>, thyme.
    INSECT—Patchouly.
    REPELLANT—Sunsation Suntan Oil; ACCELERATES TANNING in addition to
        repelling bugs. Idaho tansy may also work as a mosquito repellant. Also, Idaho
        Tansy Floral Water (used to keep flies away from horses while shoeing).
    SNAKE—Patchouly.

BULEMIA: Grapefruit. Apply to stomach and bottom of feet.

BUMPS: Frankincense, <u>Melrose</u>, <u>PanAway</u>, <u>Peace & Calming</u>.

BUNIONS: See BURSITIS.
        <u>Aroma Siez</u>, carrot,
        cypress, German
        chamomile, juniper, <u>M-
        Grain</u>.

> *Bunions are from bursitis located at the base of a toe.*

    BLEND—6 drops eucalyptus, 3 lemon, 4 ravensara, and 1 birch/wintergreen in 1 oz.
        V-6 Mixing Oil. Apply a couple drops of this blend directly on area of concern as
        often as desired.

BURDENS: See EMOTIONS. <u>Acceptance</u>, <u>Hope</u>, <u>Release</u>, <u>Valor</u>.

BURNS: Eucalyptus, geranium, helichrysum, Idaho tansy, ᶠlavender (cell renewal), melaleuca
    (Tea Tree), peppermint, ravensara (healing), Roman chamomile, rosehip, tamanu
    (mix with helichrysum).
    PERSONAL CARE—LavaDerm Cooling Mist (soothing and cooling for all burns),
        Satin Body Lotion (moisturizes and promotes healing).
    BLEND #1—Put 3 drops of lavender in some Satin Body Lotion and apply. This is
        effective for pain, healing, peeling, and sunburns.
    BLEND #2—10 German chamomile, 5 Roman chamomile, and 10 lavender. Mix
        together and add 1 drop to each square inch of burn after it has been soaked in ice
        water. If you don't have the chamomile, lavender will do great. Can top with
        LavaDerm Cooling Mist to keep skin cool and moist.

B
C

CLEANSING—Melrose.
INFECTED—Purification.
PAIN—Blend #1 (above), Mineral Essence (apply topically).
HEALING—See SCARRING. Rosehip. Blend #1 (above), ravensara or geranium mixed with helichrysum.

René-Maurice Gattefossé, Ph.D., a French cosmetic chemist who coined the phrase "Aromatherapy," severely burned his hand in a laboratory accident. The continual application of lavender oil soothed the pain, nullified the effects of gas gangrene, and healed his hand without a scar.

PEELING—Blend #1, Blend #2 (both shown above).
SUNBURN—See SUNBURN. ᶠMelaleuca (Tea Tree), tamanu (mix with helichrysum), Mineral Essence (applied topically), Blend #1 (above).
   PERSONAL CARE—LavaDerm Cooling Mist, Lavender Floral Water or Lavender Essential Water, Satin Body Lotion.
   BLEND #3—Put 10 drops of lavender in 4 oz. spray bottle of distilled water. Shake well then spray on location. This is effective for pain and healing.
SUN SCREEN—ᶠHelichrysum, tamanu, Sunsation Suntan Oil (helps filter out the ultraviolet rays without blocking the absorption of vitamin D, which is important to skin and bone development. It also accelerates tanning).

BURSITIS: Aroma Siez, cajeput, cypress, ginger, hyssop juniper, onycha (benzoin), PanAway, Roman chamomile.

Bursitis is a chronic inflammation of the fluid-filled sac that is located close to the joints. It is caused by infection, injury, or diseases like arthritis and gout. Since it can be very tender and painful, it may restrict the ability to move freely.

   BLEND—Apply 6 drops of marjoram on shoulders and arms; wait 6 minutes. Then apply 3 drops of birch/wintergreen; wait 6 minutes. Then apply 3 drops of cypress.
   MASSAGE OILS—Ortho Ease, Ortho Sport.
   TINCTURES—Arthro Plus.

CALCIUM: See HORMONAL IMBALANCE.
   SUPPLEMENTS— Allerzyme (aids the digestion of sugars, starches, fats, and proteins), Coral Sea (highly bio-available,

According to Dr. John R. Lee, processed foods, carbonated soft drinks, caffeine, and high protein, sugar and salt consumption all contribute to increased calcium deficiency in the human body (Burton Goldberg Group, Alt. Med., The Definitive Guide, pp 773-4). Sulfur cannot be metabolized if there is a calcium deficiency. This can cause poor nail and hair growth, falling hair, eczema, dermatitis, poor muscle tone, acne, pimples, gout, rheumatism, arthritis, and a weakening of the nervous system.

contains 58 trace minerals), Super Cal, Mineral Essence, Polyzyme (aids the digestion of protein and helps reduce swelling and discomfort).

CALLOUSES: Carrot, <u>Melrose</u> and oregano (callouses on feet), peppermint, Roman chamomile.

CALMING: Bergamot, ^Fcedarwood, <u>Citrus Fresh</u>, Clary sage (aromatic), <u>Gentle Baby</u>, jasmine, lavender, *Melaleuca ericifolia*, myrrh, onycha (benzoin), <u>Peace & Calming</u>, <u>Release</u>, <u>Surrender</u>, tangerine, <u>Trauma Life</u>, Western Red cedar, ylang ylang.

CANCER: See CHEMICALS, RADIATION. <u>Di-Tone</u> (rub on feet and stomach), <u>ImmuPower</u> (put on throat and all over feet, three times a day), <u>Melrose</u> (cancer sores, fights infection), clove, frankincense (diffuse), rose, sage, ^Ftarragon (anti-cancerous). Since it is very important to maintain a positive attitude while healing, it may be helpful to address the emotions using <u>Acceptance</u>, <u>Believe</u>, <u>Envision</u>, <u>Forgiveness</u>, <u>Gathering</u>, <u>Gratitude</u>, <u>Hope</u>, <u>Joy</u>, <u>Live with Passion</u>, and/or ravensara (*refer to the emotional therapies in the Science and Application section of the <u>Reference Guide for Essential Oils</u>*). One of the most common emotions cancer patients have to deal with is anger or a pattern of resentment. Others are fear, judgement, and doubt. Doubt limits God and restricts His ability to work miracles in our lives. Praying for all those with cancer can help release these emotions. Also, work on recognizing why cancer was chosen.

****COMMENTS—Refer to the chapter entitled "How to Use - The Personal Usage Reference" in the <u>Essential Oils Desk Reference</u> under "Cancer" for some excellent blend recipes, supplement recommendations, and*

> *There must be an acid condition in the body for cancer to thrive and spread. See pH Balance. VitaGreen and Power Meal contain predigested proteins and help the body move towards an alkaline balance. AlkaLime combats yeast and fungus overgrowth and helps preserve the body's proper pH balance.*
>
> *Cancer cells have a very low frequency.*

cleansing and maintenance programs for many different kinds of cancer.

*****IMPORTANT NOTICE: HEALTHCARE PROFESSIONALS ARE EMPHATIC ABOUT AVOIDING HEAVY MASSAGE WHEN WORKING WITH CANCER PATIENTS. LIGHT MASSAGE MAY BE USED, BUT NEVER OVER THE TRAUMA AREA. ALSO, THE INFORMATION IN THIS SECTION SHOULD <u>NOT</u> BE PERCEIVED AS A CURE FOR CANCER. ALWAYS CONSULT WITH YOUR HEALTHCARE PROFESSIONAL.**

C

SUPPLEMENTS—AlkaLime (acid-neutralizing mineral formulation), Body Balance (especially good for cancer), Cleansing Trio (ComforTone, Megazyme, and ICP), ImmuneTune, ImmuPro, Power Meal, Radex, Super C, VitaGreen, Wolfberry Bar (*Refer to the Wolfberry Bar in the Supplements section of the* <u>Reference Guide for Essential Oils</u> *for more information on the benefits of the Chinese Wolfberry*).

***COMMENTS—*One lady, who was receiving Chemo treatments for cancer of the spleen, used* <u>Di-Tone</u> *to promote elimination through the colon. Her doctors wondered why her Chemo treatments had not made her sick. When she felt any discomfort (light nausea or cramps in descending colon), she rubbed four to six drops of* <u>Di-Tone</u> *on her abdomen and within 10 minutes, all discomfort stopped.*

The following are recipes that some individuals have used successfully:

RECIPE #1—For the first month, supplement with the following: 6 VitaGreen three times a day, 6 Super C three times a day, 4 Radex four times a day, and 4 ImmuneTune three times a day. After remission, apply <u>ImmuPower</u> on the spine three times a day. Do a *light* full body massage with 6 clove and 15 frankincense in 1 oz. V-6 Mixing Oil.

RECIPE #2—Supplement with the following: Cleansing Trio (ComforTone, Megazyme, and ICP), 10 Radex, 12 Super C, 15 ImmuneTune, and 9 VitaGreen. Drink ½ gallon of carrot juice each day. Eliminate white flour, white sugar and red meat from the diet. Rub <u>Thieves</u> on the feet and do a *light* full body massage with frankincense.

RECIPE #3—Supplement with the following: 1 Master Formula His/Hers, 2 VitaGreen, 6 Super C, 3 Radex, and 1 ImmuneTune. Do a *light* full body massage with frankincense, clove, and V-6 Mixing Oil. Apply <u>ImmuPower</u> to the spine and feet twice a day.

BONE—Frankincense on neat, all supplements. The following is a recipe that has been used on some individuals with bone cancer:

RECIPE #1—ImmuneTune (antioxidant) and Cleansing Trio (ComforTone, Megazyme, and ICP) for a week, then JuvaTone was added for six days, then Super B was added morning and evening. Other vitamin supplements included Super C, Super Cal, and Radex. All processed foods were eliminated and a strict Vegetarian Diet was followed, including 8 glasses of water each day. Birch was applied on location for pain. Frankincense and lavender were applied on the feet.

BRAIN TUMOR—The following are recipes that some individuals have used successfully:

RECIPE #1—*Light* massage daily on spine with 1 oz. V-6 Mixing Oil, 15 drops frankincense, 6 drops clove. Rub brain stem with <u>ImmuPower</u>. Diffuse 15 drops frankincense, 6 drops clove for ½ hour three times a day.

RECIPE #2—Diffuse frankincense 24 hours a day and massage the brain stem with frankincense.

> *Frankincense contains sesquiterpenes which allow it to go beyond the blood brain barrier. Sesquiterpenes are also found in many of the emotional blends. ImmuPower builds the immune system. Clove is anti-parasitic and anti-tumoral.*

BREAST—Frankincense and clove. Often, there is an emotional issue of self-worth that must be dealt with as well. The soy solids contained in Body Balance may help prevent breast cancer.

CERVICAL—Clove, cypress, frankincense, geranium, lavender, lemon.

COLON—

SUPPLEMENTS—ICP (fiber beverage that helps prevent), CardiaCare (with *Rhododendron caucasicum* which inhibits the enzyme hyaluronidase), Coral Sea (highly bio-available, contains 58 trace minerals), Super Cal (studies have shown that taking calcium supplements at night helps protect the colon from polyps and cancer).

DIET—fast 21 days (See FASTING or CLEANSING) then have soup. See DIET.

HEART—HRT

LIVER—Frankincense (hot compress over liver), JuvaFlex and myrrh may help with liver congestion and function.

> *One woman had **cancer of the heart** which literally ate a hole in the heart. She took the tincture HRT and the tissue of her heart regenerated and the cancer disappeared!*
>
> *JuvaTone and Rehemogen build blood and hemoglobin platelets One individual had total liver regeneration by using JuvaTone, Rehemogen, and JuvaFlex.*

SUPPLEMENTS—JuvaTone was formulated to fight cancer in the liver.

LUNG—Frankincense (rub on chest or add 15 drops to 1 tsp. V-6 Mixing Oil for nightly retention enema), lavender.

BLEND #1—15 drops frankincense, 5 drops clove, 6 drops ravensara, 4 drops myrrh, and 2 drops sage. This blend can be mixed with 1 tsp. V-6 Mixing Oil if it is too strong. It is best when inserted into rectum.

LYMPHOMA—(nodes or small tumors) in neck and groin. Cleanse liver.

BLEND #2—10 drops frankincense, 5 drops myrrh, and 3 drops sage. Mix with small amount of V-6 Mixing Oil and apply daily over nodes or tumor areas and rectally. Every other day apply frankincense neat.

LYMPHOMA STAGE 4 (bone marrow)—extreme fatigue; eat vegetables and fruits, "NO MEAT". ImmuPower on the spine.

SUPPLEMENTS—Royaldophilus, Body Balance morning and night, Cleansing Trio (ComforTone, Megazyme, and ICP), 4 ImmuneTune three times a day (for one month or until remission), 4 Radex three times a day, 6 Super C three times a day,

C

6 VitaGreen three times a day. After remission, continue one more month then reduce amounts for maintenance.

MELANOMA (skin cancer)—See CORNS, WARTS. Frankincense and lavender.

OVARIAN—ImmuPower on spine three times a day.

> *BLEND #3*—15 drops frankincense, 6 drops geranium, 5 drops myrrh, ½ tsp. V-6 Mixing Oil; alternate one night in vagina (tampon to retain), next in rectum.
>
> *SUPPLEMENTS*—Body Balance three times a day, ImmuneTune six times a day, Femalin (tincture), 8 Radex a day, 6 FemiGen a day, 8 Super C a day. Those with "A" type blood should take 8 VitaGreen a day while those with "O" type blood should take 12 or more a day; VitaGreen is a mainstay, it is a predigested protein and helps maintain an alkaline balance.

PROSTATE—Anise (blend with frankincense, fennel, frankincense, ImmuPower, Mister, sage, yarrow). Apply to posterior scrotum, ankles, lower back, and bottom of feet

> *PERSONAL CARE*—Protec was designed to accompany the nightlong retention enema. It helps buffer the prostate from inflammation, enlargement, and tumor activity.
>
> *SUPPLEMENTS*—3 droppers of Male-Pro Tincture four times a day (available through Creer Labs 801-465-5423).

The following is a recipe that has been used on Prostate Cancer:

> *RECIPE #1*—Diffuse ImmuPower. Do a spinal massage and Vita Flex on the feet with ImmuPower. Blend 5 frankincense, 15 Mister, and 2 tsp. V-6 Mixing Oil together OR 15 ImmuPower with 2 tsp. V-6 Mixing Oil; insert and retain in the rectum throughout the night.
>
> *CASE HISTORY #1*—71 year old man had prostate cancer and bone metastasis. After three weeks of using frankincense, sage, myrrh, and cumin in rectal implants, he was free of cancer.

THROAT—Frankincense, lavender.

UTERINE—Geranium, ImmuPower.

> *BLEND #4*—2 to 5 drops cedarwood OR 2 to 5 drops lemon OR 2 to 5 drops myrrh in 1 tsp. V-6 Mixing Oil.

CANDIDA: See ACIDOSIS, ALKALINE, BLOOD, DIET, FOOD, THYROID, pH BALANCE. Di-Tone, cinnamon bark, clove,

> *Candida is caused by the fermentation of yeast and sugar, antibiotics, thyroid shut down, stress, chlorinated water, etc. When there is candida there is usually hypoglycemia and hypothyroidism. It is usually a digestive problem; putrefaction in the system causes candida overgrowth. Candida is a natural fungus in the stomach; we need some, but it becomes a problem when there is an overgrowth. Yeast is not the problem but the fermentation of it. The fermentation exists because of a mineral imbalance and an enzyme imbalance in the digestive system. The enzymes needed for digestion are secreted by the thyroid, so it is necessary to support both the thyroid and the digestive system. Also, maintaining a slightly alkaline state in the blood and body can help to slow the overgrowth of candida.*

EndoFlex, ᶠeucalyptus, <u>ImmuPower</u>, melaleuca (dilute with V-6 Mixing Oil for body massage), *Melaleuca quinquenervia*, <u>Melrose</u>, Mountain savory (dilute with V-6 Mixing Oil; can be hot), oregano, palmarosa (skin), peppermint (aromatic), rosemary, ᶠrosewood, ᶠspearmint, ᶠspruce, tarragon (prevents fermentation), <u>Thieves</u>. Rub on stomach area and feet or over abdomen with a hot compress.

SUPPLEMENTS—Allerzyme (aids the digestion of sugars, starches, fats, proteins), AlkaLime (combats yeast and fungus overgrowth and preserves the body's proper pH balance), Body Balance, ComforTone, Detoxzyme (helps maintain and support a healthy intestinal environment), ImmuGel (½ tsp. per day cleared up candida in the brain in one week for one individual), ICP, Megazyme (increases digestion), Mineral Essence, ParaFree, Polyzyme (aids the digestion of protein and helps reduce swelling and discomfort), Power Meal (vegetable protein), Radex, Royaldophilus (prevents overgrowth), Stevia Select (with FOS; repopulates intestines with good flora), Super C, Thyromin (to help the thyroid), VitaGreen (balances the alkaline/acid condition in the body, and provides chlorophyll and oxygen).

TINCTURES—Femalin (5-10 drops in 4 oz. of water; douche and retain for 20 minutes), Anti-Cana (creates unfriendly environment for the candida; available through Creer Labs 801-465-5423).

DIGESTIVE CANDIDA—<u>Di-Tone</u> (hot compresses over abdomen; in a retention enema at night), <u>ImmuPower</u>, <u>Thieves</u>.

VAGINAL CANDIDA—ᶠBergamot, ᶠmelaleuca, ᶠmyrrh.

BLEND—2 Tbsp. garlic oil, 8 drops lavender, 8 drops melaleuca, 1 ml. (1 softgel) Vitamin E oil. Apply to irritated area.

CANKERS: See ACIDOSIS.
Chamomile (both German and Roman), <u>Envision</u>, hyssop, laurel, melaleuca, <u>Melrose</u>, myrrh, oregano, <u>Thieves</u>.
BLEND #1—Sage with clove and lavender.
BLEND #2—Sage with Thieves.

> ***Canker sores*** *are occasionally associated with Crohn's disease, which affects the bowels. Deficiencies of iron, vitamin B12, and folic acid have been linked to this disease in some people. Stress and allergies are usually the cause of open sores in the mouth. To avoid getting canker sores, it is important to have a body chemistry that is balanced in minerals, acidity, and alkalinity (*Prescription for Nutritional Healing*, p. 126).*

SUPPLEMENTS—AlkaLime (combats yeast and fungus overgrowth and preserves the body's proper pH balance), ImmuneTune, ImmuPro, Mineral Essence, Mint Condition, VitaGreen.

C

CAPILLARIES:
BROKEN—Cypress, geranium, hyssop, lime (soothes), Roman chamomile.
BLEND—Apply 1 lavender and 1 Roman chamomile.

CARBUNCLES: Melaleuca.

CARDIOTONIC: See HEART.

CARDIOVASCULAR SYSTEM: See HEART. Anise, Aroma Life, clove, cypress, fleabane
(dilates), goldenrod, helichrysum, marjoram, onycha (benzoin), rosemary, tsuga
(opens and dilates for better oxygen exchange), ylang ylang.
SUPPLEMENTS—CardiaCare (contains ingredients that have been scientifically
tested for their abilities to support and strengthen the cardiovascular system),
Coral Sea (highly bio-available calcium, contains 58 trave minerals), ICP,
Mineral Essence, Super B, Super Cal.
TINCTURE—HRT

CARPAL TUNNEL SYNDROME: Basil, cypress, eucalyptus, lavender, lemongrass,
marjoram, oregano.
Apply oils on location
and either use massage
or Vita Flex to work
them in. First start
with basil and
marjoram on the
shoulder to help release

> *Carpal Tunnel Syndrome is a condition where inflamed carpal ligaments at the wrist press upon the median nerve. Indications include tingling or numbness in the palm or thumb and first three fingers of the hand, weak grip, or impaired finger movement.*

any energy blockages. Then lemongrass on wrist and oregano on the rotator cup
in the shoulder. Next apply marjoram and cypress on the wrist and then cypress
on the neck and down to the shoulder. Lastly, apply peppermint from the shoulder
down the arm to the wrist then out to the tips of each finger.
***COMMENTS—*Make sure it is carpal tunnel syndrome because many people that
think they have carpal tunnel syndrome (one report says up to 90%) really
have problems with muscles in the neck and shoulder that create similar
symptoms.*
MASSAGE OILS—Ortho Ease or Ortho Sport. Massage into neck, shoulder, and
wrist.
PERSONAL CARE—Prenolone/Prenolone+ (on shoulder and wrist).
SUPPLEMENTS—ArthroTune, Coral Sea (highly bio-available calcium, contains 58
trace minerals), Mineral Essence, Sulfurzyme, Super Cal.

CATARACTS: See EYES.

CATARRH (mucus): See ANTI-CATARRHAL. Cajeput, cistus, dill, ginger, hyssop (opens respiratory system to discharge mucus), jasmine, myrrh, onycha (benzoin).

CAVITIES: See TEETH.

CELIBACY (vow not to marry): Marjoram (aromatic).

CELLS: All Essential Oils restore cells to original state. Need to change the RNA and DNA to change the habit.
DNA—cell chemistry.
  SUPPLEMENTS—Super B, Thyromin, Body Balancing Trio (Body Balance, Master Formula His/Hers, VitaGreen).
FREQUENCY—Rose (enhances frequency of every cell, which brings balance and harmony to body).
LIVER—Helichrysum (stimulates cell function).
OXYGENATION—Black pepper.
REGULATING—Clary sage (removes negative programming).
RNA—cell memory.
STIMULATES—Abundance.

CELLULITE: See WEIGHT. Basil, ᶠcedarwood, cumin, cypress, fennel, geranium, ᶠgrapefruit, juniper, lavender, lemon, lime, orange, oregano, patchouly, ᶠrosemary, rosewood, sage, spikenard (increases metabolism to burn fat), tangerine (dissolves), thyme. *Refer to the chapter entitled "How to Use - The Personal Usage Reference" in the* Essential Oils Desk Reference *under "Cellulite" for some excellent blend recipes and recommendations.*
  SUPPLEMENTS—Allerzyme (aids the digestion of sugars, starches, fats, and proteins), Lipozyme (aids the digestion of fats), Power Meal (eat for breakfast).
ATTACKS FAT AND CELLULITE—Basil, grapefruit, lavender, lemongrass, rosemary, sage, thyme.
    MASSAGE OILS—Cel-Lite Magic (add grapefruit to increase activity and dissolve cellulite even faster).
    ***COMMENTS—You may try flavoring 1 gallon of water with 5 grapefruit and 5 lemon. Adjust to taste and drink. This may also improve energy. The new H2Oils packets can now be used to more easily and effectively flavor drinking water with lemon and grapefruit oils.*

CHAKRAS (Energy Centers): (*Refer to the chart at the end of the Science and Application section the* Reference Guide for Essential Oils.) Harmony (apply 1 drop on each chakra to open the energy centers and balance the electrical field of the chakras, starting at the feet and working up), lavender (brings harmony to chakras), rosemary (opens chakras), sandalwood (affects each chakra differently).

C

UNITES HEAD AND HEART—Helichrysum.
CROWN—3 Wise Men (to replace void with good/positives), sandalwood.
    OPENS—Forgiveness, Harmony.
BROW (3rd eye)—Acceptance, Awaken, and Dream Catcher (rub on lobe of ear to
    increase vision and spiritual vision), 1 drop Harmony, juniper, peppermint,
    rosemary.
    OPENS—Frankincense, Harmony.
THROAT—Sandalwood.
    OPENS—Harmony.
HEART—Sandalwood.
    OPENS A CLOSED HEART—Bergamot, Harmony.
SOLAR PLEXUS—Fennel, juniper.
    OPENS—Harmony.
SACRAL (navel)—Patchouly, sandalwood.
    BALANCING—Acceptance (balances Sacral Chakra which stores denial and sexual
    abuse), sage.
    OPENS—Harmony.
BASE—Patchouly, sandalwood.
    OPENS—Harmony.

CHANGE (Personal): See EMOTIONS. Forgiveness, Into the Future, Joy, Magnify Your
    Calling, Sacred Mountain, 3 Wise Men.

CHARLIE HORSE: See MUSCLE SPASMS. Aroma Siez, basil.
    PERSONAL CARE—Prenolone/Prenolone+.

CHEEKS: Jasmine.
    BLEND—5 Aroma Siez, 3 birch/wintergreen, and 3 spruce. Work oils between hands
    in a clockwise motion and pat on cheeks. Cup hands over nose and inhale.

CHELATION: See METALS.
    Aroma Life,
    cardamom,
    helichrysum (powerful
    chelator and anti-
    coagulant). Drink lots
    of distilled water (64
    oz. or more per day).

> *Traditional intravenous chelation therapy can cause
> scar tissue on the vascular walls. These oils,
> supplements, and tinctures provide a more natural
> approach to chelation. They may take longer to achieve
> the same results, but with minimal side effects.*

    MASSAGE OILS—Cel-Lite Magic.
    SUPPLEMENTS—Cleansing Trio (ComforTone, Megazyme, and ICP), VitaGreen
    (use with cardamom to enhance effects of Chelex tincture).

***COMMENTS—*The apple pectin that is contained in ICP helps remove unwanted metals and toxin from the body.*
  TINCTURES—AD&E, Chelex, and Rehemogen for natural cleansing.

CHEMICALS: See METALS. ᶠHelichrysum.
  SUPPLEMENTS—Chelex, Radex.

CHICKEN POX: See CHILDHOOD DISEASES.

CHIGGERS: See INSECT. Lavender.

CHILD BIRTH: See BIRTHING.

CHILDHOOD DISEASES:
  CHICKEN POX (2 weeks)—(shingles) sleep is very good. See SHINGLES. Bergamot, eucalyptus, lavender, melaleuca (Tea Tree), Roman chamomile.
    BATH—(relieves the itching) 2 drops lavender, 1 cup bicarbonate of soda, and 1 cup soda in bath and soak.
    BLEND #1—5 to 10 drops each of German chamomile and lavender to one ounce Calamine lotion. Mix and apply twice a day all over body.
    BLEND #2—10 drops lavender, 10 Roman chamomile, and 4 oz. Calamine lotion. Mix and apply twice a day all over body.
    BLEND #3—Add enough ravensara to some Green clay (from health food store) to form a paste that can be dabbed on the pox to relieve itching.
    DIFFUSE—an anti-viral oil (such as lemon) and apply the same oil all over the body twice a day. See BABIES/CHILDREN.
  MEASLES—ᶠEucalyptus, German chamomile, lavender, melaleuca. Spray or vaporize the room.
  GERMAN (3 day)—use anti-viral oils. See ANTI-VIRAL.
  RUBELLA—sponge down with one of these oils: Chamomile (Roman or German), lavender, melaleuca.
  MUMPS—Lavender, lemon, melaleuca.
  WHOOPING COUGH—Basil, cinnamon bark (diffuse or dilute well; avoid for children), Clary sage, cypress, grapefruit, hyssop, lavender, ᶠoregano, thyme.

CHILDREN: See BABIES, HYPERACTIVE CHILDREN, CHILDHOOD DISEASES.
    PERSONAL CARE—KidScents Bath Gel, KidScents Detangler, KidScents Lotion, KidScents Shampoo, KidScents Tender Tush, KidScents Toothpaste.
    SUPPLEMENTS—Mighty Mist (vitamin spray), Mighy Vites (chewable vitamin tablets).
  HYPERACTIVE—<u>Citrus Fresh</u>, <u>Peace & Calming</u>, <u>Trauma Life</u>. Diffuse.

CHILLS: Ginger, onycha (benzoin). Apply on bottom of feet and on solar plexus.

CHLOROPHYLL:
  SUPPLEMENTS—VitaGreen.

C

CHOLERA: Clove, Fravensara, Frosemary.

CHOLESTEROL: FClary sage, Fhelichrysum (regulates). Apply on Vita Flex points, over heart, and along arms.

CHOREA: See SAINT VITUS DANCE.

CHRONIC FATIGUE: See ACIDOSIS, HORMONAL IMBALANCE. Basil, Clarity, Di-Tone, ImmuPower, lavender, lemongrass, peppermint, rosemary, Thieves. (Note: Basil and peppermint are a good combination together). Combine any of the above with the Raindrop Technique.
  SUPPLEMENTS—
  AlkaLime (acid-neutralizing mineral), Body Balancing Trio (Body Balance, Master Formula His/Hers, VitaGreen), Cleansing Trio (ComforTone, Megazyme, and ICP), Coral Sea (highly bio-available calcium), ImmuneTune, ImmuPro, Mineral Essence, Power Meal, Royaldophilus, and Super Cal.

> *Chronic Fatigue* is often caused by the Epstein Barr virus. It may also be a result of chemical and metal toxicity, or conditions of high acidity.
>
> Women who are pregnant seldom have Chronic Fatigue Syndrome because of the higher amounts of natural progesterone being produced.

  PERSONAL CARE—Prenolone/Prenolone+.
  Dr. Friedmann uses the following recipe on his patients:
  RECIPE #1—1) Use the Cleansing Trio (ComforTone, Megazyme, and ICP) to detoxify. 2) Build the body and tissues with Mineral Essence and Master Formula His/Hers. 3) Build the immune system with ImmuPower and ImmuneTune or ImmuPro.

CIGARETTES:
  PURIFY AIR—Purification.
  QUIT SMOKING—See ADDICTIONS. Peace & Calming, Purification.
  SUPPLEMENTS—JuvaTone.

CIRCULATION: Aroma Life, basil, birch, cinnamon bark, Citrus Fresh, Clary sage, cumin, Fcypress, geranium, helichrysum, hyssop, nutmeg, onycha (benzoin), oregano, peppermint, <u>Peace & Calming</u>, <u>RC</u>, rosemary, thyme, wintergreen. Use in a bath, massage, or a compress.

CAPILLARY—**Cypress** (strengthens the capillary walls, and increases circulation), oregano, thyme.

PROMOTES HEALTHY—Onycha (benzoin), <u>PanAway</u>.

   MASSAGE OILS—Cel-Lite Magic dilates the blood vessels for better circulation; may add grapefruit or cypress to enhance. Also Ortho Ease and Ortho Sport.

   SUPPLEMENTS—Cleansing Trio (ComforTone, ICP, Megazyme), JuvaTone, Thyromin.

   ***COMMENTS—*Constipation affects circulation. Improving the circulation in the colon and liver improves the circulation in the blood.*

CIRCULATORY SYSTEM: See also CARDIOVASCULAR SYSTEM. <u>Aroma Life</u>, Clary sage, cypress, <u>En-R-Gee</u>, helichrysum, <u>PanAway</u>.

STIMULANT—Nutmeg, onycha (benzoin), pine.

SUPPORT—Goldenrod.

CIRRHOSIS: See LIVER.

CLARITY OF THOUGHTS: <u>Clarity</u>, rosemary.

CLEANSING: <u>Di-Tone</u> when cramping, fennel, hyssop, juniper, melaleuca (aromatic), <u>Melrose</u>, <u>Release</u> (over liver), <u>3 Wise Men</u> when trauma, put on liver to let emotions go.

> *Cleansing may help to prevent disease, improve immune function, and make the body stronger. It may also cause an emotional cleansing! DRINK LOTS OF WATER!! Any age child can go on a cleanse. Dr. Gary Young suggests that you spend two days cleansing for every year old you are. He recommends that you take ICP and Megazyme five days a week and fast once a week on distilled water and lemon juice.*

CUTS—Elemi, lavender, <u>Melrose</u> (scrapes).

BODY CLEANSE—

   SUPPLEMENTS— Cleansing Trio (ComforTone, Megazyme, and ICP). The oils contained in the Cleansing Trio will push heavy metals into the system; use <u>Sacred Mountain</u> and <u>Peace & Calming</u> to balance the system. If colon is blocked, start with ComforTone to open it. JuvaTone is the final stage of cleansing and can be taken as often as four times a day.

   TINCTURES—Rehemogen supports the body during a cleanse.

MASTER CLEANSER or LEMONADE DIET—

   2 Tbs. fresh lemon or lime juice (approx. ½ lemon), 2 Tbs. of grade C maple syrup (grades A & B are not as rich in nutrients but can be used if grade C is not available). 1/10 tsp. cayenne pepper or to taste (cayenne is a thermal warmer and

dilates the blood vessels; also has vitamin A). Combine above ingredients in a 10 oz. glass of distilled water. No substitute sugars. In the case of diabetes, use black strap molasses instead of the maple syrup. Drink between three quarts and a gallon of this lemonade each day with an herbal laxative tea first thing in the morning and just before retiring for the night.

Lemon converts to alkaline in the body. Lemons can be harmful to teeth only when in water that is not distilled because there can be a reaction with the minerals in the water. Toxins are eliminated from the bowels and bladder. Drink 6 to 12 glasses of the lemonade drink daily. When you get hungry, just drink another glass of lemonade. No other food or vitamins should be taken; the lemonade is already a food in liquid form. An herbal laxative tea may be used to help elimination. More details can be found in the book by Stanley Burroughs, Healing for the Age of Enlightenment. It will take 30 days on lemon to change the chemistry in the body. We have to change the DNA and RNA (memory or belief system) to change a habit. Then, do 30 days on carrot juice.

Refer to the book <u>Healing for the Age of Enlightenment</u> for more specific details including suggestions and specific instructions on coming off the cleanse.

CLOSED MINDED: <u>Awaken</u>, <u>Inspiration</u>.

CLOTHES: Canadian Red cedar. This oil will leave a stain so place a few drops on a cotton ball and put it in a plastic sack. Leave the sack open so the odor of the oil can do its work without it staining any clothes. Place the bag in a closet or storage box.

COCKROACHES:
   BLEND—Combine 10 peppermint and 5 cypress in ½ cup of water and spray.

COFFEE (stop drinking): (*See case study on the body's frequency reaction to coffee in the Science and Application section of the <u>Reference Guide for Essential Oils</u>*). <u>Peace & Calming</u>, <u>Purification</u>.
   SUPPLEMENTS—JuvaTone.

COLDS: Angelica, basil, cajeput, eucalyptus (in hot water, breathe deep), <u>Exodus II</u>, fir (aches and pains), ginger, Idaho tansy, lavender, ledum, ^Flemon, ^Fmelaleuca, myrtle, onycha (benzoin), orange, oregano, peppermint (relieves nasal congestion), pine, <u>Raven</u>, ravensara, <u>RC</u> (put a few drops in a box of tissue), ^Frosemary, <u>Thieves</u>, thyme. Apply <u>Raven</u> to the back and <u>RC</u> to the chest with <u>Thieves</u> on the feet. Next application rotate <u>Raven</u> and <u>RC</u>. Other oils can be diffused or applied to the forehead, temples, back of neck, and chest. *Refer to the chapter entitled "How to Use - The Personal Usage Reference" in the <u>Essential</u>*

Oils Desk Reference under "Colds and Flu" for some excellent recipes and supplement recommendations.

BLEND—Mix 6 RC and 2 ravensara. Apply to the chest, neck, throat, and sinus area. Diffuse or put 4 drops in a half cup of hot water, then place nose and mouth into cup (not in the water) and breathe deeply.

SUPPLEMENTS—Exodus, ImmuGel.

***COMMENTS—Dr. Pénoël recommends applying a trace of melaleuca alternifolia to the tip of the tongue and swallowing. This works best when done immediately upon noticing a sore throat. Repeat every minute until the throat feels better. Then apply it behind the ears and down under the jaw line. After repeating this a few times (every 5-10 minutes), massage a couple drops on the back of the neck to relieve any blockage.*

COLD SORES: See HERPES SIMPLEX. Bergamot, Blue cypress. geranium, lavender, lemon, melaleuca (Tea Tree), Melrose (fights infection), RC, Roman chamomile, Thieves.

COLIC: See BABIES. Angelica, bergamot, cardamom, carrot with fennel, coriander, cumin, dill, ginger, marjoram, melissa, Mountain savory, orange, pepper, peppermint, Roman chamomile, spearmint.

COLITIS: Anise, calamus (viral), clove (bacterial), ᶠhelichrysum (viral), ᶠtarragon, ᶠthyme (when there is infection). Redmond clay (from Redmond Minerals 1-800-367-7258) helps clean fecal matter out of pockets in the colon.
SUPPLEMENTS—AlkaLime, Cleansing Trio (ComforTone, Megazyme, and ICP).

COLON: See COLITIS and DIVERTICULITIS. Calamus may help reduce inflammation. Di-Tone and peppermint. Take 2 drops of each in distilled water 1-2 times per day. Use Redmond clay (from Redmond Minerals 1-800-367-7258) to remove fecal matter from pockets in the colon.
SUPPLEMENTS—Cleansing Trio (ComforTone, Megazyme, and ICP), Mint Condition, Royaldolphilus, Stevia Select. *Refer to the Supplements section of the Reference Guide for Essential Oils for specific usages.*

POLYPS—See POLYPS.
Cleanse the colon! Stanley Burroughs' Master Cleanse is an ideal cleansing program which affects

Polyps are tumors that arise from the bowel surface and protrude into the inside of the colon. Most polyps eventually transform into malignant cancer tumors.

the entire body. However, if fecal matter is not being eliminated from the colon 2-3 times per day, it may be necessary to start with ComforTone first until bowel movements are more frequent. Then toxins released during the Master Cleanse can be quickly eliminated from the body. (*See Master Cleanser under CLEANSING*)

SUPPLEMENTS—Cleansing Trio (ComforTone, Megazyme, and ICP). *Refer to the Supplements section of the Reference Guide for Essential Oils.*

PROLAPSED COLON—not assimilating; use Megazyme.

****COMMENTS—Stanley Burroughs recommends performing a colon lift and describes the procedure for doing so in his book Healing for the Age of Enlightenment on pages 55 to 59.*

SPASTIC—has no parasiticidal action.

SUPPLEMENTS—ComforTone then ICP (fiber beverage).

COMA: Awaken, Black pepper, cypress, frankincense, Hope, peppermint, sandalwood, Surrender, Trauma Life, Valor. Massage on brain stem, mastoids (behind ears), temples, and bottom of feet.

SUPPLEMENTS—Mineral Essence, Ultra Young.

COMFORTING: Gentle Baby.

COMPASSION: Helichrysum.

COMPLEXION: See SKIN. Apply oils to face, neck and intestines.
DULL—Jasmine, orange.
OILY—Bergamot, orange.

CONCENTRATION (POOR): Awaken, basil, Brain Power, cedarwood, Clarity, cypress, Dream Catcher, eucalyptus, Gathering, juniper, lavender, lemon, myrrh, orange, peppermint, rosemary, sandalwood, 3 Wise Men, ylang ylang.

CONCUSSION: Cypress. Rub on brain stem and bottom of feet.
****COMMENTS—One woman had a concussion with headaches and hallucinations. By applying cypress over her brain stem, her headaches left for good.*

CONFIDENCE: Jasmine, Live with Passion, sandalwood (self), Valor.

CONFUSION: Awaken, basil, Brain Power, cedarwood, Clarity, cypress, fir, frankincense, Gathering, geranium, ginger, Harmony, jasmine, juniper, marjoram, peppermint, Present Time, rose, rosemary, rosewood, sandalwood, spruce, thyme, Valor, ylang ylang.

CONGESTION: Di-Tone, cedarwood, coriander, cypress, *Eucalyptus radiata*, Exodus II, fennel, ginger, myrtle (excellent for children), Raven, RC, rosemary. To help discharge mucus, rub oil(s) on chest, neck, back, feet, and diffuse.

MASSAGE OILS—Cel-Lite Magic.
    SUPPLEMENTS—Cleansing Trio (ComforTone, ICP, Megazyme).

CONJUNCTIVITIS: *Eucalyptus radiata*, jasmine, Mixta chamomile.

CONSCIOUSNESS: Lavender. Diffusing these oils is a great way to affect consciousness.
    OPEN—Rosemary.
    PURIFYING—Peppermint.
    STIMULATING—Peppermint.

CONSTIPATION: See
        ACIDOSIS. Anise,
        Black pepper, <u>Di-Tone</u>,
        fennel, ginger, juniper,
        Fmarjoram, Forange,
        patchouly, rose,

> *Poor bowel function may be caused by enzyme deficiency, low fiber, poor bowel tone, not enough liquid in diet, stress, incorrect pH balance, and/or bad diet.*

        rosemary, sandalwood, tangerine, tarragon. Massage clockwise around abdomen
        and on Vita Flex points (feet & shins).
    SUPPLEMENTS—AlkaLime, ComforTone, Megazyme, ICP (fiber beverage),
        Sulfurzyme, and lots of water. If there is a chronic history of constipation, use
        ComforTone until the system is open, then start ICP.
    BLEND #1—Mix together 6 drops of Forange, tangerine, and spearmint and rub on
        lower stomach and colon.
    BLEND #2—15 cedarwood, 10 lemon, 5 peppermint, and 2 oz. V-6 Mixing Oil.
        Massage over lower abdomen three times a day clockwise and take supplements.
    CHILDREN—fruit juices or lots of water. Geranium, patchouly, Roman chamomile,
        rosemary, tangerine.

CONTAGIOUS DISEASES: FGinger.

CONTROL:
    OF YOUR LIFE—Cedarwood, <u>Dream Catcher</u>, <u>Envision</u>.
    SELF—<u>Motivation</u>, Roman chamomile (aromatic).

CONVULSIONS: See SEIZURE. <u>Brain Power</u>, Clary sage, lavender, neroli, Roman
    chamomile, <u>Valor</u>.
    SUPPLEMENTS—Mighty Mist/Vites, Mineral Essence, Ultra Young.

COOLING OILS: Angelica, Citrus oils, eucalyptus, lavender, melaleuca, Mountain savory,
    peppermint, Roman chamomile, spruce. Other oils that are high in aldehydes and
    esters can produce a cooling effect.

CORNS: See WARTS. Carrot, <u>Citrus Fresh</u>, clove, grapefruit, lemon, myrrh, peppermint, Roman chamomile, tangerine. Apply 1 drop of oil directly on corn.

CORTISONE: Birch, <u>EndoFlex</u>, lavender, <u>Relieve It</u>, Roman chamomile, Fspruce (is like cortisone), wintergreen.

> *BLEND*—Combine 3 drops Roman chamomile, 3 lavender, 5 spruce, and 1 birch/wintergreen and apply as a natural cortisone.

> *SUPPLEMENTS*—ProGen and Thyromin, together with <u>EndoFlex</u> are beneficial for both men and women. The three items together may also help the body produce its own cortisone.

COUGHS: Angelica, cajeput, cardamom, **cedarwood**, elemi (unproductive), Feucalyptus, fir,

> *Diffusing the oils is one of the best ways to handle a cough. It may also help to rub the oils on the throat and chest area.*

frankincense, ginger, jasmine, juniper, Fmelaleuca, Fmyrtle (helps remove mucus from lungs), myrrh, onycha (benzoin), peppermint, pine, myrrh, <u>RC</u>, ravensara, Roman chamomile, sandalwood, thyme.

> *ESSENTIAL WATERS (HYDROSOLS)*—Clary Sage (gentle enough from smaller children - spray on chest of in air). Can also diffuse using Essential Mist Diffuser.

ALLERGY—<u>Purification</u> (diffuse).

BAD—Elemi, frankincense.

> *BLEND #1*—3 drops fir, 3 lemon, 2 ravensara, 1 thyme.

> *BLEND #2*—15 drops <u>Raven</u>, 15 <u>RC</u>, 5 lemon, and 10 <u>Peace & Calming</u>. Rub on chest, throat, and neck. Can also be diffused.

SMOKERS—Myrtle.

COURAGE: Clove (aromatic), fennel (aromatic), ginger, <u>Live with Passion</u>, <u>Valor</u> (gives).

CRADLE CAP: See BABIES.

CRAMPS: See DIGESTIVE SYSTEM, HORMONAL IMBALANCE, MENSTRUATION, MUSCLES, PMS. <u>Aroma Siez</u>, basil, Fbirch, Blue cypress (abdominal), Clary sage, Fcypress, <u>Exodus II</u>, galbanum, ginger, Flavender, rosemary, Fmarjoram, wintergreen.

> *MASSAGE OILS*—Relaxation.

LEG CRAMPS—<u>Aroma Siez</u>, basil, German chamomile, lavender, marjoram, rosemary, vetiver.

> *MASSAGE OILS*—Ortho Ease, Ortho Sport, Relaxation.

> *PERSONAL CARE*—Prenolone/Prenolone+.

SUPPLEMENTS—ArthroTune, Coral Sea (highly bio-available calcium, contains 58 trace minerals), Mineral Essence, Super Cal.

MENSTRUAL CRAMPS—See DYSMENORRHEA.

    PERSONAL CARE—Prenolone/Prenolone+.

    SUPPLEMENTS—Exodus, FemiGen. Lady Flash, Lady Love (available through Creer Labs 801-465-5423).

    RECIPE #1—Take 2 FemiGen three times a day, 10 days before period. Start again two days after cycle. May take up to 6 tablets three times a day. Lady Flash and Lady Love may be applied to the ovaries, pelvis, ankles, bottom of the feet, or as a hot compress.

STOMACH CRAMPS—Di-Tone.

CREATES SACRED SPACE: Sacred Mountain.

CROHN'S DISEASE: Basil, calamus, Di-Tone, peppermint. Do Raindrop Technique on spine with ImmuPower.

    SUPPLEMENTS—AlkaLime, Body Balance, Cleansing Trio (ComforTone, ICP, and Megazyme), ImmuGel, Mineral Essence, Mint Condition, Power Meal, Royaldophilus, **Sulfurzyme**, VitaGreen.

    ***COMMENTS—*Refer to the chapter entitled "How to Use - The Personal Usage Reference" in the* Essential Oils Desk Reference *under "Crohn's Disease" for a specific regimen of supplements.*

CROWN CHAKRA:

    OPEN—3 Wise Men (releases and fills the void).

CUSHING'S DISEASE: See ADRENAL GLANDS. Basil, ImmuPower, lemon, Thieves.

    SUPPLEMENTS—Exodus, ImmuneTune, ImmuPro.

CUTS: See TISSUE. Cypress, elemi (infected), helichrysum, lavender, melaleuca, Melrose (rejuvenates tissue), onycha (benzoin), pine, ravensara, Relieve It, Roman chamomile (healing), rosewood, Thieves.

CYSTIC FIBROSIS: Alternate with Thieves, RC, lavender, and myrtle. Apply to brain stem (back of neck), temples, chest, bottom of feet, and diffuse. Raven is stronger and can replace myrtle for helping to remove mucus accumulation in the lungs. EndoFlex and helichrysum can also be used with benefit.

    BLEND—(Staphylococcus) oregano, thyme, and Melrose (up the spine using the Raindrop Technique), then 10 drops lemon, 5 drops melaleuca, and 3 drops frankincense (rub on feet, chest, and diffuse) OR 10 Raven and 5 hyssop.

    SUPPLEMENTS—VitaGreen, Megazyme, Master Formula His/Hers, all vitamins.

CYSTITIS (Bladder Infection): Basil, bergamot, cajeput, cedarwood, cinnamon bark, clove, eucalyptus, fennel, frankincense, ʳGerman chamomile, hyssop, juniper, lavender, marjoram, oregano, pine, sage, sandalwood, ʳspearmint, rosewood, ʳthyme. Massage or bathe with one of these oils.
TINCTURE—K&B.

DANDRUFF: Cedarwood, ʳlavender, melaleuca (Tea Tree), patchouly, ʳrosemary, sage, valerian.
PERSONAL CARE—Lavender Volume Hair & Scalp Wash and Lavender Volume Nourishing Rinse.

DAY DREAMING: Awaken, cedarwood, Clarity, Dream Catcher, eucalyptus, Gathering, ginger, Harmony, helichrysum, lavender, lemon, myrrh, peppermint, Present Time, rose, rosemary, rosewood, Sacred Mountain, sandalwood, spruce, 3 Wise Men, thyme, Valor, ylang ylang.

DEATH (of Loved One): See EMOTIONS: LOSS. Trauma Life.

DEBILITY: Cardamom, cumin (nervous), ʳnutmeg.

DECONGESTANT: Any of the citrus oils, ʳcypress, ʳGerman chamomile, juniper, melaleuca, patchouly.

DEFEATED: See EMOTIONS.

> *A lack of nutrients at the cellular level causes degenerative disease.* The general health condition of the body will improve if the necessary nutrients are received by the body at the cellular level. Toxins change the pH of the cell wall, which significantly reduces the ability of the cell to assimilate nutrients and oxygen. This process is the beginning of cellular starvation, which leads to degenerative disease. Then, we are hosts to viral and bacterial invasions due to our weakened or compromised immune system. Essential Oils are antimicrobial and help our immune system fight off the ravages of disease. They also have the ability to deliver nutrients to our nutritionally depleted cells. When essential oils are blended with the proper nutrients that the body requires, the essential oils act as the delivery system to take the nutrients directly into the cell and through the compromised cell wall, which has had the pH altered due to chemical toxins in the body. This process allows the body to rebuild and regain its healthful condition and allows the body's immune system to normalize. In addition, essential oils have the highest oxygenating molecules of any know substance. So, they deliver oxygen to the cells which helps in the regeneration process. (Young Living Essential Edge Newsletter — July 1996).

DEGENERATIVE DISEASE: See pH BALANCE. Citrus Fresh, Exodus II, frankincense, lavender, lemon, orange, Purification, and tangerine are excellent to diffuse in the room. Not only do these oils purify the air, but they help deliver needed oxygen to

the starving cells. All other essential oils and supplements are beneficial for
providing oxygen and nutrients to the cells of the body.. See specific ailment.
SUPPLEMENT—Power Meal.

DEHYDRATION: ImmuneTune, Mineral Essence.
   COMMENTS*—An 18-month old infant was saved from dying of dehydration when it
    was given ½ capsule of ImmuneTune in applesauce.*

DELIVERY: See PREGNANCY.

DENIAL: Roman chamomile, sage.
   OVERCOME—<u>Abundance</u>, <u>Acceptance</u>, <u>Awaken</u>.

DENTAL INFECTION: Clove and frankincense, helichrysum, melaleuca, myrrh, <u>Thieves</u>.
   Apply to jaws and gums. It may be necessary to dilute <u>Thieves</u> with V-6 Mixing
   Oil.
    PERSONAL CARE—Dentarome/Dentarome Plus Toothpaste (contains <u>Thieves</u>),
    Fresh Essence Mouthwash (contains <u>Thieves</u>), KidScents Toothpaste (for
    children).

DEODORANT: <u>Acceptance</u>, <u>Aroma Siez</u>, bergamot, citronella, cypress, <u>Dragon Time</u>,
   <u>Dream Catcher</u>, <u>EndoFlex</u>, eucalyptus, geranium, <u>Harmony</u>, <u>Joy</u>, lavender,
   melaleuca, <u>Mister</u>, myrtle, <u>Peace & Calming</u>, <u>RC</u>, <u>Release</u>, <u>White Angelica</u>.
   Apply oils neat to the skin or dilute with some V-6 Mixing Oil or Massage Oil
   Base for application under the arms. Also, 2-3 drops of an oil can be added to 4
   oz. of unscented talcum powder and 2 oz. of baking soda. Mix this well and apply
   under the arms, on the feet, or on other areas of the body.
    BATH & SHOWER GELS—Dragon Time, Evening Peace, Morning Start.
    MASSAGE OILS—Dragon Time, Relaxation.
    PERSONAL CARE—Satin Body Lotion, Sandalwood Moisture Cream. Add a couple
    drops of one of the oils listed above for additional fragrance.

DEODORIZING: Clary sage, myrrh, ᶠmyrtle, peppermint, <u>Purification</u>, sage, thyme.

DEPLETION: Cypress.

DEPRESSION: See DIET. <u>Acceptance</u>, basil, ᶠbergamot (aromatic), calamus, Clary sage,
   <u>EndoFlex</u> (apply often while taking Mineral Essence and Thyromin supplements),
   ᶠfrankincense, <u>Gathering</u>, <u>Gentle Baby</u> (on solar plexus), geranium, ginger,
   grapefruit, <u>Harmony</u>, <u>Hope</u> (on ears, especially for emotional clearing),
   <u>Inspiration</u>, jasmine, <u>Joy</u> (5 drops in palm of non-dominant hand, stir clockwise
   three times with dominant hand, then apply over heart and breathe in deeply),

juniper (over heart), lavender (aromatic), <u>M-Grain</u>, neroli, onycha (benzoin), <u>PanAway</u>, <u>Live with Passion</u>, patchouly, <u>Peace & Calming</u> (back of neck), pepper (on crown for spirit protection), ravensara (lifts emotions), <u>Release</u>, Roman chamomile, ᶠrosemary (nervous), ᶠrosewood, sage (relieves depression), sandalwood, <u>Sensation</u>, tangerine, <u>Trauma Life</u>, <u>Valor</u> (helps balance energies), ᶠylang ylang.

D

BATH AND SHOWER GELS—Sensation Bath & Shower Gel, Lemon Sandalwood or Thieves Cleansing Soaps.

MASSAGE OILS— Sensation Massage Oil.

PERSONAL CARE— EndoBalance, Prenolone/Prenolone+, Sensation Moisturizing Cream.

SUPPLEMENTS—Coral Sea (highly bio-available calcium, contains 58 trace minerals), Essential Omegas, Mineral Essence, ProMist, Thyromin, Ultra Young (helps lift depression).

> *Depression can be caused by a calcium deficiency. Stay away from carbonated soft drinks, specifically cola drinks that are high in phosphorus; they leech calcium from the body. Eating heavy protein at night does not give the body enough time to digest the food before going to sleep. The undigested food then ferments which robs the system of needed oxygen and heightens the sense of depression.*

BLEND #1—Combine 1-2 drops each of frankincense, 3 Wise Men, and Hope in the palm of your hand, rub hands together clockwise, cup hands over nose and mouth, and breathe deeply.

ANTI-DEPRESSANT—<u>Abundance</u>, <u>Awaken</u>, bergamot, <u>Christmas Spirit</u>, <u>Citrus Fresh</u>, <u>Dream Catcher</u>, frankincense, geranium, jasmine, <u>Joy</u>, lavender, lemon, melissa, <u>Motivation</u>, neroli, orange, onycha (benzoin), <u>Peace & Calming</u>, ravensara, Roman chamomile, rose, <u>Sacred Mountain</u>, sandalwood, <u>3 Wise Men</u>, <u>Valor</u>.

IMMUNE DEPRESSION—ᶠSpruce.

BATH AND SHOWER GELS—Morning Start Bath & Shower Gel, Thieves Cleansing Soap.

BLEND—5 bergamot, 5 lavender, diffuse.

SUPPLEMENTS—ImmuGel, ImmuPro.

SEDATIVES—Bergamot, cedarwood, Clary sage, cypress, frankincense, geranium, hyssop, jasmine, juniper, lavender, marjoram, *Melaleuca ericifolia*, melissa, neroli, onycha (benzoin), patchouly, Roman chamomile, rose, sandalwood, ylang ylang. Use intuition as to which one may be best for the given situation. In addition, check the safety data for each of the oils in the APPENDIX of this book.

SUICIDAL DEPRESSION—Put <u>Valor</u> then <u>Inspiration</u> on feet and hold feet for a few minutes until relaxed; this may start to release a past negative memory, start crying, etc. If not, rub <u>Present Time</u> over thymus then a drop of <u>Inner Child</u> on their thumb and have them suck the thumb, pushing the pad of the thumb to the roof of the mouth. Once the emotional release starts, put <u>Grounding</u> on the back of neck and sternum, then put <u>Release</u> on the crown of the head and wait for a while, allowing then to deal with the release. After the emotional release has subsided, rub <u>Joy</u> over the heart and <u>Hope</u> on the ears. After waking up the next morning, apply a couple drops of <u>Gentle Baby</u> on solar plexus and over the heart. <u>Magnify Your Calling</u> may also be helpful to wear as a perfume/cologne.

SUPPLEMENTS—Essential Omegas, Thyromin.

CLEANSING THE FLESH AND BLOOD OF EVIL DEITIES—Cedarwood and myrrh.

BIBLE—"Breaking the lineage of iniquity," The ancient Egyptians believed that if they didn't clear the body and mind of negative influences before dying, they could not progress into the next life and return to this world to take up the body they had left in the tomb (resurrection).

DEPROGRAMMING: <u>Forgiveness</u>, <u>Inner Child</u>, <u>Release</u>, <u>SARA</u>, <u>Trauma Life</u>.

DERMATITIS: Bergamot, chamomile (Roman and German), geranium, ᶠhelichrysum, hyssop, ᶠjuniper, lavender, *Melaleuca ericifolia*, onycha (benzoin), ᶠpatchouly, pine, ᶠthyme.

SUPPLEMENTS—Megazyme, Sulfurzyme.

****COMMENTS—Dermatitis may indicate a sulfur deficiency.*

DESPAIR: <u>Acceptance</u>, <u>Believe</u>, cedarwood, Clary sage, fir, <u>Forgiveness</u>, frankincense, <u>Gathering</u>, geranium, <u>Gratitude</u>, <u>Grounding</u>, <u>Harmony</u>, <u>Hope</u>, <u>Joy</u>, lavender, lemon, lemongrass, orange, peppermint, rosemary, sandalwood, spearmint, spruce, thyme, <u>Valor</u>, ylang ylang.

DESPONDENCY: Bergamot, Clary sage, cypress, <u>Gathering</u>, geranium, ginger, <u>Harmony</u>, <u>Hope</u>, <u>Inner Child</u>, <u>Inspiration</u>, <u>Joy</u>, orange, <u>Peace & Calming</u>, <u>Present Time</u>, rose, rosewood, sandalwood, <u>Trauma Life</u>, <u>Valor</u>, and ylang ylang.

DETOXIFICATION: ᶠHelichrysum, ᶠjuniper (detoxifier), <u>JuvaFlex</u>. Apply oils to liver area, intestines, and Vita Flex points on feet.

SUPPLEMENTS—JuvaTone, Radex, Cleansing Trio (ComforTone, Megazyme, and ICP).

DIABETES: Coriander (normalizes glucose levels), cypress, dill (helps lower glucose levels by normalizing insulin levels and supporting pancreas function), ᶠeucalyptus, fennel, ᶠgeranium, ginger, hyssop,

> *Caution: Diabetics should not use angelica Watch insulin intake carefully, may have to cut down. Keep physician informed!*

D

juniper, lavender, ᶠpine, ᶠrosemary, <u>Thieves</u>, ᶠylang ylang. Apply on back, chest, feet, and over pancreas. Diffuse.

BLEND #1—8 clove, 8 cinnamon bark, 15 rosemary, 10 thyme in 2 oz. of V-6 Mixing Oil. Put on feet and over pancreas.

BLEND #2—5 cinnamon bark and 5 cypress. Rub on feet and pancreas.

SUPPLEMENTS—Body Balance, Carbozyme (helps control blood sugar levels— can use as much as 2 capsules twice per day), Cleansing Trio (ComforTone, Megazyme, and ICP), ImmuneTune, ImmuPro, Mineral Essence, Power Meal, Stevia, Sulfurzyme (take in morning with Vitamin C before breakfast and at bed time), VitaGreen.

***COMMENTS—*Seven-year old girl took 6 VitaGreen a day (balances blood sugar), Body Balance three times a day, and ImmuneTune.*

PANCREAS SUPPORT—Cinnamon bark, fennel, geranium.

SORES (diabetic)—Do the Raindrop Technique and put <u>Valor</u> on Vita Flex points. Also lavender, <u>Melrose</u>.

DIAPER RASH: ᶠLavender.

PERSONAL CARE—KidScents Tender Tush (formulated specifically for diaper rash), Rose Ointment.

DIARRHEA: See ACIDOSIS. Cardamom, cistus, cumin, ᶠgeranium, ᶠginger, ᶠmelaleuca, ᶠmyrrh, myrtle, ᶠpeppermint, ᶠsandalwood (obstinate), spearmint (not for babies).

SUPPLEMENTS—AlkaLime, Megazyme, Mint Condition, and Royaldophilus.

ANTI-SPASMODIC—Cypress, eucalyptus, Roman chamomile.

CHILDREN—Geranium, ginger, Roman chamomile, sandalwood.

CHRONIC—Neroli, ᶠnutmeg, ᶠorange, Di-Tone (apply over stomach, colon, and Vita Flex points).

STRESS-INDUCED—Lavender.

DIET: See BLOOD, FASTING, FOOD, and CLEANSING. Diet is extremely important when trying to correct cancer, hypoglycemia, candida, etc. First, cleanse the body, drink a lot of distilled water, stay away from sugars and meats, eat vegetable protein in the mornings, carbohydrates and starches for lunch, and fruit in the evening. Hydrochloric acid and pepsin are secreted in the morning to help digest protein.

SUPPLEMENTS—Enzyme products: Allerzyme (aids the digestion of sugars, starches, fats, and proteins), Carbozyme (aids the digestion of carbohydrates), Detoxzyme (helps maintain and support a healthy intestinal environment), Fiberzyme (aids the digestion of fiber and enhances the absorption of nutrients), Polyzyme (aids the digestion of protein and helps reduce swelling and discomfort), and Lipozyme (aids the digestion of fats).

POST-DIET SAGGY SKIN: Combine 8 drops each of sage, pine, lemongrass, and 1 oz. V-6 Mixing Oil. Rub on areas.

DIGESTIVE SYSTEM: See also INTESTINAL PROBLEMS. Anise (accelerates), basil, bergamot, Black pepper, cardamom (nervous), cinnamon bark, ᶠClary sage

> *Digestive problems may indicate a mineral deficiency. Use Mineral Essence. Royaldophilus is necessary when you are detoxifying or on any type of prescription drug; you must feed the intestinal tract. If you have digestion problems, take Royaldophilus or Stevia Select (with FOS) to stop the fermentation process.*

(weak), clove, coriander (spasms), cumin (spasms and indigestion), Di-Tone (acid stomach; aids the secretion of digestive enzymes), ᶠfennel (sluggish), ginger, ᶠgrapefruit, juniper, JuvaFlex (supports and detoxifies), laurel, lemon (indigestion), ᶠlemongrass (purifier), mandarin (tonic), ᶠmarjoram (stimulates), myrrh, myrtle, neroli, ᶠnutmeg (for sluggish digestion; eases), orange (indigestion), ᶠpatchouly (stimulant), ᶠpeppermint, rosemary, ᶠsage (sluggish), spearmint, tangerine (nervous and sluggish), tarragon (nervous and sluggish). Add the oil(s) to your food, rub on stomach, or apply as a compress over abdomen.

DIFFUSION—See NEGATIVE IONS for oils that produce negative ions when diffused to help stimulate the digestive system.

ESSENTIAL WATERS (HYDROSOLS)—Peppermint or Spearmint. Spray into air, directly on abdomen, or diffuse using the Essential Mist Diffuser.

SUPPLEMENTS—AlkaLime (combats yeast and fungus overgrowth and preserves the body's proper pH balance), Body Balancing Trio (Body Balance, Master Formula His/Hers, VitaGreen), ComforTone, Essential Manna, ICP (helps speed food through digestive system; lower incidence of fermentation), Megazyme (enzymes help build the digestive system; take before meals for acid stomach), Mint Condition (take after meals; soothing to irritated stomach; reduces inflammation), Mineral Essence, ParaFree, Radex (prevention of free radicals), Royaldophilus (3 times per week to support digestive function), Stevia Select, Sulfurzyme. Other enzyme products include: Allerzyme (aids the digestion of sugars, starches, fats, and proteins), Carbozyme (aids the digestion of carbohydrates), Detoxzyme (helps maintain and support a healthy intestinal environment), Fiberzyme (aids the digestion of fiber and enhances the absorption of nutrients), Polyzyme (aids the digestion of protein and helps reduce swelling and discomfort), and Lipozyme (aids the digestion of fats).

TINCTURES—Royal Essence.

DIPHTHERIA: Frankincense, goldenrod.

DISAPPOINTMENT: Clary sage, <u>Dream Catcher</u>, eucalyptus, fir, frankincense, <u>Gathering</u>, geranium, ginger, <u>Grounding</u>, <u>Harmony</u>, <u>Hope</u>, <u>Joy</u>, juniper, lavender, orange, <u>Present Time</u>, spruce, thyme, <u>Valor</u>, ylang ylang.

DISCOURAGEMENT: Bergamot, cedarwood, <u>Dream Catcher</u>, frankincense, geranium, <u>Hope</u>, <u>Joy</u>, juniper, lavender, lemon, orange, rosewood, <u>Sacred Mountain</u>, sandalwood, spruce, <u>Valor</u>.

DISINFECTANT: Grapefruit, ᶠlemon, <u>Purification</u>, ᶠsage.
>   *BLEND*—Add the following number of drops to a bowl of water: 10 lavender (2), 20 thyme (4), 5 eucalyptus (1), 5 oregano (1). If using the larger portions, add to a large bowl of water. If using the numbers in the parentheses, add the oils to a small bowl of water. Use blend to disinfect small areas.

DIURETIC: Cardamom, ᶠcedarwood, cypress, <u>EndoFlex</u>, fennel, grapefruit (all citrus oils), juniper, ᶠlavender, lemon, ᶠlemongrass, marjoram, mugwort, onycha (benzoin), orange, oregano, ᶠrosemary, ᶠsage, **tangerine**, valerian. Apply oil(s) to kidney area on back, bottom of feet, and on location.
>   ALLEVIATES FLUIDS—Cypress, fennel, **tangerine**.
>   *BLEND*—1 fennel, 2 cypress, 5 tangerine, apply from the top of the foot to the knee.

DIVERTICULITIS: Use Redmond clay (1-800-367-7258) to get help remove fecal matter from the pockets. Rub abdomen with cinnamon bark and V-6 Mixing Oil. Anise or lavender may also help. Calamus may help with earlier stages of diverticulitis.

> *Diverticula, are like herniations through the muscular wall of the large intestine (colon), are caused by increased pressure in the bowel from constipation. The existence of these sacs that are filled with trapped fecal sludge is called **diverticulosis**. When they become infected, the rotting feces erodes the surrounding mucousa and blood vessels and bleeding, rupturing, and infection begins. This is known as **diverticulitis**.*

>   *SUPPLEMENTS*— ComforTone to open blocked colon (use daily, increasing dosage by one until bowels are eliminating waste 2-4 times per day), then ICP (fiber beverage) to cleanse colon, and Megazyme for digestive enzyme support.

DIZZINESS: Tangerine.

DNA: Chamomile strengthens positive imprinting in DNA.
>   UNLOCK EMOTIONAL TRAUMA IN DNA—<u>Acceptance</u>, <u>3 Wise Men</u> (instructs DNA to open for discharge of negative trauma), sandalwood (unlocks negative

programing in DNA and enhances the positive programming in the DNA cell to create a feeling of security and protection).

DOWN SYNDROME: Clarity, Valor. Apply to bottom of feet and diffuse.
SUPPLEMENTS—Master Formula His/Hers, Mineral Essence.

DREAM STATE: Dream Catcher dissipates negative thoughts and helps one hold onto dreams until they become reality.
INFLUENCES—Clary sage (aromatic) enhances vivid dream recall.
PROTECTION FROM NEGATIVE DREAMS (that might steal your vision)—Dream Catcher helps one achieve dreams.

DROWNING IN OWN NEGATIVITY: Grapefruit (prevent, aromatic).

DRUGS: See ADDICTIONS.

DYING: Awaken, Lazarus (available through Creer Labs 801-465-5423).

DYSENTERY: Black pepper, cajeput, cistus, clove (amoebic), cypress, eucalyptus, lemon, melissa, ᶠmyrrh, Roman chamomile. Apply on abdomen and bottom of feet.

DYSPEPSIA (IMPAIRED DIGESTION): Cardamom, coriander, cumin, tarragon, goldenrod, ᶠgrapefruit, laurel, myrrh, ᶠorange (nervous), ᶠthyme. Apply to stomach, intestines, and Vita Flex points on feet.
SUPPLEMENTS—Megazyme, Mint Condition.

EARS: Cumin (deafness following a bad viral flu infection), elemi, eucalyptus, geranium, **helichrysum** (improves certain hearing losses), Idaho tansy, juniper, marjoram, Melrose (fights infection and for earache), Purification, valerian (combine with helichrysum for added pain relief), Valor, vitex.
INSTRUCTIONS TO INCREASE AND RESTORE HEARING—

1. Rub Valor on bottom of feet, especially 2 smallest toes and smallest fingers.
2. For each ear, layer 2 drops of **helichrysum, Purification, juniper,** and **peppermint** (in that order), around the inside (not deep) and back of ear, on the mastoid bone (behind ear), along the bottom of the skull around to the back of the head, and down the brain stem. **Never drip oils directly into ear canal!
3. Then do the following ear adjustment.
    1. Pull one ear **up** then the other ear up 10 times each side; 20 times total.
    2. Pull one ear **back** then the other, 5 times each side; 10 times total.
    3. Pull one ear **down** then the other, 5 times each side; 10 times total.
    4. Pull one ear **forward** then the other, 5 times each side; 10 times total.

5. Then one quick pull with finger in each direction. Up, back, down, forward.
    4. Rub **geranium** all around back and front of ear.
    5. (Optional) Rub 2 drops **ravensara** around base of both ears.

EARACHE—1 drop of either basil, <u>Melrose</u>, or <u>ImmuPower</u>. Can also try 1 drop each of helichrysum and valerian together. Put the drop in your hand and soak a small piece of cotton (small enough to fit snugly in the ear) in the oil. Place the piece of cotton in the ear and apply the leftover oil on both the front and back of the ear with a finger.

EARACHE IN ANIMALS—(Not cats) 1 drop <u>Melrose</u> on cotton swab then around in well of ear. **Do not put oils directly into ear canal**.

HEARING IN A TUNNEL—<u>Purification</u>, ravensara.

INFECTION—<u>ImmuPower</u>, melaleuca, <u>Melrose</u> (inside well of ear, down and around ear on the outside and under chin). <u>Purification</u> inside well of ear, *Melaleuca ericifolia* and lavender all around outside of ear.

> *Ear infections can be caused by food allergies!*
>
> **Caution:** *When working on the ears, <u>do not put the oils directly into the ear canal</u>. Apply only 1-2 drops of oil to the ear by rubbing on the inside, outside, and on the mastoid bone directly behind the ear.*

INFLAMMATION—Eucalyptus,

PIMPLES (in ears)—ImmuPower.

TINNITUS (ringing in the ears, block in eustachian tube)—**Helichrysum** (rub on inside and out of ears), juniper.

EATING DISORDERS:

    ANOREXIA—<u>Citrus Fresh</u>, coriander, grapefruit.
    BULIMIA—<u>Citrus Fresh</u>, grapefruit.
    OVEREATING—Ginger, lemon, peppermint, spearmint.

ECZEMA: Bergamot, eucalyptus, geranium, ᶠGerman chamomile, ᶠhelichrysum, ᶠjuniper, lavender, *Melaleuca ericifolia*, melissa, ᶠpatchouly, ᶠrosewood, sage.
    SUPPLEMENTS—Sulfurzyme.
    ***COMMENTS—*Eczema may indicate a sulfur deficiency.*
    DRY—Bergamot, geranium, ᶠGerman chamomile, hyssop, rosemary.
    WET—ᶠGerman chamomile, hyssop, juniper, lavender, myrrh.

EDEMA: See HORMONAL IMBALANCE. ᶠCypress (alleviates fluids), fennel (breaks up fluids), juniper, geranium, ᶠgrapefruit, ledum, ᶠlemongrass, rosemary, **tangerine** (alleviates fluids). *Drink water every 3 hours.*
    BLEND—1 fennel, 2 cypress, 5 tangerine. Apply from the top of the foot to the knee.

ANKLES—5 cypress, 3 juniper, and 10 tangerine or use equal parts of cypress and tangerine. Apply from ankles to knees and on Vita Flex bladder points on feet.
DIURETIC—ᶠCedarwood, cypress, EndoFlex, fennel, grapefruit, juniper, ᶠlavender, lemon, ᶠlemongrass, onycha (benzoin), orange, oregano, ᶠrosemary, ᶠsage.
***COMMENTS—*For water retention in the legs, Dr. Friedmann rubs tangerine, cypress, and juniper on inside of ankle(s) and leg(s) and on the kidney and heart Vita Flex points. He also has his patients inhale the oils as they are rubbed on.*

ELBOW: See TENNIS ELBOW.

ELECTRICAL PROBLEMS IN THE BODY: See BALANCE for methods of balancing the electrical energies of the body. Frankincense, Harmony, Valor.

ELECTROLYTES:
BALANCING—Citrus Fresh (increases absorption of Vitamin C).
*SUPPLEMENTS—*Super C, Mineral Essence.
*TINCTURES—*Royal Essence.

EMERGENCY OILS: The following oils are recommended by Dr. Daniel Pénoël as ones that everyone should have with them for any emergency:
Melaleuca (Alternifolia)—Colds, coughs, cuts, sore throat, sunburn, wounds.
Ravensara—Powerful antiviral, antiseptic. Respiratory problems, viral infections, wounds.
Peppermint—Analgesic (topical pain reliever) for bumps and bruises. Also for fever, headache, indigestion, motion sickness, nausea, nerve problems, spastic colon, vomiting.
Basil—Earache, fainting, headaches, spasms (can substitute fennel), poisonous insect or snake bites, malaria.
Lavender—Burns (mix with melaleuca), leg cramps, herpes, heart irregularities, hives, insect bites and bee stings, sprains, sunstroke. *If in doubt, use lavender!*
Geranium—Bleeding (increases to eliminate toxins, then stops; can substitute cistus), diarrhea, liver, regenerates tissue and nerves, shingles.
Helichrysum—Bruises, bleeding (stops on contact), hearing, pain, reduce scarring, regenerate tissue.
***COMMENTS:** Dr. Pénoël also recommends including Melaleuca ericifolia because it is more suited to children then Melaleuca alternifolia, and also elemi because it has similar properties to frankincense and myrrh but is less expensive.*

EMOTIONS: *See EMOTIONAL RELEASE in the Science and Application section at the beginning of the <u>Reference Guide for Essential Oils</u>. Refer to the Auricular Emotional Therapy chart in the Basic Information section of this book for points on the ears where the oils can be applied.* <u>Acceptance</u>, <u>Aroma Siez</u>, <u>Awaken</u> (supports spiritual emotions), <u>Citrus Fresh</u> and spruce (on the chest and breathe in <u>Sacred Mountain</u>), cypress (aromatic, healing), <u>Envision</u> (support and balance), <u>Gathering</u> (to help with feelings and thoughts), geranium (women), German chamomile (stability), goldenrod (relaxing and calming), <u>Gratitude</u>, <u>Humility</u> and <u>Forgiveness</u> (to help with forgiveness), Idaho balsam fir (balancing), lavender (men), melissa (supports mind and body), <u>Live with Passion</u> (balancing, uplifting, strengthening, and stabilizing), ravensara (lifts emotions), <u>Release</u> (soothing), rose (brings balance and harmony to the body), <u>Surrender</u> (calming and balancing), <u>3 Wise Men</u>, <u>Trauma Life</u>, valerian (helps replace emotions), <u>White Angelica</u> (balances and protects), White lotus.

BLEND—Layer the oils listed below. Wait 10 minutes between each oil to allow the emotions to be released more gently. The individual releasing the emotions should shut their eyes and should have no sounds, music, or candles in the room to distract them. They need to shut down their senses to get into their subconscious deep seated emotions. Breathe synergistically with their breathing.

> *For **EMOTIONS**, see other topics such as: ABUSE, AGITATION, ANGER, APATHY, ARGUMENTATIVE, BOREDOM, CONFUSION, DAYDREAMING, DESPAIR, DESPONDENCY, DISAPPOINTMENT, DISCOURAGEMENT, FEAR, FORGETFULNESS, FRUSTRATION, GRIEF/SORROW, GUILT, IRRITABILITY, JEALOUSLY, MOOD SWINGS, OBSESSIVENESS, PANIC, POOR CONCENTRATION, RESENTMENT, RESTLESSNESS, and SHOCK.*
>
> *For more information on using essential oils to help release stored emotions, read <u>Releasing Emotional Patterns using Essential Oils</u> by Carolyn Mein.*
>
> *For some exciting information about how emotions and feelings affect one's physical health, you may want to read Karol K. Truman's books, <u>Feelings Buried Alive Never Die . . .</u> and <u>Healing Feeling from Your Heart</u>.*

1. Rub <u>Valor</u> on feet.
   If there are 2 helpers, have one person hold the individual's feet (your right hand to their right foot, left to left; cross arms if necessary) during the entire procedure. Be sure not to break the energy.
2. Rub <u>Peace & Calming</u> on navel, feet, and on the forehead (from left to right).
3. Put <u>Harmony</u> on each chakra in clockwise direction, on wrists, shoulders and inside ankles.
4. Put <u>3 Wise Men</u> on crown.

BATH AND SHOWER GELS—Evening Peace or Sensation Bath & Shower Gel, Sacred Mountain, Lavender Rosewood, or Peppermint Cedarwood Moisturizing Soaps.

MASSAGE OILS—Relaxation or Sensation Massage Oil.

PERSONAL CARE—Prenolone/Prenolone+, Sensation Hand & Body Lotion.

SUPPLEMENTS—ProMist.

*****APPLICATION**—*The oils listed here under Emotions can either be diffused, worn as perfume/cologne, applied behind ears and across forehead, applied directly on the ears as specified, or applied to locations as listed in the Emotional Release part of the Science and Application section of the <u>Reference Guide for Essential Oils</u>.*

ACCEPTANCE (Self-Acceptance)—<u>Acceptance</u>, <u>Forgiveness</u>, and <u>Joy</u>. Layer oils on the specific ear point (*refer to the Auricular Emotional Therapy chart in the Basic Information section of this book for location of the HEART point to use for Acceptance*).

ANGER and HATE—<u>Joy</u> (apply to pituitary Vita Flex points on feet and hands as well), <u>Release</u>, and <u>Valor</u>. Layer oils on the specific ear point (*refer to the Auricular Emotional Therapy chart in the Basic Information section of this book for location of the point to use for Anger & Hate*). Other oils that my be useful include <u>Acceptance</u>, <u>Forgiveness</u>, helichrysum (with deep-seated anger for strength to forgive), and <u>Humility</u>.

BALANCE—<u>Forgiveness</u>, frankincense, geranium, <u>Grounding</u>, <u>Harmony</u>, <u>Hope</u>, <u>Inner Child</u>, <u>Joy</u>, juniper, lavender, orange, <u>Present Time</u>, <u>Release</u>, Roman chamomile, sandalwood, <u>SARA</u>, <u>3 Wise Men</u>, <u>Trauma Life</u>, <u>Valor</u>, vetiver, <u>White Angelica</u>.

PERSONAL CARE—Prenolone/Prenolone+.

SUPPLEMENTS—ProMist.

BLOCKS—Cypress, frankincense, <u>Harmony</u>, helichrysum, <u>Release</u> (over liver), sandalwood, spearmint, spikenard, spruce, <u>3 Wise Men</u>, <u>Trauma Life</u>, and <u>Valor</u> help to release emotional blocks. <u>Acceptance</u> can help one accept the change.

BURDENED (Bearing Burdens of the World)—<u>Release</u> and <u>Valor</u>. Layer oils on the specific ear point (*refer to the Auricular Emotional Therapy chart in the Basic Information section of this book for the location of the point to use for Bearing Burdens of the World*). <u>Acceptance</u> may also be good to use.

CHILDHOOD ISSUES—<u>SARA</u>. Apply to the HEART point on the ears.

FEAR (relating to Childhood Issues)—<u>Gentle Baby</u>, <u>Inner Child</u>, <u>SARA</u>. Apply to the FEAR point on the ears.

FATHER or MOTHER—<u>Gentle Baby</u> and/or <u>Inner Child</u>. Apply to the FATHER or MOTHER point on the ears (*refer to the Auricular Emotional Therapy chart in the Basic Information section of this book for the location of the HEART, FEAR, FATHER, or MOTHER points to use for Childhood Issues*).

CLEARING—<u>Forgiveness</u>, <u>Grounding</u>, <u>Harmony</u> (use <u>Hope</u> when emotional clearing), <u>Inner Child</u>, <u>Joy</u>, juniper, <u>Present Time</u>, <u>Release</u> (massage a couple drops on both ears for a general clearing), <u>SARA</u>, <u>3 Wise Men</u>, <u>Valor</u>, <u>White Angelica</u>. *For some simple instructions on how to do emotional clearing, refer to the page on Emotional*

> *The emotions of the mind are the most elusive part of the human body. People are extremely handicapped emotionally and are continually looking for ways to clear these negative emotions. Many of the emotional blends referred to in this book were created from the research of the ancient Egyptian rituals of clearing emotions. They were created with the intent of helping people overcome the trauma of emotional and physical abuse enabling them to progress and achieve their goals and dreams. The Egyptians took three days and three nights to clear emotions. In order to create a very peaceful setting, they would put the person in a room with 10 to 12 inch thick walls of solid cement and close the door so there would be no sight or sound.*

Release in the Science and Application section of the <u>Reference Guide for Essential Oils</u>. Another good reference for information on clearing negative emotions is the book, "Releasing Emotional Patterns" by Carolyn L. Mein, D.C.

COLDNESS (Emotional)—Myrrh, ylang ylang.

CONFIDENCE—<u>Envision</u>, jasmine (euphoria), Live with <u>Passion</u>.

DEFEATED—<u>Acceptance</u>, cypress, fir, <u>Forgiveness</u>, <u>Inspiration</u>, <u>Joy</u>, juniper, spruce, <u>3 Wise Men</u>, <u>Valor</u>.

DEPRESSION—Most of the single oils and blends help with depression as they tend to lift by raising one's frequency. Some of the best include <u>Christmas Spirit</u>, <u>Citrus Fresh</u>, <u>Gentle Baby</u>, <u>Hope</u>, <u>Joy</u>, <u>Peace & Calming</u>, <u>Valor</u>, and <u>White Angelica</u>. Use whichever blend(s) work best for you. Layer oils on the specific ear point (*refer to the Auricular Emotional Therapy chart in the Basic Information section of this book for the location of the point to use for Depression*). Other oils that may be good to use include <u>Humility</u>, <u>Inner Child</u>, lavender, and <u>SARA</u>.
  SUPPLEMENTS—Essential Omegas.

EMOTIONAL TRAUMA—Sandalwood, <u>Trauma Life</u>.

EXPRESSION (Self-Expression)—<u>Motivation</u> and <u>Valor</u> (for courage to speak out). <u>Joy</u> may be added to encourage enjoying life to its fullest. Apply to the SELF-EXPRESSION point on the ears. Take deep breaths to help express oneself.
  EXCESSIVE—<u>Surrender</u>. Apply to the SELF-EXPRESSION point on the ears.
  FOCUSED—<u>Release</u>, then <u>Acceptance</u> or <u>Gathering</u>. Layer oils on the SELF-EXPRESSION point on the ears.
  LOST IDENTITY—<u>Inner Child</u>. Apply to the SELF-EXPRESSION point on the ears (*refer to the Auricular Emotional Therapy chart in the Basic Information section of this book for the location of the SELF-EXPRESSION point*).

EYES—See EYES for oils that help with eyesight.

    VISION OF GOALS—<u>Believe</u>, <u>Dream Catcher</u>, <u>Acceptance</u>, <u>3 Wise Men</u>. Layer on the EYES & VISION point on the ears (*refer to the Auricular Emotional Therapy chart in the Basic Information section of this book for the location of the EYES & VISION point*). <u>Envision</u> and <u>Into the Future</u> may also help.

FATHER—Lavender. Apply to the FATHER point on the ears. Another oil that may be helpful to layer on top of lavender is helichrysum, especially when deep-seated anger is present.

    CHILDHOOD ISSUES—<u>Gentle Baby</u> or <u>Inner Child</u>. Apply to the FATHER point on the ears.

    MALE ABUSE—Helichrysum and lavender. Layer oils on the FATHER point on the ears.

    SEXUAL ABUSE—Lavender, <u>Release</u>, and ylang ylang. Layer oils on the FATHER point on the ears. <u>SARA</u> may also be helpful (*refer to the Auricular Emotional Therapy chart in the Basic Information section of this book for the location of the FATHER point to use for Father related issues*).

FEAR—<u>Valor</u>, <u>Release</u>, and <u>Joy</u>. Layer on the FEAR point on the ears. <u>Acceptance</u> and <u>Harmony</u> may also be helpful.

    CHILDHOOD ISSUES—<u>Gentle Baby</u>, <u>Inner Child</u>, or <u>SARA</u>. Apply to the FEAR point on the ears.

    FUTURE—<u>Into the Future</u>. Apply to the FEAR point on the ears (*refer to the Auricular Emotional Therapy chart in the Basic Information section of this book for the location of the FEAR point*).

FEMALE ISSUES—See MOTHER.

GRIEF—Bergamot. Apply to the HEART point on the ears (*refer to the Auricular Emotional Therapy chart in the Science and Application section for the location of the HEART point to use for Grief*). Another oil that may be helpful is tangerine (when diffused, increases optimism and releases emotional stress).

HEART (Broken or Heavy Heart)—Refer to both GRIEF and LOSS as well. <u>Acceptance</u>, <u>Forgiveness</u>, and <u>Joy</u>. Layer oils on the HEART point on the ears (*refer to the Auricular Emotional Therapy chart in the Science and Application section for the location of the point to use for Heart*). <u>Release</u> and <u>Valor</u> may also be good to use.

LOSS (Eases the Feeling)—<u>Joy</u>, <u>Sensation</u>, tangerine (stability).

MALE ISSUES—See FATHER.

MIND (Open)—<u>3 Wise Men</u>. Apply to the OPEN THE MIND point on the ears as well as the crown of the head and the navel (*refer to the Auricular Emotional Therapy chart in the Basic Information section of this book for the location of the OPEN THE MIND point*). <u>Acceptance</u>, <u>Believe</u>, <u>Clarity</u>, frankincense, <u>Gathering</u>, <u>Magnify Your Purpose</u>, <u>Motivation</u>, <u>Release</u>, and sandalwood may also be helpful.

MOTHER—Geranium. Apply to the MOTHER point on the ears. Inner Child and SARA
    may also be helpful.
    ABANDONMENT—Geranium, Acceptance, and Forgiveness. Layer oils on the
        MOTHER point on the ears.
    SEXUAL ABUSE—Geranium and ylang ylang. Layer oils on the MOTHER point on
        the ears (*refer to the Auricular Emotional Therapy chart in the Basic
        Information section of this book for the location of the MOTHER point to use
        for Mother related issues*).
OVERWHELMED—Acceptance and Hope. Layer on the OVERWHELMED point on
    the ears (*refer to the Auricular Emotional Therapy chart in the Science and
    Application section for the location of the OVERWHELMED point*). Grounding
    and Valor may also be helpful.
PITY (Self-Pity)—Acceptance. Apply to the SELF PITY point on the ears. Forgiveness
    and Joy may also be helpful.
    COURAGE (to move beyond feeling)—Release then Valor. Layer on the SELF-PITY
        point on the ears.
    PAINFUL—Can feel like heaviness in the chest. PanAway. Apply to the SELF-PITY
        point on the ears (*refer to the Auricular Emotional Therapy chart in the Basic
        Information section of this book for the location of the SELF-PITY point*).
PROTECTION FROM NEGATIVE EMOTIONS—Magnify Your Purpose (empowering
    and uplifting), grapefruit, 3 Wise Men (release), White Angelica. Apply oils to
    the forehead and over the heart.
REJECTION—Forgiveness and Acceptance. Layer on the REJECTION point on the ears.
    Grounding and Valor may also be helpful.
    FROM FATHER—Use lavender first then Forgiveness and Acceptance. Layer on the
        REJECTION point on the ears.
    FROM MOTHER—Use geranium first then Forgiveness and Acceptance. Layer on
        the REJECTION point on the ears (*refer to the Auricular Emotional Therapy
        chart in the Science and Application section for the location of the
        REJECTION point*).
RELEASE—ᴿRoman chamomile.
STRESS—Believe, Clary sage, Evergreen Essence, Live with Passion, Surrender.
SUICIDAL—Gathering, Hope, Joy, Live with Passion, Release, Trauma Life.
SYMPATHY & GUILT—Joy and Inspiration. Layer on the SYMPATHY & GUILT
    point on the ears (*refer to the Auricular Emotional Therapy chart in the Basic
    Information section of this book for the location of the SYMPATHY & GUILT
    point*). Release, PanAway, and/or Acceptance may also be helpful.
UPLIFTING—Valor (on feet), birch, Dream Catcher, En-R-Gee, Gratitude, lemon,
    orange, wintergreen.
VISION—See EYES.

EMPHYSEMA: Eucalyptus, Exodus II, Raven (Hot compress on chest). May use Raven
   rectally, RC on chest and back. Reverse each night. Thieves on feet, ImmuPower
   on spine.
   SUPPLEMENTS—Exodus.
   ***COMMENTS—Dr. Terry Friedmann used Exodus on a 68-year-old male who had
   emphysema. He was on oxygen 24 hours a day. He gave him four per day for
   one week. When the man came back in, Dr. Friedmann used an oxymeter to
   test his concentration of blood oxygen. His concentration of blood oxygen,
   without his oxygen tank, was higher after taking Exodus than it was when he
   just had his oxygen tank.*

EMPOWERMENT: Magnify Your Purpose, Sacred Mountain.

ENDOCRINE SYSTEM: See
   ADRENAL CORTEX,
   THYROID,
   PITUITARY, LUPUS,
   etc. Black pepper,
   cinnamon bark, dill,
   EndoFlex, Frosemary.
   PERSONAL CARE—
   EndoBalance,
   Prenolone/ Prenolone+.
   SUPPLEMENTS—
   Thyromin and

> *The adrenal glands, pituitary gland, thyroid gland,
> parathyroid glands, thymus gland, pineal gland,
> pancreas, ovaries, and testes are all a part of the
> endocrine system. The endocrine glands secrete
> hormones, transmitted via the bloodstream, which are
> responsible for regulating growth, metabolism, enzyme
> activity, and reproduction. Essential oils may either act
> as hormones or stimulate the endocrine glands to
> produce hormones. This production of hormones has a
> regulating effect on the body.*

   FemiGen (women) or ProGen (men), Power Meal (pre-digested protein). ProMist
   and ThermaMist may also help.
   TINCTURES—Femalin.

ENDOMETRIOSIS: See
   HORMONAL
   IMBALANCE. Clary
   sage, cypress,
   eucalyptus, geranium,
   Melrose (hot compress
   on abdomen), nutmeg, Thieves (on feet).

> ***Endometriosis*** *is the growth of endometrial tissue in
> abnormal locations as on ovaries or peritoneal
> (abdominal) cavity.*

   SUPPLEMENTS—Cleansing Trio (ComforTone, Megazyme, and ICP), Super C,
   FemiGen.
   RECIPE #1—Combine bergamot, lavender, and Clary sage and use with a hot
   compress over the abdomen or add 2 drops of each to 1 Tbsp. V-6 Mixing Oil and
   insert into the vagina. Use a tampon to retain overnight. This may help rebuild
   the normal tissue.

ENDURANCE:
  PHYSICAL—
     SUPPLEMENTS—Be-Fit, CardiaCare (with *Rhododendron caucasicum* which has been shown clinically to enhance physical endurance by increasing blood supply to the muscles and brain), Power Meal, WheyFit.

ENERGY: <u>Abundance</u>, <u>Awaken</u>, basil (when squandering energy), Black pepper, <u>Clarity</u>,
    cypress, <u>En-R-Gee</u>, <u>Envision</u> (balances), eucalyptus (builds), ᶠfir, <u>Hope</u>, <u>Joy</u>,
    juniper, lemon, lemongrass, <u>Motivation</u>, myrtle (supports adrenal glands to
    increase energy), nutmeg (increases), orange (aromatic), peppermint, rosemary,
    thyme (aromatic; gives energy in times of physical weakness and stress), <u>Valor</u>
    (balances), <u>White Angelica</u>.

     BATH AND SHOWER GELS—Morning Start Bath & Shower Gel or Lemon Sandalwood Cleansing Soap gives you a fresh start with a surge of energy.
     ESSENTIAL WATERS (HYDROSOLS)—Basil, Mountain Essence, Peppermint, Thyme. Spray into air or directly on face (don't spray directly in eyes or ears) or diffuse using the Essential Mist Diffuser.
     SUPPLEMENTS—VitaGreen (gives energy), Radex (increases energy), Master Formula His/Hers (Multi-Vitamin), Mineral Essence, Thyromin, Super B, Royal Essence (under tongue for quick energy boost).
  ELECTRICAL ENERGY (frequency)—<u>Forgiveness</u> (high frequency), rose.
  INCREASE—<u>Brain Power</u>, <u>Clarity</u>, <u>En-R-Gee</u>, eucalyptus, grapefruit, peppermint, rosemary.
     DIFFUSION—See POSITIVE IONS for oils that produce positive ions when diffused to help increase energy.
     TINCTURES—Royal Essence.
     SUPPLEMENTS—Ultra Young.
  INTEGRATES ENERGY FOR EQUAL DISTRIBUTION—Patchouly.
  MAGNETIC—<u>Abundance</u>, <u>Joy</u> (enhances and attracts magnetic energy of prosperity and joy around the body).
  NEGATIVE—<u>White Angelica</u> (frequency protects against bombardment of), ginger, juniper (clears negative energy).
  PHYSICAL—Bergamot, cinnamon bark (aromatic), lemon (aromatic), patchouly (aromatic).
  SEXUAL ENERGY—Ylang ylang (aromatic; influences).
     TINCTURES—Royal Essence (increases energy).

ENERGY CENTERS: See CHAKRAS.

ENLIGHTENING: Helichrysum.

ENTERITIS: Cajeput.

ENZYMES: Fresh carrot juice has one of the largest concentrations of enzymes. Drink 8 oz. per day. Add apple and lemon to help with detoxification.

SUPPLEMENTS—Enzyme products: Allerzyme (aids the digestion of sugars, starches, fats, and proteins), Carbozyme (aids the digestion of carbohydrates), Detoxzyme (helps maintain and support a healthy intestinal environment), Fiberzyme (aids the digestion of fiber and enhances the absorption of nutrients), Polyzyme (aids the digestion of protein and helps reduce swelling and discomfort), and Lipozyme (aids the digestion of fats).

EPILEPSY: See SEIZURE. Brain Power, Clary sage. Apply to back of neck and brain Vita Flex points on bottom of feet.

SUPPLEMENTS— Cleansing Trio (ComforTone, Megazyme, ICP).

> **OILS TO AVOID IF EPILEPTIC**
>
> *There are several oils that should not be used if prone to epilepsy. Please see the APPENDIX for safety data on the oils and products mentioned in this book. For further contraindication information, please consult the following books:*
>
> *Essential Oil Safety—A Guide for Health Care Professionals by Robert Tisserand and Tony Balacs and Aromatherapy for Health Professionals by Shirley and Len Price.*

EPSTEIN BARR: See CHRONIC FATIGUE, HYPOGLYCEMIA. Eucalyptus, ImmuPower, Thieves. Do RAINDROP TECHNIQUE on spine with the addition of ImmuPower.

SUPPLEMENTS—AlkaLime, ComforTone, Exodus, ICP, ImmuGel, ImmuneTune, ImmuPro, JuvaTone, Megazyme, Mineral Essence, Radex, Super C, Thyromin, VitaGreen.

EQUILIBRIUM: Surrender (emotional), ylang ylang.

NERVE—Petitgrain.

ESSENTIAL OILS: Essential oils function as a catalyst to deliver nutrients to starving cells. SENSITIVE TO SKIN (caustic, high in phenols, may need to dilute)—Cinnamon bark, clove, fennel, grapefruit, lemon, nutmeg, orange, oregano, peppermint. Test the oil first in a small, sensitive area. If irritation occurs, dilute with 1 drop of above oil to 20 drops lavender or mix with V-6 Mixing Oil.

ESTROGEN: Clary sage and Mister help the body produce estrogen. Anise (increases).

***COMMENTS—*Some sugar sweeteners block estrogen. Honey goes into blood stream quickly, which affects the pancreas and the production of estrogen.*

PERSONAL CARE—Prenolone/Prenolone+ (pregnenolone is the master hormone; used to balance estrogen and progesterone, whichever is needed).

SUPPLEMENTS—2 FemiGen three times a day, ten days before period. Start again two days after cycle. May take up to 6 tablets three times a day. CortiStop (Women's) can also help increase estrogen levels by lowering cortisol levels.

TINCTURE—1 dropper of Estro three times a day in water.

EUPHORIA: Clary sage (aromatic), jasmine.

EXHAUSTION: First, work with one or more of the following nervous system oils to calm and relax: Bergamot, Clary sage, coriander, cumin, elemi, frankincense, lavender, pine. Secondly, use basil, ginger, grapefruit, lavender, lemon, Roman chamomile, rosemary, or sandalwood.

TINCTURE—Royal Essence. Take 1-2 droppers in 4 oz. of water.

EXPECTORANT: Black pepper, elemi, eucalyptus, frankincense, helichrysum, ᶠmarjoram, mugwort, pine, ᶠravensara. Apply oils to throat, lungs, and diffuse.

EXPRESSION (Self Expression): Helichrysum, Into the Future, Joy (when unable to express physically), Motivation, Raven, RC, Valor.

EYES: Thieves on feet (especially 2 big toes), M-Grain on thumb prints, layer Mister, Dragon Time and EndoFlex on Vita Flex points, ankles, and pelvis. Carrot is good around eye area, cypress (also helps circulation), fennel, frankincense, German chamomile, lavender, lemon, lemongrass (improves eyesight).

> **NEVER PUT OILS DIRECTLY IN THE EYES!**
>
> *Be careful when applying oils near the eyes. Be sure to have some V-6 Mixing Oil handy for additional dilution if irritation occurs. Never use water to wash off an oil that irritates.*

BASE OILS (good blends of)—Almond or hazelnut.

SUPPLEMENTS—Essential Manna, Power Meal, Sulfurzyme, Wolfberry Bars.

TINCTURES—Add AD&E drops for all eye problems.

***COMMENTS—Refer to the chapter entitled "How to Use - The Personal Usage Reference" in the Essential Oils Desk Reference under "Eye Disorders" for additional recipe, oil, and supplement recommendations.

EYE DROP RECIPE—Combine 5 parts distilled water, 2 parts honey, and 1 part apple cider vinegar (do not use white vinegar). Mix together and store in a bottle. Does not need to be refrigerated. This special eye drop formula is found in Stanley Burroughs' book, *Healing for the Age of Enlightenment* and has proven over the years to be superior to most commercial eye drops. These drops have been successful for helping to clear glaucoma, cataracts, spots, film, and growths of various kinds. Apply drops one at a time to each eye several times a day until condition has cleared.

CATARACTS—
>   *BLEND #1*—8 lemongrass, 6 cypress, and 3 eucalyptus. Apply around the eye area two times a day. Don't get in the eyes.

DRY-ITCHY—Melaleuca (in humidifier).

EYE LID DROP (or DROOPING EYELIDS)—
>   *BLEND #2*—<u>Aroma Life</u>, 1 helichrysum, 5 lavender.
>   *BLEND #3*—Helichrysum and peppermint (don't get in the eyes).
>   *MASSAGE OILS*—Cel-Lite-Magic (around eyes).
>   *SUPPLEMENTS*—3 VitaGreen four times a day. After massaging Vita Flex points, eat 2 whole oranges a day with the white still on the orange. It is very important to eat all the white you can plus Super C, ComforTone, and ICP (fiber beverage) after meals.
>   *VITA FLEX POINTS*—Fingers, toes, and around the eyes.

IMPROVE VISION—<u>Dragon Time</u>, <u>EndoFlex</u>, frankincense, juniper, lemongrass, <u>Mister</u>, <u>M-Grain</u>, <u>Thieves</u>. Apply oils to feet, Vita Flex eye points, thumbs, ankles, pelvis, eye area (not in eyes), eyebrows. According to Dr. Mercola, just about any oil can be used if it is consistently rubbed around each eye for several minutes twice a day. This must be continued for at least 3 weeks before any improvement can be seen. He recommends using **frankincense and lavender**.
>   *BLEND #4*—10 lemongrass, 5 cypress, 3 *Eucalyptus radiata*, in 1 oz. V-6 Mixing Oil. Apply around eyes morning and night to improve eyesight. Can also be applied to Vita Flex eye points on fingers and toes, and also on the ears *(refer to the Auricular Emotional Therapy chart in the Basic Information section of this book for the Eyes and Vision point on the ears)*.
>   *BLEND #5*—5 lemongrass, 3 cypress, 2 eucalyptus, in 1 oz. of V-6 Mixing Oil. Apply as a blend or layer the oils on the eye area (not in eyes).
>   *TINCTURES*—AD&E to take the pressure off the liver and intestines and to improve the vision.
>   ****COMMENTS*—One individual, who was not able to see color and had no peripheral vision, rubbed frankincense on his eyelids and just above his eyebrows. Soon thereafter he was able to see color and his peripheral vision returned.*

IRIS, INFLAMMATION OF—Eucalyptus.

RETINA (Bleeding)—
>   *BLEND #6*—5 tangerine, 5 orange, and 5 grapefruit. Mix and apply 2 drops on fingers and toes. Massage Vita Flex points two times a day or more. Diffuse and let vapor mist around eye. Rub Cel-Lite Magic around the eyes too. Then, eat two whole oranges a day with the white still on the orange. Eat all of the white you can.

SUPPLEMENTS—Super C.

RETINA (Strengthen)—Cypress, lavender, lemongrass, helichrysum, juniper, peppermint, sandalwood. Apply oil(s) around eye area.

    BLEND #7—5 juniper, 3 lemongrass, 3 cypress. Rub on brain stem twice a day.

SPIRITUAL EYES (3rd eye, brow chakra)—<u>Acceptance</u>, <u>Awaken</u>, <u>Dream Catcher</u>. Rub oil on ear lobe to increase both physical and spiritual vision.

SWOLLEN EYES—Cypress and helichrysum. Lavender (antiseptic) is also safe around eyes. If swollen eyes are due to allergies, try putting peppermint on the back of the neck.

F

FACIAL OILS: Refer to the Personal Care section of the <u>Reference Guide for Essential Oils</u> for many other beneficial skin care products.

BROKEN CAPILLARIES—Cypress, geranium, hyssop, Roman chamomile.

DEHYDRATED—Geranium, lavender.

DISTURBED—Clary sage, geranium, hyssop, juniper, lavender, lemon, patchouly, Roman chamomile, sandalwood.

DRY—Geranium, German chamomile, hyssop, lemon, patchouly, rosemary, sandalwood.

ENERGIZING—Bergamot, lemon.

HYDRATED—Cypress, fennel, geranium, hyssop, lavender, lemon, patchouly, sandalwood.

NORMAL—Geranium, lavender, lemon, Roman chamomile, sandalwood.

OILY—Cypress, frankincense, geranium, jasmine, juniper, lavender, lemon, marjoram, orange, patchouly, Roman chamomile, rosemary.

REVITALIZING—Cypress, fennel, lemon.

SENSITIVE—Geranium, German chamomile, lavender.

FAINTING: See SHOCK. Nutmeg. Hold one of the following under the nose: Basil, Black pepper, <u>Brain Power</u>, <u>Clarity</u>, lavender, neroli, peppermint, rosemary, spearmint, <u>Trauma Life</u>.

FAITH: <u>Hope</u> (increases).

FASTING: Fasting is the avoidance of solid foods altogether, while liquid consumption ranges between nothing (complete avoidance of all liquids as well) to fresh juices with just water being somewhere in the middle. **Complete avoidance fasting (no food or liquid) should only be done when feeling good**, while fasting on fresh juices can be very healing when sick. The Master Cleanser Lemonade fast (see CLEANSING) is one of the most beneficial juice fasts. While it takes 30 days on this cleanse to change the chemistry in the body (such as eliminating the need or desire for animal proteins), very effective health results can be achieved after only 10 days. To enhance the effectiveness of the change in body chemistry, the 30-day lemon juice fast can be followed by a carrot juice fast for another 30 days. Body

Balance and VitaGreen may be taken two times a day for two weeks but should then be stopped so changes can be made at the cellular level; protein prevents this change. When a mother fasts, the breast fed baby gets the benefits as well (the mammary glands filter the toxins so they are not harmful to the baby).

FAT: See CELLULITE, DIET and WEIGHT.

> *Ultra Young may help stimulate the pituitary for increased production of the human growth hormone. This hormone is one of the most powerful side-effect-free agents for rejuvenating the body, restoring lean body mass, and reducing fat.*

BATH (ATTACK FAT)— Add 6 drops of blend to the bath water and soak in tub.

BLEND—8 grapefruit, 5 cypress, 4 lavender, 4 basil, and 3 juniper.

SUPPLEMENT—Allerzyme (aids the digestion of sugars, starches, fats, and proteins), Lipozyme (aids the digestion of fats), ThermaMist (blocks fat synthesis and regulates appetite with HCA, spray before meals or when cravings occur), Power Meal (eat for breakfast as a meal replacement), Ultra Young (improves fat-to-lean ratios by stimulating production of the human growth hormone).

***COMMENTS—Eat more grapefruit to dissolve fat faster.

FATHER (Problems with): Acceptance, lavender, Valor. Apply to ears (*refer to the Auricular Emotional Therapy chart in the Basic Information section of this book*).

FATIGUE: Clove, En-R-Gee, pine, ᶠravensara (muscle), ᶠrosemary (nervous), ᶠthyme (general).

MENTAL—Basil, Clarity, lemongrass, Peace & Calming. Basil and lemongrass together are a good combination. Apply on temples, back of neck, feet and diffuse.

OVERCOMING—Thyme or En-R-Gee on spine, wait a few minutes, then Awaken all over the back and spine; OR En-R-Gee on feet and Awaken on temples and cheeks.

PHYSICAL—See ENERGY. Clarity, Peace & Calming. Apply on liver, feet, diffuse, and as a body massage.

SUPPLEMENTS—AlkaLime (acid-neutralizing mineral formulation), ImmuGel, Power Meal, Sulfurzyme, Thyromin, VitaGreen.

TINCTURE—Royal Essence. Take 1-2 droppers with 4 oz. of water.

FATTY DEPOSITS: See CELLULITE and WEIGHT.

DISSOLVE—Basil, cypress, grapefruit, juniper, lavender.

SUPPLEMENTS—Allerzyme (aids the digestion of sugars, starches, fats, and
proteins), Body Balancing Trio (Body Balance, Master Formula His/Hers,
VitaGreen), Lipozyme (aids the digestion of fats), Power Meal.

FEAR: Bergamot, Clary sage, cypress, fir, geranium, Hope, juniper, marjoram, Motivation
(releases emotional and physical fears), myrrh, orange, Present Time, Roman
chamomile, rose, sandalwood, spruce, Valor, White Angelica, ylang ylang.
****COMMENTS—Fear causes the blood vessels to tighten, restricting the amount of
oxygen and nutrients that can reach the cells.*

F

FEET: Fennel, lavender, lemon, pine (excessive sweating), Roman chamomile.
CALLOUSES—
CLUB FOOT—Massage with one of the following—Ginger (see below), lavender, Roman
chamomile, rosemary (see below).
CORNS—See CORNS.
NOT TO BE USED ON BABIES EXCEPT FOR CLUB FOOT—Ginger, rosemary.
ODOR—Mix 1 Tbs. baking powder with 2 drops of sage and put in a plastic bag. Shake
and eliminate lumps with a rolling pin and put in shoes. Rub calamus of feet.

FEMALE PROBLEMS: See HORMONAL IMBALANCE, INFERTILITY,
MENOPAUSE, MENSTRUATION, OVARIES, PMS, PREGNANCY,
UTERUS, ETC. Anise, Mister (during time of month when you are out of sorts),
Clary sage, Sacred Mountain (female balance).
SUPPLEMENTS—Body Balancing Trio Hers (Body Balance, Master Formula Hers,
VitaGreen), FemiGen, Prenolone/Prenolone+.
ABNORMAL PAP SMEARS—
RECIPE #1—Add 10 drops ImmuPower and 5 drops frankincense to 1 Tbsp. V-6
Mixing Oil and insert into vagina. Use tampon to retain overnight. In the
morning, douche with 3 drops of Femalin in 6 oz. of distilled water. Take Master
Formula Hers to support nutrient levels and ImmuneTune and Radex to support
the body. May continue daily for as long as necessary.
BALANCE FEMALE HORMONES—Bergamot, ylang ylang.
BATH AND SHOWER GELS—Dragon Time Bath & Shower Gel for that time of
month which leaves women with lower back pain, stress, and sleeping difficulties.
Pour 1 tsp. to 1 oz. of the gel in water while filling your tub.
SUPPLEMENTS—Three times a day one week before cycle starts, take 2 droppers
full of F.H.S. (available through Creer Labs 801-465-5423) in water after
starting. One week after the cycle, take Master Formula Hers four times a day
and 6 VitaGreen a day. CortiStop (Women's) can also help reduce cortisol levels
and balance hormones.
HEMORRHAGING—See HEMORRHAGING.

MASSAGE OILS—Combine 10 helichrysum with 1 tsp. V-6 Mixing Oil and massage around ankles, lower back, and stomach.

INFECTION—ᶠBergamot (general), frankincense, and <u>Melrose</u> (may mix and insert in vagina at night; may alternate with the blend below).

BLEND #1— 8 juniper, 8 melaleuca, and 8 <u>Purification</u>. Put in water and douche OR 3 drops of each in 1 tsp. V-6 Mixing Oil and insert at night using a tampon to retain.

BLEND #2—8 juniper, 8 lavender, and 8 <u>Melrose</u>. Alternate with Blend #1 and follow same instructions.

INFERTILITY (FEMALE)—See FERTILITY. Clary sage, cypress, fennel, geranium, melissa, nutmeg, Roman chamomile, thyme. Before the cycle, rub 10 drops <u>Dragon Time</u> around ankles, lower back, and lower stomach. During the cycle, rub 4 drops basil in the same places as before.

PERSONAL CARE—Prenolone/Prenolone+.

SUPPLEMENTS—Essential Manna, FemiGen, Master Formula Hers, ProMist, VitaGreen.

OVARIES—See OVARIES.

PMS—See PMS.

MASSAGE OILS—Dragon Time.

PERSONAL CARE—Prenolone/Prenolone+.

SUPPLEMENTS—Body Balancing Trio Hers (Body Balance, Master Formula Hers, VitaGreen), Essential Omegas, FemiGen.

TINCTURES—Femalin (glandular functions and reproductive organs).

POSTPARTUM

DEPRESSION— Basil, Clary sage, <u>Gentle Baby</u>, <u>Harmony</u>, <u>Joy</u>, nutmeg (see the safety data in the APPENDIX of this book), <u>Peace & Calming</u>, <u>Valor</u>, <u>White Angelica</u>.

> ***Natural Progesterone or Pregnenolone may help prevent postpartum depression.*** *Just before a woman has a baby her body produces about 400 mg of progesterone each day to help hold the placenta in place. When the baby is born, the production of progesterone falls dramatically. The body's inability to produce high doses of progesterone can help induce postpartum depression.*

PERSONAL CARE— Prenolone/Prenolone+.

SUPPLEMENTS—Essential Omegas.

Some women have had wonderful results with the following recipe:

RECIPE #1—<u>Valor</u> first (2-5 drops on each foot and hold to balance energies), <u>Harmony</u> (use finger to dab small amount on each energy center (chakra)), <u>Joy</u> (apply a drop between and just above the breasts), and <u>White Angelica</u> (on the crown of the head and over the top of the shoulders).

REPRODUCTIVE SYSTEM— Femalin (may help protect from candida and
degeneration), FemiGen (may help build and balance the reproductive system and
maintain better hormonal balance for developmental years all the way through
menopause).

FERTILITY: Bergamot, Clary sage, <u>Dragon Time</u>, fennel, geranium, melissa, <u>Mister</u>, sage,
<u>Sensation</u>, yarrow. Apply on reproductive Vita Flex areas on feet, particularly
around front of ankle, in line with ankle bone, on each side of ankle under ankle
bone, and up along the Achilles tendon. Women: on lower back and on lower
abdomen near pubic bone. Can also dilute with V-6 Mixing Oil and use as
vaginal retention implant. Men: on lower abdomen near pubic bone, on area
between scrotum and rectum, and as a rectal implant (diluted with V-6 Mixing
Oil).

PERSONAL CARE—Prenolone/Prenolone+, Protec (as rectal or vaginal implant).
SUPPLEMENTS—AlkaLime, Essential Manna, ProMist, Ultra Young, VitaGreen.
FemiGen (women) and ProGen (men).

***COMMENTS—An accumulation of petrochemicals in the body can cause sterility in
both men and women. Do the MASTER CLEANSER (See CLEANSING) for 10
to 20 days consecutively. After coming off the cleanse, focus on alkaline-ash
foods. When the body is acidic, it can be hard to conceive.*

FEVER: Basil, bergamot, ᶠeucalyptus, fennel (breaks up), fir, ginger, ImmuPower (rub on
spine), lavender, ledum, ᶠlemon (reduces–1 or 2 drops in rice milk or water and
sip slowly), melaleuca, ᶠpeppermint (reduces–1 or 2 drops in rice milk or water
and sip slowly), rosemary cineol, spearmint (not on babies). Peppermint can also
be diffused in the room or applied to the bottom of feet.

PERSONAL CARE—Cinnamint Lip Balm.
SUPPLEMENTS—AlkaLime, ImmuGel, Mineral Essence, Radex, Super C.
TINCTURE—Royal Essence.

TO COOL THE SYSTEM—Bergamot, *Eucalyptus radiata*, peppermint (or Peppermint
Floral Water).
TO INDUCE SWEATING—Basil, cypress, fennel, lavender, melaleuca, peppermint,
Roman chamomile, rosemary.

FIBER: ICP is a fiber beverage, designed to bulk up in liquid and flush out the intestines.
SUPPLEMENTS—Cleansing Trio (ComforTone, Megazyme, and ICP).

FIBROCYSTS: See HORMONAL IMBALANCE.

FIBROIDS: See HORMONAL IMBALANCE. Cistus, <u>EndoFlex</u>, frankincense,
helichrysum, Idaho tansy, lavender, oregano, pine, <u>Valor</u>. Put 3 drops of either oil
in douche. Also apply to Vita Flex points of feet.

MASSAGE OILS—Cel-Lite Magic.
PERSONAL CARE—Protec.
SUPPLEMENTS—AlkaLime, Megazyme, Power Meal, Thyromin, Ultra Young, VitaGreen.

FIBROMYALGIA: See ACIDOSIS, HORMONAL IMBALANCE. May need to detoxify the liver. ImmuPower; massage with PanAway

> *Fibromyalgia is a condition of high acid and generalized pain all over the body; tiny movement brings on pain; extra low pain threshold. Since there are very few positive findings, it is difficult to diagnose. Some sources say that natural progesterone may be beneficial.*

adding birch/wintergreen & spruce for an additional cortisone response. It may be helpful to use some anti-inflammatory oils like birch, helichrysum, lavender, myrrh, patchouly, rosemary, rosewood, spruce, thyme, or wintergreen.
MASSAGE OILS—Ortho Ease or Ortho Sport (for full body), and do the Raindrop Technique.
SUPPLEMENTS— Allerzyme (aids the digestion of sugars, starches, fats, and proteins), AlkaLime (combat yeast and fungus overgrowth and preserve the body's proper pH balance), Body Balance (for vitamins and minerals), Coral Sea (highly bio-available calcium, contains 58 trace minerals), Essential Manna, ImmuneTune (four days), JuvaTone, Mineral Essence, Power Meal, Royaldophilus, Stevia Select, **Sulfurzyme**, Super C, Super Cal (no more than 1 per day, because of the poor ability to utilize minerals), VitaGreen (to get alkaline balance).
***COMMENTS—Dr. Bernard Jensen suggested that people with fibromyalgia should eliminate all refined sugars from their diet. Refer to the chapter entitled "How to Use - The Personal Usage Reference" in the Essential Oils Desk Reference under "Fibromyalgia" for an excellent supplement regimen.*

FIBROSITIS: See HORMONAL IMBALANCE.
BLEND—Combine 2 cinnamon bark, 10 eucalyptus, 10 ginger, 6 nutmeg, 10 peppermint, and 3 rosemary with 2 Tbs. V-6 Mixing Oil and massage chest and back once a day.

FINGER:
MASHED—Geranium (for the bruising), helichrysum (to stop the bleeding), lavender (to help for all things), lemongrass (for tissue repair), and PanAway (for the pain).

FLATULENCE (gas): Angelica, anise, bergamot, cardamom, coriander, cumin, eucalyptus, fennel, ᶠginger, juniper, ᶠlavender, myrrh, nutmeg, onycha (benzoin), peppermint,

Roman chamomile, rosemary, spearmint (not for babies), ᶠtarragon. Apply oil(s) to stomach, abdomen, and Vita Flex points of feet.

FLU: Clove, <u>ImmuPower</u>, <u>RC</u>, <u>Raven</u> (apply to thymus area, Vita Flex points on feet, chest, back, and on any place where the flu has settled), *Eucalyptus radiata*, <u>Exodus II</u>, fir (aches and pains), goldenrod, ginger, Idaho tansy (on bottom of feet), lavender, ledum, ᶠmelaleuca, *Melaleuca ericifolia*, ᶠmyrtle, onycha (benzoin), orange, oregano, ᶠpeppermint, pine, ᶠrosemary, <u>Thieves</u>, thyme (apply to thymus point on feet and where flu has settled), tsuga.

F

   ****COMMENTS—According to the <u>Essential Oils Desk Reference</u>, "[Idaho] tansy should be applied topically on stomach and bottom of feet." (EDR-June 2002; Ch. 28; Flu) It may be best to dilute Idaho tansy first in one teaspoon V-6 Mixing Oil or Massage Oil before topical application.*

   BATH—2 Tbs. Evening Peace Bath & Shower Gel with drops of the following oils: 1 birch/wintergreen, 20 eucalyptus, 5 frankincense, 3 helichrysum, 15 ravensara, and 6 spruce. Mix together and put mixture under the faucet while running HOT bath water. SOAK until cool. Also consider using Thieves Cleansing Soap to wash hands with, especially during cold and flu season.

   SUPPLEMENTS—Exodus, ImmuneTune, ImmuGel, Master Formula His/Hers, Megazyme, Mint Condition, ParaFree, Radex, Super C.

FLUIDS: See EDEMA or DIURETIC.

FOCUS: <u>Brain Power</u> (during strenuous mental activity), <u>Clarity</u>, <u>Gathering</u> (for greater focus), <u>Surrender</u> (balancing; clears the mind).
   SUPPLEMENTS—Sulfurzyme.

FOOD: See pH BALANCE. Use basil for soups and stuffing. Use cinnamon bark, clove, orange, tangerine, and thyme for flavorings.

> *The body secretes pepsin, protease and hydrochloric acid in the morning for the digestion of protein. If you eat fruit in the morning you have almost instant putrefaction (fermentation). Sub-acid fruits (like strawberries) are the only fruit that can be eaten with protein.*

   ****COMMENTS—According to the <u>Essential Oils Desk Reference</u>, "They are so concentrated that only 1-2 drops of an essential oil is equivalent to a full bottle (1-2 oz. size) of dried herbs. . . . For a recipe that serves six to ten people, add 1 to 2 drops of an oil and stir in after cooking and just before serving, so the oil does not evaporate." (EDR-June 2002; Ch. 4; Other Uses; Cooking) Refer to that same section in the <u>Essential Oils Desk Reference</u> for more ideas on cooking with essential oils.*

BREAKFAST—Proteins (meat, fish, eggs), mixed grains, sunflower seeds, nuts, Power Meal, and Body Balance. Fruit in the morning will cause candida overgrowth, hypoglycemia, and dysfunction of the thyroid gland. Take Megazyme or Polyzyme to help with the digestion, especially when animal protein has been eaten. Also, 8 oz. of carrot juice per day with apple and lemon helps detoxify the body and provides necessary enzymes.

LUNCH—Eat salads, complex carbohydrates like rice, beans, soup, steamed vegetables, bread (Jack Sprout Bread is good) that is toasted (reduces gluten content), baked potatoes, yams, squash, Body Balance.

AFTER 3:00 p.m.—Refrain from eating animal proteins. Body Balance and Power Meal are predigested proteins and can be eaten with fruit. Foods that are easier on the digestive system at night are fruit, soups, lightly steamed vegetables, and salads.

ASSIMILATION OF—
   SUPPLEMENTS—Enzyme products: Allerzyme (aids the digestion of sugars, starches, fats, and proteins), Carbozyme (aids the digestion of carbohydrates), Detoxzyme (helps maintain and support a healthy intestinal environment), Fiberzyme (aids the digestion of fiber and enhances the absorption of nutrients), Polyzyme (aids the digestion of protein and helps reduce swelling and discomfort), and Lipozyme (aids the digestion of fats). Megazyme.

FIBER—ICP (fiber beverage).

OIL—V-6 Mixing Oil (six different vegetable oils) is excellent for cooking and making salad dressings.

SUGAR SUBSTITUTE—Stevia, Stevia Select.

FOOD POISONING: Flavor a cup of water with 6 drops <u>Di-Tone</u>, swish around in mouth, and swallow. <u>Exodus II</u>, patchouly, rosemary cineol, tarragon, <u>Thieves</u>.
   SUPPLEMENTS—Detoxzyme, Exodus, Megazyme.

FOREHEAD: Jasmine.

FORGETFULNESS: See MEMORY. <u>Acceptance</u> (over heart and liver), <u>Brain Power</u> (1 drop under tongue), cedarwood, <u>Clarity</u>, cypress, <u>Dream Catcher</u>, <u>Hope</u>, fir, <u>Gathering</u>, geranium, juniper, marjoram, myrrh, orange, <u>Present Time</u>, Roman chamomile, rose, sandalwood, <u>3 Wise Men</u>, rose, <u>Valor</u>, <u>White Angelica</u>, ylang ylang. Wear as perfume/cologne or put a couple drops in hands, rub together, cup over nose and mouth, and breathe deeply.
   SUPPLEMENTS—Essential Manna, Royal Essence, Ultra Young/Ultra Young+, VitaGreen.

FORGIVE (and FORGET): <u>Acceptance</u>, <u>Forgiveness</u>, <u>3 Wise Men</u>, <u>Valor</u>, <u>White Angelica</u>.

FORMALDEHYDE: <u>Purification</u> (removes).

FORMULA FOR BABIES: See BABIES.
> *SUPPLEMENTS*—BODY BALANCE (⅓ scoop to 10 oz. water).

FORTIFYING: Cypress.

FRECKLES: Idaho tansy. Mix 2-3 drops with lotion and spread over face. Can be used two or three times per week.

FREE RADICALS:
ELIMINATE—
> *SUPPLEMENTS*—Chelex, ImmuGel, and Radex help eliminate and prevent the build up of free radicals.

FRIGIDITY: See LIBIDO, SEX STIMULANT. ᶠClary sage, jasmine, nutmeg (overcome frigidity and impotence), rose, ᶠylang ylang (helps balance male/female energies).
> *SUPPLEMENTS*—EndoBalance, Prenolone/Prenolone+, ProMist.

FRUSTRATION: Acceptance, Clary sage, frankincense, Gathering, ginger, Hope, Humility, juniper, lavender, lemon, orange, peppermint, Present Time, Roman chamomile, spruce, 3 Wise Men, thyme, Valor, ylang ylang.

FUNGUS: Abundance, cajeput, clove, fennel, geranium, ImmuPower, lavender, lemongrass, melaleuca, Melrose, RC, Raven, Roman chamomile, rosemary verbenon, Thieves. Apply topically (dilution with V-6 Mixing Oil may be necessary depending on the oil) or add to bath water. Do the RAINDROP TECHNIQUE to help purge the body of pathogenic fungi that may exist along the spinal cord or in the lymphatic system. May also try the MASTER CLEANSER (See CLEANSING) to clean out the intestinal tract and re-alkalinize the body.
> *BLEND*—2 myrrh, 2 lavender. Put on location.
> *SUPPLEMENTS*—AlkaLime (designed to combat yeast and fungus overgrowth and preserve the body's proper pH balance), ImmuGel, Megazyme, Radex, Royaldophilus, Stevia Select (with FOS - combats overgrowth of bad bacteria), Super C, Thyromin, VitaGreen.
> ***COMMENTS**—Refer to the chapter entitled "How to Use - The Personal Usage Reference" in the Essential Oils Desk Reference under "Fungal Infections" for some excellent blends and tips for combating systemic fungal infections.*
FUNGAL INFECTIONS—*Eucalyptus citriodora*, geranium, melaleuca (Tea Tree), patchouly.
PREVENTS GROWTH OF—Melrose (two times a day for seven days), Purification.

GALLBLADDER: ᶠGeranium, ᶠGerman chamomile, juniper, <u>JuvaFlex</u> (stimulates), lavender, rosemary (supports). Apply over gallbladder area (can use a hot compress) and vita Flex points on feet.
    SUPPLEMENTS—Megazyme, Mint Condition, Sulfurzyme (aids bile secretion and magnifies effects of vitamins).
INFECTION IN—ᶠHelichrysum.
STONES—Geranium, grapefruit, lime, ᶠnutmeg, rosemary.

GANGRENE: Cistus, elemi, <u>Exodus II</u>, <u>ImmuPower</u>, lavender (used by Dr. Gattefossé to recover from gas gangrene), <u>Melrose</u>, Mountain savory, ravensara, <u>Thieves</u>, thyme.
    SUPPLEMENTS—Exodus, ImmuGel, ImmuneTune, ImmuPro, Radex, Super C.

GAS: See FLATULENCE. ᶠLavender, nutmeg, onycha (benzoin), tarragon. Apply to large intestine Vita Flex points on the feet.

GASTRITIS: (Inflammation of the stomach lining). See ANTI-INFLAMMATORY. Calamus, <u>Di-Tone</u>, fennel, laurel, peppermint, pine, sage, spikenard, tarragon, yarrow. Apply over stomach area with hot compress. One drop of oil in rice or almond milk taken as a dietary supplement (*NOTE: use only those oils approved for internal use by FDA. Look for GRAS or FA designations in "Single Oil Summary Information" in the Appendix*).
    SUPPLEMENTS—AlkaLime, Cleansing Trio (ComforTone, Megazyme, and ICP), Mineral Essence, Mint Condition, Royaldophilus.

GENERAL TONIC: Grapefruit, lemon, Mountain savory, ᶠspruce.

GENITALS: ᶠClary sage.

GENTLENESS: Rosewood (aromatic).

GERMS: See BACTERIA.
AIRBORNE—Fir.
GERMICIDAL—ᶠLemon, <u>RC</u>.

GINGIVITIS: <u>Forgiveness</u>, <u>Harmony</u>, helichrysum, melaleuca, <u>Melrose</u>, myrrh, <u>Present Time</u>, rose, rosemary, ᶠsage, <u>Thieves</u>. Apply on throat and gums.
    PERSONAL CARE—Dentarome/Dentarome Plus Toothpaste (contains <u>Thieves</u>), Fresh Essence Mouthwash (contains <u>Thieves</u>), KidScents Toothpaste (for children).

GLANDULAR SYSTEM: ᶠSage, spearmint, spruce. Blue cypress may help stimulate the amygdala, pineal gland, pituitary gland, and hypothalamus.
SUPPLEMENTS—EndoBalance. ProGen (male) or FemiGen (female) for glandular nutrients.

GLAUCOMA: See EYES.
SUPPLEMENTS—Sulfurzyme (to help regulate the fluid pressure in the eye), Super C, Super B, Megazyme (to help relieve stress on the pancreas, if congested).

GOITER: See ENDOCRINE SYSTEM, LYMPHATIC SYSTEM. Cleanse the lymphatic system. Balance the endocrine system with EndoFlex.
PERSONAL CARE—EndoBalance.

G

GOUT: Basil, birch, calamus, ᶠfennel, geranium, hyssop, JuvaFlex, ᶠlemon, nutmeg, onycha (benzoin), PanAway, pine, thyme, wintergreen, yarrow. Cleanse with MASTER CLEANSER (See CLEANSING) and drink lots of fluids (water, juices, etc.).
MASSAGE OILS—Ortho Ease and Ortho Sport.
SUPPLEMENTS—ArthroTune, Cleansing Trio (ComforTone, Megazyme, and ICP), CardiaCare (with *Rhododendron caucasicum* which helps increase uric acid elimination), Cleansing Trio (ComforTone, Megazyme, and ICP), Coral Sea (highly bio-available calcium, contains 58 trace minerals), Essential Manna, JuvaTone, Mineral Essence, Sulfurzyme, Super C, Super Cal, Thyromin, VitaGreen.
***COMMENTS*—*Refer to the chapter entitled "How to Use - The Personal Usage Reference" in the* Essential Oils Desk Reference *under "Gout" for some excellent blend recipes and supplement recommendations.*

GRAVES DISEASE: See THYROID: HYPERTHYROIDISM. Blue tansy, EndoFlex, lemongrass, myrrh, spruce.
SUPPLEMENTS—ImmuPro, Mineral Essence, Sulfurzyme (helps mitigate effects of autoimmune diseases), Thyromin, VitaGreen.

GRIEF/SORROW: Bergamot (turns grief into joy), Clary sage, eucalyptus, Forgiveness, Gentle Baby (massage whole body), Hope, Joy (over the heart), juniper, lavender, Present Time, Release, Roman chamomile, Sacred Mountain (back of the neck), 3 Wise Men (rub on crown), Valor (on the feet), White Angelica (on the forehead or shoulders).

GROUNDING: Fir, Grounding, Hope, Joy, patchouly, spruce, 3 Wise Men, tsuga.
FEELING OF—cypress (aromatic).

GUILT: <u>Acceptance</u>, <u>Awaken</u>, cypress, <u>Forgiveness</u>, frankincense, <u>Gathering</u>, geranium, <u>Harmony</u>, <u>Inner Child</u>, <u>Inspiration</u>, juniper, lemon, marjoram, <u>Peace & Calming</u>, <u>Present Time</u>, <u>Release</u>, Roman chamomile, rose, sandalwood, spruce, thyme, <u>Valor</u>, <u>White Angelica</u>.

GULF WAR SYNDROME: Exodus II.

GUM DISEASE: See GINGIVITIS. <u>Forgiveness</u>, <u>Harmony</u>, ^Fmelaleuca, <u>Melrose</u> (fights infection), myrrh, <u>Present Time</u>, tsuga.
    PERSONAL CARE—Dentarome/Dentarome Plus Toothpaste (contains <u>Thieves</u>), Fresh Essence Mouthwash (contains <u>Thieves</u>).

GUMS: See GINGIVITIS. Lavender, <u>Melrose</u> (fights infection), myrrh (infection), Roman chamomile.
    PERSONAL CARE—Dentarome/Dentarome Plus Toothpaste (contains <u>Thieves</u>), Fresh Essence Mouthwash (contains <u>Thieves</u>), KidScents Toothpaste (for children).
  SURGERY ON GUMS—For one individual, helichrysum was applied with a Q-tip every 15 minutes to kill the pain. No other pain killer was used.

HABITS: See ADDICTIONS. <u>Acceptance</u>, lavender.
    ***COMMENTS—To break bad habits, you need to change the DNA and RNA. sandalwood and frankincense help with this.

HAIR: *Refer to the Personal Care Products section of the <u>Reference Guide for Essential Oils</u> for a list of ingredients and more details on chemical-free shampoos and conditioners.*
    TINCTURES—AD&E
    ***COMMENTS—Refer to the chapter entitled "How to Use - The Personal Usage Reference" in the <u>Essential Oils Desk Reference</u> under "Hair and Scalp Problems" for some excellent blend recipes.
  BEARD—Cypress, lavender, lemon, rosemary, thyme.
  BODY—Cedarwood (gives the hair shaft more body, more strength, and more life), tamanu.
  CHILDREN—Lavender Volume Hair & Scalp Wash with Lavender Volume Nourishing Rinse or KidScents Shampoo with KidScents Detangler.
  COLOR—(keep light) 1 Mixta chamomile, 1 lemon, and 1 quart of water. Rinse hair.
  DAMAGED (perms, color-treated, bleached)—Tamanu.
    PERSONAL CARE—Lemon Sage Clarifying Hair & Scalp Wash and Lemon Sage Clarifying Nourishing Rinse (leave on hair for about 10 minutes) together helps remove buildup of styling products and recondition hair. Rosewood Moisturizing Hair & Scalp Wash and Rosewood Moisturizing Nourishing Rinse (leave on hair

for about 10 minutes) together may restore manageability and shiny, healthy look. Also KidScents Shampoo.

DANDRUFF—Basil, birch, Canadian Red cedar, cedarwood, cypress, ᶠlavender, rosemary, sage, thyme, wintergreen.

> *PERSONAL CARE*—KidScents Shampoo, Lavender Volume Hair & Scalp Wash, Lavender Volume Nourishing Rinse.

DRY—Birch, geranium, lavender, rosemary, sandalwood, wintergreen.

> *PERSONAL CARE*—Rosewood Moisturizing Hair & Scalp Wash and Rosewood Moisturizing Nourishing Rinse (leave on hair for about 10 minutes) together may restore manageability and shiny, healthy look.

ESTROGEN BALANCE—Clary sage in Lavender Volume Hair & Scalp Wash and Lavender Volume Nourishing Rinse help promote estrogen balance in the membrane tissue around the hair follicle. This serves to balance testosterone levels and prevent the thickening of the tissue around the follicle that results in hair loss.

> *BLEND #1*—1 lavender, 6 patchouly in 2-5 oz. Rosewood Moisturizing Hair & Scalp Wash.
>
> *BLEND #2*—Mix together 2 cinnamon bark, 4 cypress, 4 geranium, 2 juniper, 5 lavender, and 3 rosemary. Then put one drop of the blend into ¼ tsp of water and rub on bald area and entire scalp. A gentle night treatment.
>
> *PERSONAL CARE*—Lavender Volume Hair & Scalp Wash and Lavender Volume Nourishing Rinse with Clary sage (see ESTROGEN BALANCE above).
>
> *SUPPLEMENTS*—VitaGreen, ComforTone, Megazyme, Thyromin, Super B (for stress).

FRAGILE HAIR—Birch, Clary sage, lavender, Roman chamomile, sandalwood, thyme, wintergreen.

> *PERSONAL CARE*—KidScents Shampoo, Lavender Volume Hair & Scalp Wash and Lavender Volume Nourishing Rinse.

GREASY—Petitgrain.

GROWTH (stimulate)—Basil, Canadian Red cedar, cedarwood, cypress, geranium, ginger, grapefruit, hyssop, lavender, lemon, rosemary, sage, thyme, ylang ylang (promotes).

> *PERSONAL CARE*—Lavender Volume Hair & Scalp Wash and Lavender Volume Nourishing Rinse.
>
> *SUPPLEMENTS*— Sulfurzyme. A deficiency in sulfur can result in hair loss or poor hair growth.

ITCHING—Lavender and ᶠpeppermint (skin).

LOSS—Birch, Canadian Red cedar, ᶠcedarwood, Clary sage, cypress, ᶠlavender, laurel (after infection), lemon, Roman chamomile, ᶠrosemary, sage, thyme, wintergreen, ᶠylang ylang.

G

H

ALOPECIA AREATA
(inflammatory hair loss disease) thyme (CT thymol), rosemary (CT cineol), lavender, cedarwood. Add any or all of these oils to jojoba and grapeseed carrier oils and massage into scalp daily.

> *In males, hair loss can often be blamed on heredity, hormones (high levels of testosterone), and aging. Other reasons for hair loss may include poor circulation, hypertension, acute illness, surgery, radiation, Scarlet Fever, Syphilis, stress, sudden weight loss, iron deficiency, diabetes, hypothyroidism, drugs, poor diet, and vitamin deficiency.*
>
> *Avoid hair products that are not natural on the hair. Avoid chlorinated swimming pools or polluted seas. Chemical products may also leave a residue build-up which can cause hair loss. Correcting a hormonal imbalance or hypertension (dilate blood vessels and stimulate cell division) may help.*

PERSONAL CARE—
Lavender Volume Hair & Scalp Wash and Lavender Volume Nourishing Rinse.
SUPPLEMENTS—
Sulfurzyme, Super B, Thyromin.
***COMMENTS*—Refer to the chapter entitled "How to Use - The Personal Usage Reference" in the <u>Essential Oils Desk Reference</u> under "Hair Loss" for some excellent blend recipes.

SILKY AND SHINY—Tamanu.
PERSONAL CARE—KidScents Shampoo, Rosewood Moisturizing Hair & Scalp Wash and Rosewood Moisturizing Nourishing Rinse (leave on hair for about 10 minutes) together may help maintain manageability and shiny, healthy look.

SPLIT ENDS—
PERSONAL CARE—KidScents Shampoo with KidScents Detangler, Rosewood Moisturizing Hair & Scalp Wash and Rosewood Moisturizing Nourishing Rinse (leave on hair for about 10 minutes) together may restore manageability and shiny, healthy look.

HALITOSIS: Cardamom, lavender, ᶠnutmeg, ᶠpeppermint, <u>Thieves</u>.
SUPPLEMENTS—
AlkaLime.
PERSONAL CARE—
Dentarome/Dentarome Plus Toothpaste (contains <u>Thieves</u>),

> *Don't you just love the feel of clean teeth and fresh breath! Try putting a drop of Thieves on your toothbrush instead of toothpaste. At first, it is a little warm, but it sure feels refreshing. If this doesn't work for you, try putting a drop on your toothpaste or put 10 drops of Thieves in a small spray bottle full of distilled water and mist in your mouth before brushing your teeth.*

Fresh Essence Mouthwash (contains <u>Thieves</u>), KidScents Toothpaste (for children).

HANDS: Eucalyptus, geranium, lavender, lemon, patchouly, rosemary, sandalwood.
DRY—Geranium, patchouly, sandalwood.
PERSONAL CARE—Genesis Hand & Body Lotion, Rose Ointment, Sunsation Suntan Oil.
NEGLECTED—Geranium, lemon, patchouly.
TINGLING IN—Lemongrass in Genesis Hand & Body Lotion.

HANGOVERS: Fennel, grapefruit, lavender, lemon, rose, rosemary, sandalwood.
SUPPLEMENTS—Super C.

HAPPINESS: Christmas Spirit, Joy.

HARMONY IN BODY SYSTEMS: Acceptance, clove (aromatic), geranium (harmonizing), Harmony, Inspiration, Roman chamomile.
MASSAGE OILS—Sensation Massage Oil creates an exotic arousal and increases sexual desire. The fragrance creates a peaceful and harmonious feeling that is helpful in easing relationship stress. Relaxation Massage Oil also creates a peaceful and harmonious feeling.
PERSONAL CARE—Sensation Hand & Body Lotion.
OF MIND AND BODY—Release.

HARSHNESS: Jasmine.

HASHIMOTO'S DISEASE: See THYROID: HYPERTHYROIDISM. Blue tansy, EndoFlex, lemongrass, myrrh, spruce.
SUPPLEMENTS—ImmuPro, Mineral Essence, Sulfurzyme (helps mitigate effects of autoimmune diseases), Thyromin, VitaGreen.

HATE: Acceptance, Forgiveness, Release.

HAY FEVER: Cajeput, eucalyptus, lavender, Roman chamomile, rose.

HEADACHES: See MIGRAINE HEADACHES. Basil, Aroma Life (massage on arteries in neck), Aroma Siez, calamus, cardamom, Clarity,

> *Clarity may cause headaches when chemicals or metals are in the brain. To break this blockage put Aroma Life or helichrysum on arteries in the neck.*

clove, eucalyptus, Dragon Time, frankincense, Gentle Baby, lavender, marjoram, Mister, M-Grain, ᶠpeppermint, Relieve It, ᶠrosemary. Apply to temples, back of neck, forehead, and diffuse.

***COMMENTS—*According to the* <u>Essential Oils Desk Reference</u>, *"For headaches, put one drop [*<u>Thieves</u>*] on tongue and push tongue against the roof of the mouth." (EDR-June 2002; Ch. 8; Thieves; Application) Also, Refer to the chapter entitled "How to Use - The Personal Usage Reference" in the* <u>Essential Oils Desk Reference</u> *under "Headaches" for some excellent blend recipes and supplement recommendations for several different types of headaches.*

> *ESSENTIAL WATERS (HYDROSOLS)*—Clary Sage, Spearmint (cooling and soothing). Spray into air or directly on face (don't spray directly in eyes or ears) or diffuse using Essential Mist Diffuser.

COLD/FLU HEADACHES—Cumin.

EMOTIONAL HEADACHES—<u>Joy</u>.

MENSTRUAL MIGRAINES—See HORMONAL IMBALANCE.

CHILDREN'S MIGRAINES—

> *BLEND*—5 drops Mixta chamomile, 10 grapefruit, 5 peppermint, 3 rosemary, and 4 oz. V-6 Mixing Oil for children under seven and 2 oz. V-6 Mixing Oil for children over seven.

MIGRAINE HEADACHES—(may be caused by problems in the colon. Cleanse the colon using supplements). <u>Aroma Siez</u>, ᴿbasil, birch, marjoram, <u>M-Grain</u>, <u>PanAway</u>, <u>Peace & Calming</u>, ᴿpeppermint, <u>Relieve It</u>, <u>Release</u>, Roman chamomile, spearmint, wintergreen, ylang ylang.

> *SUPPLEMENTS*—AlkaLime (if caused from acidosis), Cleansing Trio (ComforTone, Megazyme, and ICP). Do not use ComforTone and JuvaTone together (*See ComforTone in Supplement section of the* <u>Reference Guide for Essential Oils</u>).

STRESS HEADACHES—<u>M-Grain</u>, Roman chamomile.

SUGAR HEADACHES—<u>Thieves</u> for low blood sugar headaches.

> *SUPPLEMENTS*—Allerzyme (aids the digestion of sugars, starches, fats, and proteins), AlkaLime, Carbozyme, Mineral Essence.

HEALING: <u>Acceptance</u>, Clary sage (aromatic), clove, cypress, eucalyptus (aromatic), frankincense, <u>Humility</u>, lemon (aromatic), melaleuca, <u>PanAway</u>, sage.

HEALTH: <u>Abundance</u>, lavender (aromatic), lemon (aromatic).
IMPROVE—
> *SUPPLEMENTS*—Cleansing Trio (ComforTone, Megazyme, and ICP).

PROMOTES—Eucalyptus, juniper (aromatic).

HEARING: See EARS.

HEART: <u>Aroma Life</u> on heart and all Vita Flex heart points, <u>Citrus Fresh</u>, <u>Clarity</u>, cypress, <u>Dragon Time</u>, fleabane, <u>Forgiveness</u>, <u>Gentle Baby</u>, geranium, ginger, <u>Harmony</u>, <u>Hope</u>, hyssop, <u>Joy</u>, lavender, <u>Mister</u>, <u>M-Grain</u>, <u>PanAway</u>, <u>Relieve It</u>, rosemary, <u>Valor</u> on feet, <u>White Angelica</u>, ylang ylang (balances heart function). Apply oils to carotid arteries, heart, feet, under left ring finger, above elbow, behind ring toe on left foot, and Vita Flex points on the feet.

    SUPPLEMENTS—CardiaCare, Mineral Essence, Power Meal, Sulfurzyme, Ultra Young (may help reverse heart disease), Wolfberry Bars.

    TINCTURES—HRT and Rehemogen.

ANGINA—<u>Aroma Life</u>, ^Fginger, laurel, ^Forange (for false angina). Apply to heart and Vita Flex heart point.

    TINCTURES—HRT.

ARRHYTHMIA—<u>PanAway</u> on heart and <u>Relieve It</u> on left foot Vita Flex heart point (rotate each application).

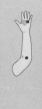

> **HEART PUMP FOR HEART STRESS**
>
> *Using your thumbs, apply pressure in an alternating "pumping" fashion between the following two heart points: (1) on the left hand at the lifeline under the ring finger; and (2) just inside the elbow. Also apply <u>Aroma Life</u> to the chest, hand, and heart points. And of course, GET HELP FAST!*

    Goldenrod and lavender are also good. Research done by Dr. Pénoël indicates that ylang ylang may be beneficial in preventing or correcting an irregularity in the force or rhythm of the heart.

    TINCTURES—HRT.

BRINGS JOY TO HEART—<u>Christmas Spirit</u>, <u>Citrus Fresh</u>, <u>Joy</u>.

CARDIOTONIC—Lavender, thyme.

    SUPPLEMENTS—CardiaCare (strengthens and supports).

CARDIOVASCULAR SYSTEMS—See CARDIOVASCULAR SYSTEM. <u>Aroma Life</u> (cardiac spasms), cinnamon bark (strengthens), cypress (strengthens the capillary walls and increases circulation), fennel, fleabane (dilates), <u>Joy</u>, ^Forange (cardiac spasms), palmarosa (supports), sandalwood (strengthens).

    SUPPLEMENTS—CardiaCare (strengthens and supports).

    TINCTURES—1-2 droppers of HRT two to three times per day.

CORONARY ARTERY—Prenolone/Prenolone+.

    ***COMMENTS**—Research has shown that natural progesterone protects the coronary artery from going into spasms. Provera, a synthetic progestin, offers no protection from coronary artery spasms. In fact, it promotes the spasm to the point of completely shutting off the flow of blood. This may explain the increase in heart attacks in women 5 to 10 years after menopause, many of whom are on synthetic progestin.*

    SUPPLEMENTS—CardiaCare (contains Hawthorne Berry which helps dilate the coronary arteries and increase blood circulation to the heart).

HEART TISSUE—Marjoram has been found to help rejuvenate smooth muscle tissue of the heart.

    TINCTURES—HRT.

    ***COMMENTS—*One woman had cancer of the heart which literally ate a hole in her heart. She used HRT and the heart tissue regenerated itself and the cancer disappeared. One man had a heart attack and was awaiting a heart transplant, he used <u>Aroma Life</u>, <u>Valor</u>, and lavender topically and HRT orally. After four weeks of using the oils, he was told by his doctor that he was doing too well to have a heart transplant.*

HYPERTENSION (high blood pressure)—See BLOOD.

LARGE VALVE—<u>Aroma Life</u> (shortness of breath).
    TINCTURES—HRT.

PALPITATIONS (rapid and forceful contraction of the heart)—<u>Aroma Life</u>, lavender, melissa, ᶠorange, peppermint, ᶠylang ylang.
    SUPPLEMENTS—CardiaCare (strengthens and supports).
    TINCTURES—HRT.

PROLAPSED MITRAL VALVE—Marjoram.

STIMULANT—Coriander, cumin.

STRENGTHENS HEART MUSCLE—Lavender, marjoram, peppermint, rose, rosemary (<u>Alternative Medicine—A Definitive Guide</u>, p. 722).

STRENGTHENING—Cinnamon bark.
    SUPPLEMENTS—CardiaCare (strengthens and supports).

TACHYCARDIA (accelerated rhythm of the heartbeat)—Goldenrod, ᶠlavender, orange, spikenard, ylang ylang.
    SUPPLEMENTS—CardiaCare (strengthens and supports), Power Meal, Wolfberry Bars.
    TINCTURES—HRT.

HEARTBURN: Cardamom, <u>Di-Tone</u> (over stomach and colon), <u>Gentle Baby</u>, ᶠlemon, ᶠpeppermint (over thymus).
    BLEND—2 lemon, 2 peppermint, 3 sandalwood, and ½ oz. V-6 Mixing Oil. Apply to breast bone. Using palm of hand, massage in a clockwise motion applying pressure. Do Vita Flex on feet.
    SUPPLEMENTS—AlkaLime, Megazyme, Mint Condition.

HEMATOMA (swelling or tumor filled with diffused blood): <u>Aroma Life</u>, German chamomile, ᶠhelichrysum.

HEMORRHAGING: Helichrysum, rose, ylang ylang. Massage around ankles, lower back, and stomach. Cayenne pepper may also help.

HEMORRHOIDS: <u>Aroma Life</u>, basil, ᶠClary sage, ᶠcypress, frankincense, helichrysum, juniper, myrrh, ᶠpatchouly, ᶠpeppermint, ᶠsandalwood. Put cypress and helichrysum inside on location.

HEPATITIS: Cinnamon bark, cypress, eucalyptus, JuvaFlex (over the liver), ImmuPower (on spine and liver), melaleuca, myrrh, oregano, patchouly, Release (on feet and liver), Roman chamomile, rosemary, thyme.

> *SUPPLEMENTS*—Cleansing Trio (ComforTone, Megazyme, and ICP) for 1 week, 4 Royaldophilus a day, Master Formula His/Hers, 1 VitaGreen a day, 4 Super C three times a day, 1/4 tsp. ImmuGel three times a day. Add JuvaTone on the 3rd day.

> ****COMMENTS—Refer to the chapter entitled "How to Use - The Personal Usage Reference" in the Essential Oils Desk Reference under "Liver" subcategory "Hepatitis" for a specific daily program using supplements and blends.*

> DETOXIFY LIVER—Ledum and JuvaTone together.

> VIRAL—FMyrrh and JuvaFlex, ledum, Fravensara, Frosemary. Apply to spine, compress over liver area, and Vita Flex points on feet. Alternate oils.

>> *SUPPLEMENTS*—Super C.

HERNIA: Apply oil(s) on location, lower back, and Vita Flex points on feet.

> HIATAL HERNIA—Basil, cypress, fennel, geranium, ginger, hyssop, lavender, peppermint, rosemary, vitex. Drink water. Put the first two fingers of each hand just below the sternum (under center of rib cage), press in firmly, and brush down quickly and firmly. This can also be done after raising up on toes and while dropping down on heels to more firmly emphasize the effect.

>> *SUPPLEMENTS*—Megazyme before meal, Mint Condition, ComforTone, ICP (fiber beverage) after meal.

> INCISIONAL HERNIA (usually caused by scar tissue failing to heal from an abdominal wound or incision)—Basil, geranium, ginger, helichrysum, lavender, lemon, lemongrass, melaleuca.

> INGUINAL—Lavender, lemongrass.

HERPES SIMPLEX: Blue cypress, bergamot with *Eucalyptus radiata*, eucalyptus, geranium, Flavender, lemon, melissa, Fravensara, rose.

> *Jean Valnet, M.D., a French physician, recommends a blend of lemon and geranium. Tisserand suggests eucalyptus and bergamot. Dr. Wabner says that a one-time application of either true rose oil or true melissa oil led to complete remission of herpes simplex lesions. Apply the oil directly on the lesions at the first sign of an outbreak. (Alternative Medicine—The Definitive Guide, p. 56).*

HICCOUGHS: Sandalwood, Ftarragon.

HIGH BLOOD PRESSURE: See BLOOD.

HIVES: See ACIDOSIS, pH BALANCE. Hives may be the result of too much acid in the blood or the result of a niacin flush (vitamin B3 taken on empty stomach). Patchouly (may relieve itching), peppermint, Roman chamomile.

  SUPPLEMENTS—AlkaLime (combat yeast and fungus overgrowth and preserve the body's proper pH balance), Coral Sea (highly bio-available calcium, contains 58 trace minerals), Super Cal (may prevent), VitaGreen.

  ***COMMENTS—One woman broke out in hives over her entire body, she used peppermint oil diluted with V-6 Mixing Oil for a body massage. Almost instantly, her body cooled off and the hives diminished until gone.*

HODGKIN'S DISEASE: Clove. Apply to liver, kidney, and Vita Flex points on feet.

HOPE: Hope (restores).

HORMONAL IMBALANCE:
  Anise, ylang ylang.
  PERSONAL CARE—
  Prenolone/Prenolone+.
  SUPPLEMENTS—Exodus,
  FemiGen, Mineral
  Essence, Sulfurzyme
  (lowered libido).
  TINCTURES—Femalin.

HORMONAL SYSTEM:
  Acceptance, Aroma
  Life, Clarity, davana,
  Dragon Time,
  EndoFlex, fennel,
  goldenrod, Gentle
  Baby, Mister, M-Grain,
  myrrh, myrtle,
  peppermint, Relieve It,
  sandalwood, ᶠspearmint
  (hormone-like), ylang
  ylang. The most
  common places to
  apply oils for hormonal
  balance are the Vita
  Flex points on ankles,

A hormonal imbalance can cause many problems including, PMS, pre- and post-menopausal conditions, depression, endometriosis, fibromyalgia, fibrocysts, infertility, insomnia, irregular menstrual cycles, lowered libido, menstrual migraines, osteoporosis, ovarian cysts, unexplained first-trimester miscarriages, water retention, etc. Carbonated water can cause hormone deficiency. But, most often, it is a result of estrogen dominance; that is, not enough progesterone to balance out the amount of estrogen. Estrogen is manufactured in several places of the body, even after menopause, and is also found in much of our food, especially animal and dairy products. Progesterone is secreted by the corpus luteum, by the placenta, and in small amounts by the adrenal glands. If the ovaries are not functioning properly, have been removed, or if they have atrophied because of menopause or hysterectomy, the woman is undoubtedly estrogen dominant. Therefore, she is a candidate for the problems listed above. One successful approach for the above problems is NATURAL PROGESTERONE (obtained from the Wild Yam or SOY). Two good books to read about natural progesterone are What Your Doctor May Not Tell You About Premenopause and What Your Doctor May Not Tell You About Menopause. Both books were written by John R. Lee, MD.

lower back, thyroid, liver, kidneys, gland areas, the center of the body and along both sides of the spine, and the clavicle area. It may also help to diffuse them.

ESSENTIAL WATERS (HYDROSOLS)—Clary Sage (contains natural scleral - helps stimulate production of estrogen). Spray into air of diffuse using Essential Mist Diffuser.

BALANCE—Bergamot, FClary sage, clove (aromatic), <u>EndoFlex</u>, fennel, geranium, <u>Legacy</u>, <u>Mister</u> (creates greater balance), nutmeg, sage, ylang ylang.

MASSAGE OILS—Dragon Time.

PERSONAL CARE—Prenolone/Prenolone+.

SUPPLEMENTS—Coral Sea (highly bio-available calcium, contains 58 trace minerals), CortiStop (Men's and Women's), Exodus, FemiGen (female), ProGen (male), ProMist, Super B, Super Cal, Thyromin, Ultra Young+, VitaGreen.

TINCTURES—Estro, Femalin, Royal Essence.

DISTURBANCES—

SUPPLEMENTS—ProGen (male) or FemiGen (female).

FEMALE—<u>Mister</u> (for estrogen).

SUPPLEMENTS—CortiStop (Women's), FemiGen, ProMist, Ultra Young+.

TINCTURES—Estro, Femalin.

MALE—<u>Mister</u>.

SUPPLEMENTS—CortiStop (Men's), ProGen, ProMist, Ultra Young+.

SEXUAL ENERGY—Goldenrod (shows more potential for impotence than Viagra!), ylang ylang.

SUPPLEMENTS—ProMist.

HOT FLASHES: See HORMONAL IMBALANCE. Bergamot (estrogen), Clary sage (estrogen), <u>Dragon Time</u>, <u>EndoFlex</u>, fennel, <u>Mister</u> (estrogen) works for women in Canada, or Fpeppermint. Apply these oils on the ankles at the ovary and uterus Vita Flex points. If hypoglycemic, use <u>Aroma Siez</u> with <u>M-Grain</u>.

***COMMENTS—*Some women have had success using a drop of <u>EndoFlex</u> under their tongues three times a day. Be cautious as it contains nutmeg and an overdose could cause problems.*

PERSONAL CARE—Prenolone/Prenolone+.

SUPPLEMENTS—CortiStop (Women's), FemiGen, Mineral Essence.

TINCTURES—AD&E, Femalin (estrogen).

OTHER—Lady Flash & Lady Love (available through Creer Labs 801-465-5423). Apply on ovaries, pelvis, ankles, bottom of feet.

HOUSECLEANING: Put a few drops of oil on your dust cloth or put 10 drops in a spray bottle of water and mist.

BATHROOMS/KITCHENS—Fir, lemon, or spruce for cleaning and disinfecting.

CARPETS—<u>Purification</u>, lemon (has been used to remove black shoe polish)

DISHES—A couple of drops of <u>Melrose</u> or lemon in the dishwater make for sparkling dishes and a great smelling kitchen.

FURNITURE POLISH—Fir, lemon, or spruce work well for polishing furniture.

GUM/GREASE—Lemon oil is terrific for dissolving gum and grease.

LAUNDRY—Adding oils to the washer can increase the anti-bacterial benefits, provide greater hygiene, and the clothes come out with a fresh, clean smell.

MOLD/FUNGUS—<u>Purification</u>.

HYPERACTIVITY: <u>Citrus Fresh</u>, lavender, <u>Peace & Calming</u> (gets them off Ritalin), Roman chamomile, <u>Trauma Life</u> (calming), <u>Valor</u> (sometimes works

> *Hyperactivity* may indicate a trace mineral deficiency. Get off Prozac and Ritalin and use Mineral Essence. It is interesting to note that 48 out of 49 death row inmates were tested and found to be deficient in the same trace minerals.

better than <u>Peace & Calming</u>). Apply to Vita Flex points on the feet and diffuse.

SUPPLEMENTS—ComforTone, ICP, Megazyme, Mineral Essence, healthy diet.

HYPERPNEA (abnormal rapid breathing): ᶠYlang ylang. Apply to lung area and Vita Flex points.

HYPERTENSION (high blood pressure): See BLOOD.

HYPOGLYCEMIA: See PROTEIN. Cinnamon bark, clove, ᶠeucalyptus, <u>Gentle Baby</u>, <u>Thieves</u>, thyme.

SUPPLEMENTS— Allerzyme (aids the digestion of sugars, starches, fats, and proteins), AlkaLime, Body Balance, Polyzyme (aids the

> *Protein deficiency causes* **hypoglycemia**. *Honey enters the blood stream faster than sugar and can cause hypoglycemia. When flu and virus enter the body and mix with problems of hypoglycemia, it can cause candida, Epstein barr virus, allergies, etc. There is a progressive deterioration from hypoglycemia. Signs of hypoglycemia are: headaches, fatigue, PMS, ornery, moody, weak, light headed, not hungry in the morning because body is still digesting its food from the night before.*

digestion of protein and helps reduce swelling and discomfort), Power Meal, Stevia, Stevia Select, Sulfurzyme, VitaGreen, WheyFit (lactose-free protein from three sources; provides highest ranking protein for digestibility), Wolfberry Bars.

HYSTERIA: Lavender, melaleuca, neroli. Apply to heart, bottom of feet, and diffuse.

IMMUNE SYSTEM: <u>Abundance</u>, cistus, clove, cumin, <u>Exodus II</u>, frankincense, geranium, Idaho tansy, <u>ImmuPower</u>, lavender, ledum (supports), lemon, melaleuca, Mountain savory, <u>Raven</u>, ravensara, rosemary (supports), <u>Thieves</u> (enhances; massage on feet and body), thyme (immunological functions), White lotus.

SUPPLEMENTS—AlkaLime (designed to combat yeast and fungus overgrowth and preserve the body's proper pH balance), Body Balancing Trio (Body Balance, Master Formula His/Hers, VitaGreen), Cleansing Trio (ComforTone, Megazyme, and ICP), Essential Manna, Exodus, ImmuGel, ImmuneTune, ImmuPro, Mineral Essence, Power Meal, Radex, Super B, Super C, Thyromin, Ultra Young (may help raise levels of cytokines, interleukin 1 & 2, and tumor necrosis factor), VitaGreen, Wolfberry Bar (*Refer to the Wolfberry Bar in the Supplements section of the* <u>Reference Guide for Essential Oils</u> *for more information on the benefits of the Chinese Wolfberry*).

TINCTURES—AD&E.

STIMULATES—ᶠCinnamon bark, ᶠfrankincense, <u>ImmuPower</u>, lavender (for nervous immune system), ᶠmelaleuca, Mountain savory, ᶠoregano, <u>Thieves</u>. Apply oil(s) to bottom of feet, along spine, under arms, dilute for massage, and diffuse for ½ hour at a time.

BOOSTING IMMUNE DEFENSE—Cumin, ledum.

IMPETIGO: Lavender, myrrh. Boil 4 ounces water, cool, add 5 to 10 drops lavender and wash. You may also use myrrh (cover for an hour). Do hot compress on site.

> *Impetigo is an infection of the outer layers of the skin. It is caused by an infected scratch or insect bite. It starts as tiny red spots, then it turns into blisters that can fill with pus. It is contagious to self and others. Approach the problem and handle it as it is noticed.*

ESSENTIAL WATERS (HYDROSOLS)—Lavender or Lavender Floral Water.

IMPOTENCY: ᶠClary sage, ᶠclove, goldenrod (shows more potential in clinical trials at the University of Montreal, Canada than the drug Viagra), ᶠginger, jasmine, mister, nutmeg, rose, ᶠsandalwood, ylang ylang.

***COMMENTS—*Some men have had success using Natural Progesterone creams (or a pregnenolone cream such as Prenolone or Prenolone+) for this problem.*

SUPPLEMENTS—CortiStop (Men's - reduces the levels of cortisol and enhances the production of testosterone), ProMist.

INCONTINENCE: See BLADDER.

INDIFFERENCE: Jasmine.

INDIGESTION: Angelica, cumin, ginger, <u>JuvaFlex</u>, ᶠlavender, ᶠpeppermint, nutmeg, valerian (nervous indigestion).

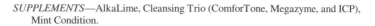

SUPPLEMENTS—AlkaLime, Cleansing Trio (ComforTone, Megazyme, and ICP), Mint Condition.

INFECTION: See ANTI-INFECTIOUS. ᶠBergamot, cajeput (urethra), ᶠcinnamon bark, clove, ᶠClary sage, cypress, elemi (chest/bronchial infections), Idaho tansy, jasmine (bacterial infection), juniper, fennel, lavender, lemongrass, *Melaleuca quinquenervia* (viral), <u>Melrose</u> (prevents growth of all infections), myrrh (fungal infection), oregano, peppermint, ᶠpine (severe), raven, ravensara, rosemary (oral infection), <u>Thieves</u>, thyme (urinary infection).

FUNGICIDAL—Cedarwood.

INFECTED WOUNDS—Frankincense, melaleuca, patchouly.

    BLEND (to draw infection out)—1 thyme. Apply hot compress twice daily. Mix together 3 lavender, 2 melaleuca, and 2 thyme with 1 tsp. V-6 Mixing Oil. After the infection and pus have been expelled, apply a little of the mixture twice daily on the infected area.

    SUPPLEMENTS—Body Balance, ImmuGel, ImmuneTune, ImmuPro, Radex, Super C.

INFECTIOUS DISEASE: Bergamot, cinnamon bark, clove, <u>Exodus II</u>, ginger, hyssop (viral infections), <u>ImmuPower</u>, juniper (viral infections), lemon, melaleuca, myrtle, <u>Raven</u>, <u>RC</u>, and thyme (bacterial infection).

    ****COMMENTS—Dr. Young uses <u>Raven</u>, <u>RC</u>, and <u>ImmuPower</u> together for infectious diseases.*

INFERIORITY:

    OVERCOMING—Peppermint.

INFERTILITY: See HORMONAL IMBALANCE. Anise, bergamot, Clary sage, cypress, <u>Dragon Time</u> (place on ankles, lower abdomen, and in vagina for women), fennel, geranium, melissa, <u>Mister</u> (for men, place in rectum, across lower back, around and under ankles), nutmeg, Roman chamomile, sage, thyme, yarrow, ylang ylang. Feed the thyroid.

    SUPPLEMENTS—ProGen (male) or FemiGen (female), Prenolone/Prenolone+, and 1-3 VitaGreen three times a day.

INFLAMMATION: See ANTI-INFLAMMATORY. Birch, calamus (intestines and colon), clove, elemi (breast and uterus), frankincense, helichrysum, juniper, lavender, myrrh, <u>PanAway</u>, <u>Peace & Calming</u>, <u>Relieve It</u>, Roman chamomile, spruce, wintergreen.

    MASSAGE OILS—Ortho Sport.

***COMMENTS—*Refer to the chapter entitled "How to Use - The Personal Usage Reference" in the* Essential Oils Desk Reference *under "Inflammation" for some excellent blend recipes.*

INFLUENZA: See FLU or COLDS.

INJURIES: See TISSUE, SCARRING. Melrose (regenerates tissue), helichrysum (reduces scarring and discoloration).
SPORT—Helichrysum, Melrose, PanAway.
MASSAGE OILS—Ortho Ease, Ortho Sport.

INNER KNOWING: Inner Child (reconnects you with your inner child), SARA.

INSANITY: Hope (ears), Release (liver), Relieve It.

INSECT:
BITES—See BITES. Cajeput, bergamot cajeput, Idaho tansy.

> Dr. Jean Valnet says that basil, cinnamon, garlic, lavender, lemon, onion, sage, savory, and thyme are effective against insect bites because of their antitoxic and anti-venomous properties.

BLEND #1—Combine 3 drops Roman chamomile, 4 eucalyptus, 10 lavender, and 1 thyme with 1 Tbs. V-6 Mixing Oil.
***COMMENTS—*Refer to the chapter entitled "How to Use - The Personal Usage Reference" in the* Essential Oils Desk Reference *under "Insect Bites" for some excellent blend recipes for bites/stings from different types of insects.*
POISONS FROM BROWN RECLUSE SPIDER OR WASPS—Purification (removes poisons from the body).
INSECTICIDAL—Citronella.
ITCHING—Lavender.
PERSONAL CARE—Satin Body Lotion with lavender.
REPELLENT—Bergamot, Purification.
FLORAL WATERS—Idaho Tansy (has been used with success as a fly and mosquito repellent on horses and other animals).
PERSONAL CARE—Sunsation Suntan Oil.
BLEND #2—Combine 5 lavender, 5 lemongrass, 3 peppermint, and 1 thyme and put on feet or add to cup of water and spray on.
BLEND #3—Clove, lemon, and orange.
BLEND #4—Put 5 lemon and 5 Purification in a little spray bottle of water and mist on your skin to protect yourself against insects, flies, and mosquitos.

I

PERSONAL CARE—Sunsation Suntan Oil helps filter out the ultraviolet rays without blocking the absorption of vitamin D, which is important to skin and bone development. ACCELERATES TANNING.

***COMMENTS—*Dr. Friedmann came in contact with a person who had bugs growing on their face and scalp. Somehow they were subjected to a fungus to which the bugs were attracted. They established their nests, laid and hatched their eggs on her skin. She had been using many products and was only able to suppress the problem but not correct it. Dr. Friedmann applied <u>Melrose</u>, helichrysum, lavender, and <u>ImmuPower</u> on her Thymus. She stopped using all other chemicals and several weeks later the bugs were almost gone.*

INSOMNIA: Angelica, basil, ᶠbergamot, <u>Citrus Fresh</u>, Clary sage, ᶠcypress, ᶠlavender, lemon, ᶠmarjoram, *Melaleuca ericifolia*, ᶠmyrtle (for hormone-related insomnia), neroli, nutmeg (small amount), ᶠorange, <u>Peace & Calming</u>, petitgrain, ᶠravensara, Roman chamomile (small amount), rosemary, sandalwood, <u>Surrender</u> (behind the ears), valerian, ᶠylang ylang.

    BLEND #1—Combine 6 <u>Citrus Fresh</u> with 6 lavender or 6 <u>Peace & Calming</u>. Apply blend to big toes, bottom of feet, 2 drops around navel, 3 drops on back of neck.

    BLEND #2—2 drops Roman chamomile, 6 geranium, 3 lemon, and 4 sandalwood. Mix together and add 6 drops in your bath at bedtime and 5 drops with 2 tsp. V-6 Mixing Oil for a massage after bath.

    SUPPLEMENTS—ImmuPro.

    ***COMMENTS—*Refer to the chapter entitled "How to Use - The Personal Usage Reference" in the <u>Essential Oils Desk Reference</u> under "Insomnia" for some excellent blend recipes.*

FOR CHILDREN—12 months to 5 years—lavender, Roman chamomile; 5 to 12 years—Clary sage, geranium, *Melaleuca ericifolia*, ylang ylang (infection).

INTESTINAL PROBLEMS: See ACIDOSIS, COLITIS, COLON, CONSTIPATION, DIGESTIVE SYSTEM, DIVERTICULITIS, PARASITES, etc. ᶠBasil, cajeput, calamus (reduces inflammation and detoxifies), ginger, ᶠmarjoram, patchouly (aids in the digestion of toxic waste), rosemary, tarragon.

    SUPPLEMENTS—AlkaLime, Cleansing Trio (ComforTone, Megazyme, and ICP), ParaFree, JuvaTone, Royaldophilus.

ANTISEPTIC—Nutmeg.

CRAMPS—ᶠClary sage, <u>Di-Tone</u>.

FLORA—Royaldophilus.

PARASITES—ᶠBergamot, ᶠclove, <u>Di-Tone</u>, ᶠfennel, ᶠlemon, peppermint, ravensara, ᶠRoman chamomile.

    SUPPLEMENTS—AlkaLime, Cleansing Trio (ComforTone, Megazyme, and ICP), and ParaFree assist in cleansing the intestinal tract of toxic debris and parasites, which are hosts for many diseases.

    SOOTHE—Spearmint.
    SPASM—ᶠTarragon, ᶠfennel.

INVIGORATING: Birch/wintergreen.
    IN SUMMER—Eucalyptus, peppermint.

IONS:
    INCREASE NEGATIVE IONS—Bergamot, citronella, lemongrass, orange.
    INCREASE POSITIVE IONS—Cajeput, frankincense, helichrysum, juniper, *Melaleuca quinquenervia,* pine, ravensara, ylang ylang.

IRON: Important for learning. Raisins are good natural source.
    SUPPLEMENTS—Master Formula Hers/His, Mighty Vites (chewable).

IRRITABILITY: Forgiveness, Hope, Humility, Inspiration, lavender, myrrh, Present Time, Surrender, Valor. All single oils EXCEPT: Eucalyptus, pepper, peppermint, and rosemary.
    SUPPLEMENTS—AlkaLime.

IRRITABLE BOWEL SYNDROME: Calamus, Di-Tone, peppermint. Take 2 drops of each in distilled water 1-2 times per day. Anise may also help.
    SUPPLEMENTS—Mint Condition (works with Megazyme and Di-Tone).

ITCHING: Lavender, Peace & Calming (ears), peppermint (ears). Apply on location too.
    BLEND—6 lavender and 3 rosemary with Satin Body Lotion.
    PERSONAL CARE—Rose Ointment, Satin Body Lotion.

JAUNDICE (liver disease): ᶠGeranium, lemon, rosemary.

JEALOUSY: Bergamot, eucalyptus, Forgiveness, frankincense, Harmony, Humility, Joy, lemon, marjoram, orange, rose, rosemary, Sacred Mountain, sandalwood, thyme, Valor, White Angelica.

JET LAG: Brain Power, Clarity, En-R-Gee, eucalyptus, geranium, grapefruit, ImmuPower (for protection), lavender, lemongrass, peppermint, Present Time, Valor. Apply to temples, thymus, and bottom of feet. It is best not to eat heavy foods and to drink as much water as possible.
    SUPPLEMENTS—Power Meal, Radex, Sulfurzyme, Super C.

JOINTS: Birch (discomfort), cajeput (stiff), Douglas fir (calming to tired and overworked joints), Idaho balsam fir (pain from exercising), nutmeg, Roman chamomile (inflamed), spruce (aching), wintergreen.

****COMMENTS—Refer to the chapter entitled "How to Use - The Personal Usage
Reference" in the <u>Essential Oils Desk Reference</u> under "Joint Stiffness and
Pain" for some excellent blend recipes.*

JOYOUS: <u>Abundance</u>, bergamot (turns grief to joy), <u>Christmas Spirit</u>, <u>Citrus Fresh</u> (brings
joy to children), <u>Joy</u>, orange (aromatic).

KIDNEYS: <u>Aroma Life</u>, calamus (reduces congestion after intoxication), Clary sage,
<u>EndoFlex</u>, geranium, grapefruit, juniper (for better function of kidneys), <u>JuvaFlex</u>,
ledum (strengthen), ⁺lemongrass (combine with juniper for greater synergistic
effect). Apply over kidneys as a hot compress. Drink plenty of distilled water (3-
4 quarts each day). When kidneys start producing ammonia, it can go to the brain
and people have died from that alone. Do the MASTER CLEANSER (See
CLEANSING).
SUPPLEMENTS—VitaGreen (turns blood back to alkaline).
TINCTURES—K&B.
****COMMENTS—Refer to the chapter entitled "How to Use - The Personal Usage
Reference" in the <u>Essential Oils Desk Reference</u> under "Kidney Disorders" for
some excellent blend recipes and supplement recommendations.*
BLOCKAGE—
MASSAGE—kidney points on feet twice a day.
SUPPLEMENTS—Cleansing Trio (ComforTone, Megazyme, and ICP), JuvaTone
(First week: 2 tablets a day; Second week: 3 tablets a day for 90 days).
CAPILLARIES BEING ATTACKED IN KIDNEYS—
SUPPLEMENTS—Need to support the body and cleanse the blood with VitaGreen,
Cleansing Trio (ComforTone, Megazyme, and ICP).
INFECTION IN—Rosemary. Apply to kidneys and Vita Flex points.
BLEND #1—Cypress, marjoram, and <u>Thieves</u> or <u>JuvaFlex</u>. Apply as a hot compress.
FOOD—Drink one gallon of distilled water and 2 quarts cranberry juice in a day.
INFLAMMATION (Nephritis)—<u>Aroma Life</u>, juniper, <u>JuvaFlex</u>. Do a colon cleanse (see
CLEANSING).
FOOD—Drink one gallon of distilled water and 2 quarts cranberry juice in a day.
SUPPLEMENTS—ImmuneTune, Power Meal, Radex, Super C, VitaGreen.
TINCTURES—K&B, Rehemogen.
****COMMENTS—Refer to the chapter entitled "How to Use - The Personal Usage
Reference" in the <u>Essential Oils Desk Reference</u> under "Kidney Disorders"
subcategory "Inflammation in the Kidneys (Nephritis)" for a very specific
regimen of supplements and blends.*
MUSCLES THAT WON'T WORK IN THE KIDNEYS—<u>Aroma Siez</u> and <u>EndoFlex</u>.
BLEND #2—8 fennel and 10 juniper.
STONES—Eucalyptus, hyssop, juniper.

BLEND #3—10 juniper and 10 geranium. Apply as a hot compress over kidneys once a day.

SUPPLEMENTS—After being on the Cleansing Trio (ComforTone, Megazyme, and ICP) for 10 days, add ImmuneTune, Radex, and Super C.

PASS (without edges)—Drink 4 oz. distilled water with juice from ½ lemon every 30 minutes for 6 hours straight. Then take 2 Tbsp. extra light virgin olive oil with the juice from 1 full lemon. Repeat daily until stone passes.

KNEE CARTILAGE INJURY:
BLEND—8 clove, 12 ginger, 10 nutmeg with 2 oz. V-6 Mixing Oil. Massage three times a day. Apply ice for swelling and inflammation. Wrap knee and elevate when sitting. Use the ice method three times a day and alternate with a hot compress and the oils.

MASSAGE OILS—Ortho Ease, Ortho Sport.

PERSONAL CARE—Regenolone.

LABOR: See PREGNANCY. Gentle Baby, jasmine (pain).

LACTATION (secretion of breast milk): See NURSING. ᶠFennel or basil (increase flow), peppermint with cold compress (decrease flow). Apply above the breasts on the lymph area and 2-3 drops on the spine, about breast level.

SUPPLEMENTS—PD 80/20, Prenolone/Prenolone+, ProMist.

LACTOSE INTOLERANCE: Lemongrass (reported to help eliminate lactic acid from fermentation of lactose in milk).

SUPPLEMENTS—Power Meal, WheyFit.

LARYNGITIS: Jasmine, ledum, Melrose, onycha (benzoin), sandalwood.

DIFFUSE—Frankincense, lavender, sandalwood, thyme.

BLEND—Add one drop each of Melrose and lemon to 1 tsp. honey. Swish around in mouth for a couple of minutes to liquify then swallow.

LAUNDRY: Lemon, Purification.

****COMMENTS—Adding oils to the washer can increase the anti-bacterial benefits, provide greater hygiene, and the clothes come out with a fresh, clean smell. A few drops of oil can also be placed on a washcloth and put in the dryer with laundry or added to a bottle of water, shook well, and sprayed into the dryer before drying the laundry.*

LAXATIVE: Hyssop, jasmine, tangerine.

SUPPLEMENTS—Cleansing Trio (ComforTone, Megazyme, and ICP).

LETHARGY: Jasmine.

LIBIDO (Low): See FRIGIDITY, SEX STIMULANT. Dragon Time, Joy, Mister, nutmeg, Live with Passion, rose, Sensation, ylang ylang. Do the MASTER CLEANSER (See CLEANSING).
    SUPPLEMENTS— PD 80/20, Prenolone/Prenolone+, ProMist, Sulfurzyme.
  MEN—Additional oils include Black pepper, cinnamon, ginger, myrrh, and pine. See also PROSTATE.
    PERSONAL CARE—Protec (combine with frankincense to decongest the prostate).
  WOMEN—Additional oils include Clary sage, geranium, and jasmine.

LICE: Eucalyptus, geranium, lavender, lemon, pine (repels), rosemary. Apply oil(s) to bottom of feet and rub over scalp three times a day.

LIGAMENTS: See MUSCLES. **Lemongrass** (torn or pulled; combine with marjoram to stimulate torn ligaments).
    ESSENTIAL WATERS (HYDROSOLS)—German Chamomile (relaxing and soothing). Spray directly on area of concern.
  TORN—Birch, clove, helichrysum, marjoram, PanAway, wintergreen.
    MASSAGE OILS—Ortho Sport.

LIPOMA: See TUMORS.

LIPS: German chamomile, lavender, lemon, melaleuca.
  DRY LIPS—
    BLEND—2 to 5 drops geranium and 2 to 5 drops lavender.

LISTLESSNESS: Jasmine.

LIVER: Acceptance, cypress, dill, Di-Tone, fleabane, ᶠgeranium (cleanses and detoxifies the liver), ᶠGerman chamomile, goldenrod (supports liver function), grapefruit (liver disorders), ᶠhelichrysum, JuvaFlex (detoxification), ledum (powerful detoxifier), myrrh, Peace & Calming, ravensara, ᶠsage (for liver problems), Release (apply to liver and Vita Flex points), Roman chamomile, 3 Wise Men (on crown).
    SUPPLEMENTS—JuvaTone.
  ***COMMENTS—*When the liver is toxic, it makes the mind lethargic and slows the emotions. For those who have liver problems, be careful about the oils used and the amounts. Ease into a liver cleanse!*
  CIRRHOSIS OF LIVER—Frankincense, geranium, juniper, lavender, myrrh, Roman chamomile, rosemary, rose.
    SUPPLEMENTS—JuvaTone, Body Balance, Super C.
  CLEANSING—JuvaFlex, ledum (with JuvaTone), and/or myrrh.

      SUPPLEMENTS—Sulfurzyme may help detoxify the liver.
FUNCTION (improve)—JuvaFlex, goldenrod, and myrrh. Do a compress over the liver
    and alternate the oils on the liver Vita Flex points.
HEPATITIS—See HEPATITIS. JuvaFlex, **ravensara** (viral).
JAUNDICE (liver disease)—ᴿGeranium.
REGENERATION—
    ****COMMENTS—One individual had total liver regeneration using JuvaTone,*
      Rehemogen, and JuvaFlex.
SPOTS—Idaho Tansy Floral Water, Prenolone/Prenolone+.
STIMULANT FOR LIVER CELL FUNCTION—ᴿHelichrysum, ledum (combine with
    JuvaTone).
    SUPPLEMENTS—Cleansing Trio (ComforTone, Megazyme, and ICP), Megazyme,
    JuvaTone (helps increase digestion in the liver).

LONGEVITY: Fennel (aromatic), Longevity (can be taken internally as dietary supplement).
    SUPPLEMENTS—Berry Young Delights (cookies that are loaded with antioxidant
    ingredients like Chinese Wolfberry), Berry Young Juice [a delicious blend of
    powerful antioxidant fruit juices - measures higher on the ORAC (oxygen radical
    absorbent capacity) scale than ever Tahitian Noni Juice], CardiaCare (with
    Rhododendron caucasicum), Longevity Capsules.

LOSS OF LOVED ONE: Basil, cedarwood, cypress (diffuse), fir, Forgiveness, jasmine, Joy,
    rose, spruce, Valor, ylang ylang.
    BATH & SHOWER GELS—Sensation Bath & Shower Gel.
    MASSAGE OIL—Sensation Massage Oil.
    PERSONAL CARE—Sensation Hand & Body Lotion.

LOSS OF SMELL: Basil.

LOVE: Forgiveness, Joy, juniper, lavender, Sensation, ylang ylang.
    BATH & SHOWER GELS—Sensation Bath & Shower Gel contains oils used by
    Cleopatra to enhance love and increase the desire to be close to that someone
    special.
    MASSAGE OILS—Sensation Massage Oil.
    PERSONAL CARE—Sensation Hand & Body Lotion.
ATTRACTS—Joy.
SELF LOVE—Joy.

LOU GEHRIG'S DISEASE: See ALZHEIMER'S DISEASE, BRAIN, MULTIPLE
    SCLEROSIS, PARKINSON'S DISEASE, PINEAL GLAND, PITUITARY
    GLAND. Use the same oils as you would if you were handling Multiple
    Sclerosis, Alzheimer's, and Parkinson's Disease. Drink steam distilled water.

Acceptance (may help to oxygenate the pineal and pituitary glands), Brain Power, Clarity (for brain function), cypress (circulation), Peace & Calming, Valor.
SUPPLEMENTS—Cleansing Trio (ComforTone, Megazyme, and ICP), JuvaTone, Sulfurzyme.

LUMBAGO: See BACK PAIN. Sandalwood.

LUNGS: See RESPIRATORY SYSTEM. Aroma Life, ᶠeucalyptus, Raven (stronger than RC), RC (diffuse to open lungs and to send oxygen to red blood cells), frankincense (stimulates), hyssop (diffuse to clear lungs of mucus), ravensara. Apply on chest with hot compress or on Vita Flex lung points on the feet.
BLEND—Equal parts *Melaleuca ericifolia* and either RC or Raven (depending on strength desired). Add to 1 oz. V-6 Mixing Oil and insert into rectum for retention (at least 15 min. if not overnight). Rectal implant is one of the quickest ways to affect the lungs.

PULMONARY—Aroma Life, cypress, eucalyptus, pine (antiseptic), ᶠsage, ᶠsandalwood.

> *The pulmonary is the designated artery conveying blood from the right ventricle of the heart to the lungs or any of the veins conveying oxygenated blood from the lungs to the left atrium of the heart.*

LUPUS: See ADRENAL CORTEX, DIGESTIVE SYSTEM, ENDOCRINE SYSTEM IMMUNE SYSTEM, THYROID. Acceptance, clove, EndoFlex, ImmuPower (alone has cleared up Lupus), Joy, Present Time (key oil for Lupus), Thieves (every 2 hours on the feet), Valor (always use first on the feet for courage to overcome fear and build self esteem).
BATH—Put 30 drops EndoFlex in softened Bath Gel Base (to

> *Lupus is a collagen break-down that may effect the skin, joints, and other systems of the body. It occurs because of thyroid and adrenal malfunction. The immune system cells malfunction and some of the good immune cells turn and destroy other good immune cells. This attack leads to an allergic reaction. The immune cells go crazy and attack whatever is convenient for them. The endocrine systems are usually affected and may shut down. In order to heal Lupus, it is necessary to cleanse the body, reduce the toxins, increase blood circulation, and nutritionally support the endocrine functions. When this happens, the adrenal glands can secrete the cortisone that is necessary for connective tissue repair and maintenance.*
>
> *To determine whether or not the thyroid needs help, you must monitor your basal cell temperature. Place a mercury thermometer under your arm pit and leave it there for 10 minutes. If your temperature is below 97.6° you need to work on the thyroid (See RECIPE #1).*

soften, put in small container and set in hot water) and shake 30 times. Bathe 30 minutes every day. Bath Gel Base cleanses the pores of the skin.

MASSAGE—Thieves (every 2 hours on feet).

PERSONAL CARE—Regenolone (may help reverse symptoms).

SUPPLEMENTS—ComforTone, ICP, and Megazyme (cleanses the body of toxins and supports the digestive function), Thyromin (is a main stay for Lupus as it feeds and regulates the thyroid), ImmuneTune (immune support), ImmuPro, Power Meal (pre-digested protein that contains wolfberry), and VitaGreen (high in chlorophyll; contains melissa which supports the connective tissue and the immune function). Carrot juice is also very supportive.

****COMMENTS—Refer to the chapter entitled "How to Use - The Personal Usage Reference" in the Essential Oils Desk Reference under "Lupus" for a specific daily regimen using supplements and blends.*

ADRENAL GLANDS—Nutmeg has adrenal cortex properties and is contained in EndoFlex. EndoFlex or Blend #1 can be applied over the adrenal gland area using a hot compress. It would also help to apply and massage the Vita Flex points.

BLEND #1—3 drops clove (rub in), 5 drops nutmeg (rub in), 7 drops rosemary (rub in), and 20 drops V-6 Mixing Oil. Apply a hot compress.

BLEND #2—30 cypress, 30 lemongrass, and 30 EndoFlex in 4 oz. V-6 Mixing Oil. Massage whole body every day.

FLUID RETENTION (caused by steroids)—EndoFlex.

ENDOCRINE SYSTEM SUPPORT—See ENDOCRINE SYSTEM, EndoFlex.

PERSONAL CARE—EndoBalance.

The following is a recipe that has been used for individuals with Lupus:

RECIPE #1—If your basal cell temperature is below 97.6° F (36.5° C), you need to work on the thyroid. Take 2 Thyromin at bedtime. If your temperature doesn't come up in three days, you will need to increase the amount of Thyromin you are taking. Take 1 upon arising along with the 2 at bedtime. When your temperature gets back up to 97.6° F, stop taking the one in the morning. Gradually go off the 2 at night. Check regularly to see that your temperature continues to stay at 97.6° F. In addition, choose one of the following oils to work as tissue generators: Acceptance, Joy, Present Time, or Valor; apply to Vita Flex points and thyroid. To support the adrenal glands, use Blend #1. To determine the adrenal area, lay a yard stick across the back from elbow to elbow and go up 2". Apply ImmuPower on the spine and Vita Flex points. Finally, supplement with Super C, 2 Thyromin or more if needed, and ImmuneTune.

CASE HISTORY #1—After doing the following for two months, one individual was totally free from Lupus: Thyromin 2 caps morning, 2 evening until temperature stayed down for three days, then increased to 3 morning and 3 evening. Also, oils used included ImmuPower, and Valor among others.

CASE HISTORY #2—Nurse in a hospital in the east gave ImmuPower to a patient as she was leaving the hospital from another serious bout with Lupus. She had

Lupus for 22 years. She felt better very soon after she used <u>ImmuPower</u>. No symptoms of Lupus were found after eight days.

CASE HISTORY #3—After suffering from systemic lupus for some time, one lady decided there was nothing left to try from the doctors. She turned to the oils and started applying <u>ImmuPower</u>, <u>EndoFlex</u>, and <u>Joy</u> over her thymus and on her feet over the Vita Flex points for the pineal and pituitary glands. She also began taking Thyromin supplements. After only a day and a half of applying <u>EndoFlex</u> to her toes, she began to have some feeling return. After a while (specific time unknown), the "butterfly" on her face disappeared and blood tests returned "just fine".

THOUGHT PATTERNS AND EMOTIONS—Feelings experienced may be those you are not aware of or patterns you brought forward from your ancestors in the DNA. A feeling of giving up. Better to die than stand up for one's self. Anger and a need to be punished. Feelings of deep grief. Laughing on the outside, but crying on the inside. Self destructive programming, an internal cannibalism, a loss of self worth. (Remember it may not have begun with you, we carry in our cells the programming of our ancestors for 4 generations back). May feel one or more of the above. Reprogram your cells by claiming your power, loving and approving of yourself in every way (no judgment). You are free and safe; speak up for yourself freely and easily. Righteous judgment is seeing only the good we do; God's judgment. Visualize your body healed or healing. Learn the reason you chose this lesson and learn from it so you can get past it and be healed. Put as little energy as possible into your affliction.

LYME DISEASE: <u>Clarity</u> (back of ears), <u>Joy</u> (over heart), <u>RC</u> (on chest and inhale), <u>Sacred Mountain</u> (on back of neck), <u>Thieves</u> (on feet and thymus), <u>White Angelica</u> (on forehead).
SUPPLEMENTS—Cleansing Trio (ComforTone, Megazyme, and ICP), Radex, ArthroTune.

LYMPHATIC SYSTEM: See IMMUNE SYSTEM. ᶠCypress (aromatic), <u>Di-Tone</u>, <u>JuvaFlex</u> (detoxifying), ledum (inflamed lymph nodes), ᶠsage, sandalwood (supports), tangerine.
BALANCE AND LONGEVITY—Aroma Life, <u>Mister</u>.
BLEND—5 drops Roman chamomile, 5 lavender, and 5 orange in 2 Tbs. V-6 Mixing Oil. Apply a few drops of blend and massage.
CLEANSING—Lemon, lime.
ESSENTIAL WATERS (HYDROSOLS)—Idaho Tansy (supports cleansing). Spray into air, directly on area of concern, or diffuse using the Essential Mist Diffuser.
DECONGESTANT FOR—Aroma Life, <u>Citrus Fresh</u>, cumin, ᶠcypress, ᶠgrapefruit, helichrysum, lemongrass, myrtle, orange, rosemary, tangerine, thyme.
MASSAGE OILS—Cel-Lite Magic.

SUPPLEMENTS—Body Balance.
DRAINAGE OF—ʳHelichrysum, ʳlemongrass.
ELIMINATES WASTE THROUGH—ʳLavender.
INCREASE FUNCTION OF—Lemon.
    MASSAGE OILS—Cel-Lite Magic (stimulates lymph), Relaxation.
    SUPPLEMENTS—Body Balancing Trio (Body Balance, Master Formula His/Hers,
       VitaGreen), ImmuGel, Power Meal.

MALARIA: Lemon with honey in water to prevent.

MALE: See AFTERSHAVE or SKIN. Awaken.
    PERSONAL CARE—PD 80/20, Prenolone/Prenolone+, Satin Body Lotion
      (moisturizes skin leaving it soft, silky, and smooth), Sensation Hand and Body
      Lotion (moisturizes and protects skin with an alluring fragrance). KidScents
      Lotion makes a great aftershave as it soothes and rehydrates the skin.
    GENITAL AREA—
      INFECTION—Eucalyptus, lavender, melaleuca, oregano, patchouly.
      INFLAMMATION—Hyssop, lavender, Roman chamomile.
      SWELLING—Cypress, eucalyptus, hyssop, juniper, lavender, rosemary.
    HORMONAL SYSTEM (male)—Mister (balances).
    INFERTILITY (male)—Basil, cedarwood, Clary sage, sage, thyme.
      SUPPLEMENTS—ProMist, Body Balancing Trio His (Body Balance, Master
      Formula His, VitaGreen).
    JOCK ITCH—Cypress, lavender, melaleuca, or patchouly. Put 2 drops of any one of
      these oils in 1 tsp. V-6 Mixing Oil and apply to area morning and night OR put 2
      drops of any one of these oils in a small bowl of water and wash and dry area well.
      SUPPLEMENTS—ProGen, Body Balancing Trio His (Body Balance, Master
      Formula His, VitaGreen).

MASSAGE: Any of the different Massage Oils - Ortho Ease and Ortho Sport are excellent.
    BLEND—5 drops Mixta chamomile, 5 lavender, 5 orange with 2 Tbs. V-6 Mixing Oil.
    Apply as a relaxing massage.

MEASLES: See CHILDHOOD DISEASES. Eucalyptus.

MEDICATION:
    SUPPLEMENTS—Super C.

MEDITATION: Canadian Red cedar, Dream Catcher (also for sweat lodges), elemi
    (aromatic), Gratitude, Humility, Inspiration, myrrh (aromatic), Roman
    chamomile, sandalwood, Sacred Mountain, tsuga (uplifting and grounding).

L

M

MELANOMA: See CANCER.
  OF SKIN—Frankincense and lavender.

MEMORY: See AMNESIA. <u>Aroma Life</u>, basil (for poor memory), bergamot, calamus,
    <u>Clarity</u>, clove (memory deficiency), <u>Dragon Time</u>, <u>En-R-Gee</u>, <u>Gentle Baby</u>,
    ginger, grapefruit, <u>Joy</u> (of love), lavender, lemon (improves), lemongrass, <u>Mister</u>,
    Mountain savory (may bring back good memories), <u>M-Grain</u>, <u>Relieve It</u>, rose,
    rosemary. Wear as a perfume, apply to temples, and diffuse.
      BLEND #1—Add a drop of lemongrass to 1-3 drops of <u>Clarity</u>. May be best to dilute
        with a few drops of V-6 Mixing Oil. Apply to forehead, temples, behind ears, and
        on back of neck. Cup hands over nose and mouth and breathe deeply.
      BLEND #2—Add a drop of rosemary to 1-3 drops of <u>M-Grain</u>. Apply as described in
        Blend #1.
    IMPROVE—Clary sage (aromatic), ꟳclove, lime.
      BLEND #3—5 basil, 2 peppermint, 10 rosemary, and 1 oz. V-6 Mixing Oil.
    RELEASES NEGATIVE—<u>Forgiveness</u> (has high frequencies), geranium (aromatic), <u>3</u>
        <u>Wise Men</u>.
    RETENTION—<u>Clarity</u>.
    STIMULATE—Calamus, rosemary (aromatic).
      BLEND #4—2 drops Blue tansy, 2 Roman chamomile, 3 geranium, 4 lavender, 3
        rosemary, 3 rosewood, 1 spearmint, 2 tangerine, and 1 oz. V-6 Mixing Oil. Apply
        a few drops of blend to back of neck, wrist, and heart.

MENOPAUSE: See HORMONAL IMBALANCE. Angelica, basil, bergamot, cardamom,
    Clary sage, ꟳcypress, <u>Dragon Time</u> (add V-6 Mixing Oil and use in douche,
    enema, or in rectum), <u>EndoFlex</u> (on throat, parathyroid, and thyroid), ꟳfennel,
    geranium, jasmine, ꟳlavender, <u>Mister</u>, neroli, nutmeg (balances hormones),
    ꟳorange, Roman chamomile, rose, rosemary, ꟳsage, thyme. Apply oil(s) to feet,
    ankles, lower back, groin, and pelvis.
      BATH & SHOWER GELS—Add 1 tsp. - 1 oz. Dragon Time Bath & Shower Gel to
        bath while filling tub with water. Soaking helps relieve lower back pain, stress,
        and sleeping difficulties that are associated with a woman's cycle.
      MASSAGE OILS—Dragon Time.
      SUPPLEMENTS—CortiStop (Women's), FemiGen, PD 80/20, Prenolone/
        Prenolone+.
      TINCTURES—Femalin.
    ****COMMENTS**—The possibility for heart attacks in women increase by 5 to 10%
        following menopause.*
    PRE-MENOPAUSE—ꟳClary sage, <u>EndoFlex</u>, ꟳfennel, lavender, <u>Mister</u>, nutmeg (balances
        hormones), tarragon.

MENSTRUATION: See
    HORMONAL
    IMBALANCE and
    PMS.

> *Amenorrhea is the absence of menstruation. The oils listed are those which induce menstrual flow (emmenagogic).*
>
> *Emmenagogue is an agent that induces or hastens menstrual flow. Many of these oils should be avoided during pregnancy. Please see PREGNANCY for safety data.*

AMENORRHEA—ᶠBasil,
    carrot, cistus, Clary
    sage, <u>Dragon Time</u>,
    fennel, hyssop, juniper,
    lavender, marjoram,
    myrrh, peppermint,
    Roman chamomile, rose, rosemary, sage.

DYSMENORRHEA—Clary
    sage then basil, cypress,
    <u>Dragon Time</u>, fennel,
    jasmine, juniper,
    lavender, marjoram,
    peppermint, Roman
    chamomile, rosemary,
    sage, ᶠtarragon, yarrow.

> *Dysmenorrhea is painful menstruation. Apply one or more of these oils to the abdomen. It may also help to use a hot compress. Each of us have different body chemistries so if one oil doesn't work, try a different one.*
>
> *Menorrhagia is abnormally heavy or extended menstrual flow. It may also refer to irregular bleeding at any time. This situation may be a sign of a more serious condition so please see your doctor.*

*BATH & SHOWER
    GELS*— Add 1 tsp. - 1
    oz. Dragon Time Bath
    & Shower Gel to bath
    while filling tub with water. Soaking helps relieve lower back pain, stress, and
    sleeping difficulties that are associated with a woman's cycle.

M

GENERAL CARE—
    BLEND—Before and during cycle, combine 10 drops <u>Dragon Time</u> with 4 basil and
        rub around ankles, lower back, and lower stomach.
    MASSAGE OILS—Dragon Time (uncomfortable days and irregularity)
    PERSONAL CARE—PD 80/20 or Prenolone/Prenolone+ may help to regulate the
        hormones which should alleviate many of the problems associated with
        menstruation. See HORMONAL IMBALANCE.
    SUPPLEMENTS—Three times a day one week before cycle starts, take 2 droppers
        full of F.H.S. (available through Creer Labs 801-465-5423) in water. One week
        after the cycle, take Master Formula Hers four times a day and 6 VitaGreen a day.
        Also FemiGen (for PMS), Exodus.
IRREGULAR—Clary sage, fennel, lavender, melissa, ᶠpeppermint, Roman chamomile,
    rose, ᶠrosemary, ᶠsage.
MENORRHAGIA—Cypress, geranium, Roman chamomile, rose.
SCANTY—Jasmine, lavender, melissa, peppermint. See oils listed under
    AMENORRHEA.

MENTAL: <u>Brain Power</u> (increases capacity and clarity by dissolving petrochemicals),
ᶠoregano (mental diseases), sage (strain, aromatic), vitex (unrest).

ACCURACY—<u>Clarity</u>, peppermint. Diffuse or inhale.

ALERTNESS—<u>Clarity</u>, <u>En-R-Gee</u>.

   ***COMMENTS—*These oils are good for night driving.*

FATIGUE—<u>Aroma Life</u>, <u>Awaken</u>, ᶠbasil, cardamom, <u>Clarity</u>, <u>Dragon Time</u>, <u>Gentle Baby</u>,
lemongrass, <u>Mister</u>, <u>M-Grain</u>, <u>Relieve It</u>, ᶠrosemary, sage (diffuse), ᶠylang ylang.
Basil and lemongrass together are a good combination.

IMPAIRMENT—Sulfurzyme.

RETARDATION—Can be due to a mineral deficiency. Essential Manna, Mighty
Mist/Vites, Mineral Essence.

STRESS—Clary sage, <u>Evergreen Essence</u>, pine (aromatic), <u>Surrender</u>.

   *SUPPLEMENTS—*ImmuPro.

METABOLISM:
BALANCE—Clove (aromatic), <u>EndoFlex</u> (increases), oregano, spearmint, <u>Valor</u>.

INCREASE (over all)—Spearmint, spikenard.

LIPID—Hyssop (regulates).

STRENGTHEN (vital centers)—Sage.

   *SUPPLEMENTS—*Thyromin (regulates metabolism), ThermaBurn (tablets),
ThermaMist (oral spray), Power Meal.

METALS: See CHELATION.
Helichrysum, <u>Peace &
Calming</u>, <u>Sacred
Mountain</u>, <u>Valor</u>.

*SUPPLEMENTS—*Chelex,
Cleansing Trio
(ComforTone,
Megazyme, and ICP),
JuvaTone, Radex.

PULL OUT—Drink steam
distilled water. The

> *Heavy metals in the system give off toxic gases and can
> create allergic symptoms and hormonal imbalances. For
> example, cadmium can create hyperactivity and learning
> disabilities in children. Cigarette smoke and caffeine all
> contain cadmium. Ridding the body of heavy metals is
> extremely important for proper immune function. Cast-
> iron cookware leaves heavy iron deposits in the body.
> Aluminum cookware leaves aluminum deposits in the
> body. Glass or Stainless Steel cookware is best.*

absence of minerals in distilled water creates a vacuum-like action that pulls
metals and toxins from the body.

   *BLEND #1—*Combine 10 cypress, 10 juniper, 10 lemongrass with 1 oz. V-6 Mixing
Oil and massage under arms, over kidneys, and on bottoms of feet.

   *BLEND #2—*Add 2-4 drops <u>Thieves</u> and 1-3 drops helichrysum to a rolled gauze and
place between cheek and gums to pull out dental mercury. Leave in one place
during the night and throw away the gauze roll in the morning. Next night place a
new gauze roll with oil in a different place. Continue in like manner until all

areas have been affected. ***NOTE: Dilute with V-6 Mixing Oil for use on very sensitive gums or on children.***

MICE (REPEL): Purification.

MIGRAINE HEADACHES: See HEADACHES. Aroma Siez, ᶠbasil, cumin, ᶠeucalyptus, German chamomile, grapefruit, lavender, M-Grain, ᶠmarjoram, ᶠpeppermint, spearmint, valerian.
SUPPLEMENTS—Cleansing Trio (ComforTone, Megazyme, and ICP).

MILDEW: Purification (put a few drops in a squirt bottle and spray into the air to neutralize mildew).

MIND: Basil (absent minded), Believe (stimulates), Surrender (clearing), Western Red cedar (powerful effects on subconscious and unconscious mind).
ESSENTIAL WATERS (HYDROSOLS)—Western Red Cedar. Spray into air or diffuse using the Essential Mist Diffuser.

MINERALS (deficiency):
SUPPLEMENTS—Cleansing Trio (ComforTone, Megazyme, and ICP).
TINCTURES—Royal Essence, Mineral Essence.

MISCARRIAGE: See PREGNANCY.

MOLD: Purification.

M

MOLES: Frankincense, geranium, lavender, Melrose.

MOMENT:
BEING IN—Present Time.

MONO (MONONUCLEOSIS): ImmuPower, RC, Thieves.
BLEND—3 oregano, 3 Thieves, and 3 thyme. Rub on feet.
INFECTIOUS—ᶠRavensara.
SUPPLEMENTS—Build immune system. Cleansing Trio (ComforTone, Megazyme, and ICP), ImmuneTune, ImmuGel, ImmuPro, Power Meal, Super C.

MOOD SWINGS: See HORMONAL IMBALANCE. Can be due to a Vitamin B deficiency. Acceptance, bergamot, Clary sage, Dragon Time or Mister, fennel, Gathering, geranium, Harmony, jasmine, Joy, juniper, lavender, lemon, Peace & Calming, peppermint, Present Time, rose, rosemary, sage, sandalwood, spruce, Trauma Life, Valor, yarrow, ylang ylang.

SUPPLEMENTS—AlkaLime (may help if the mood swing is a result of over acidification), Super B.

MORNING SICKNESS: See PREGNANCY.

MOSQUITOS: See INSECT. Frequent mosquito bites could be due to a Vitamin B deficiency.
    SUPPLEMENTS—Super B.

MOTHER (Problems with): <u>Acceptance</u>, geranium, <u>Valor</u>. Apply to ears (*refer to the Auricular Emotional Therapy chart in the Basic Information section of this book*).

MOTION SICKNESS: <u>Di-Tone</u>, ginger, <u>M-Grain</u>, nutmeg, ᶠpeppermint, spearmint. Apply to feet, temples, and wrists. Can also apply a drop or two of <u>Di-Tone</u> to the hands, stir in a clockwise motion, apply behind both ears, rub hands together, cup over nose and mouth and breathe deeply.
  ***COMMENTS—*According to the Essential Oils Desk Reference, "Mix 4 drops peppermint and 4 drops ginger in 1 ounce V-6 Mixing Oil or Massage Oil Base. Rub on chest and stomach before traveling." (EDR-June 2002; Ch. 28; Digestion Problems; Travel Sickness)*

MOTIVATION:
    TO MOVE FORWARD—<u>Envision</u> (emotional support), <u>Magnify Your Purpose</u> (empowering and uplifting), <u>Motivation</u>, myrrh, <u>Live with Passion</u>.
    SUPPLEMENTS—Sulfurzyme.

MUCUS: See ANTI-CATARRHAL.
    ᶠCypress, helichrysum (discharge), goldenrod (discharges respiratory mucus), hyssop (opens respiratory system and discharges toxins and mucus), mugwort (expels), onycha (benzoin), ᶠrosemary.

MULTIPLE SCLEROSIS (M.S.): See MYELIN SHEATH. Aroma

> *Multiple Sclerosis is a chronic degenerative disorder of the central nervous system where the myelin sheath, which covers the nerves, is gradually destroyed throughout the brain and/or spinal cord. Eventually it causes muscular weakness, loss of coordination, speech and visual disturbances, and bladder and bowel problems. It may be caused by a virus or a defect in the immune system.*
>
> *According to D. Gary Young, progesterone is absolutely necessary in manufacturing, building, repairing, and rejuvenating the myelin sheath. Progesterone is naturally produced from pregnenolone.*

Siez, birch, Clarity, cypress, elemi, frankincense, geranium, helichrysum, Idaho tansy, juniper, oregano, Peace & Calming, peppermint, rosemary, sage, sandalwood, thyme, wintergreen. Do the Raindrop Technique.

PERSONAL CARE—PD 80/20, Prenolone/Prenolone+.

SUPPLEMENTS—ArthroTune, Body Balance, Cleansing Trio (ComforTone, Megazyme, and ICP), Essential Omegas, ImmuneTune, ImmuPro, JuvaTone, Mineral Essence, Power Meal, Sulfurzyme, Super B, Super C, VitaGreen.

The following are recipes that have been used successfully:

RECIPE #1—Supplement with VitaGreen, Cleansing Trio (ComforTone, Megazyme, and ICP), Radex, ImmuneTune, and Super C. Blend 10 cardamom, 10 peppermint, and 10 rosemary with 1 oz. V-6 Mixing Oil for a full body massage. Finally, diffuse Acceptance and Awaken.

RECIPE #2—Supplement with 8 Super Cal, 2 Super B (after breakfast), 6 Super C, 6 VitaGreen four times a day, 4 ImmuneTune, Master Formula His/Hers, and ArthroTune. Apply juniper and peppermint, one at a time, on the spine. If the M.S. is in the neck, work up the spine. If it is in the legs, work down the spine. Do a cold compress and wait for 30 minutes. Remove the compress and repeat again.

RECIPE #3—Take 2 droppers full of Mineral Essence morning and evening to conduct current to reconnect the nerve tissues. Take ½ Super B in the morning and evening with meals for the first week. Then increase the dosage. Use juniper, geranium, and peppermint on the bottom of the feet and up the legs and spine. Apply oils in the direction of the paralysis. Apply juniper and cypress on the base of the neck, then add Aroma Siez. Next do the Raindrop Technique on the spine using oregano and thyme. Use Peace & Calming and Clarity for brain function and cypress for circulation. Use the Cleansing Trio (ComforTone, Megazyme, and ICP) and JuvaTone for six days. Also use ArthroTune and Super C for six days. Then start on Super B morning and evening, Body Balance or meal, 6 VitaGreen four times a day, 4 ImmuneTune two times a day.

BLEND—6 juniper, 4 sandalwood, 2 peppermint, 12 geranium. Mix and massage into neck, spine, and bottom of feet.

***COMMENTS**—*Avoid hot baths, etc. Heat is the worst thing you can do. If anything, insulate the body with ice packs. Lowering the body temperature with cold packs helps to regenerate the myelin sheath. The person can be kept in the cold packs either for as long as they can stand it or until their body temperature drops 3 degrees. The body temperature must be monitored closely to avoid lowering it to far. This process can be repeated until the person can only stand being in the cold packs for 20 minutes. It is also best to avoid diet foods, especially those that contain aspartame as it is known to cause MS, brain damage, and other problems.*

MUMPS: See CHILDHOOD DISEASES. Lavender, melaleuca.

MUSCLES: Aroma Siez, basil, birch, cypress, Idaho balsam fir, lavender, lemongrass, **marjoram**, peppermint, White fir, wintergreen.

ESSENTIAL WATERS (HYDROSOLS)—Basil (relaxing), German Chamomile (relaxing and soothing for sore muscles). Spray directly on area on concern.

MASSAGE OILS—Ortho Ease, Ortho Sport, Relaxation (these oils are great for all problems associated with muscles).

SUPPLEMENTS—AminoTech (enhances muscle building and body toning), Arthro Plus, Be-Fit (enhances strength and endurance), CardiaCare, Coral Sea (highly bio-available calcium, contains 58 trace minerals), Essential Manna, Mineral Essence, Power Meal, Sulfurzyme, Super Cal, WheyFit, Wolfberry Bar (*Refer to the Wolfberry Bar in the Supplements section of the Reference Guide for Essential Oils for more information on the benefits of the Chinese Wolfberry*).

***COMMENTS—One professional trainer for body builders used Be-Fit, Power Meal, and Wolfberry Bars to increase muscle mass and strength beyond anything he had previously achieved!

ACHES AND PAINS—Aroma Siez, ᶠbirch, ᶠclove, Douglas fir, ginger, helichrysum, Idaho balsam fir, lavender, lemongrass (especially good for ligaments), **marjoram**, nutmeg, oregano, PanAway, peppermint, Relieve It, Roman chamomile, rosemary, spearmint, thyme, vetiver, White fir (with inflammation), wintergreen.

SUPPLEMENTS—Sulfurzyme.

***COMMENTS—Refer to the chapter entitled "How to Use - The Personal Usage Reference" in the Essential Oils Desk Reference under "Muscles" for some excellent blends to help with sore and tight muscles.

ANTI-INFLAMMATORY—Basil, peppermint, White fir. See ANTI-INFLAMMATORY and INFLAMMATION for additional oils.

***COMMENTS—Refer to the chapter entitled "How to Use - The Personal Usage Reference" in the Essential Oils Desk Reference under "Muscles" for an excellent blend to help reduce inflammation.

CARDIAC MUSCLE—Goldenrod, lavender, marjoram, neroli, peppermint, rose, rosemary.

SUPPLEMENTS—CardiaCare (strengthen and support).

CRAMPS/CHARLEY HORSES—Aroma Siez, basil, Clary sage, coriander, cypress, grapefruit, jasmine, lavender (aromatic), **marjoram**, pine, Roman chamomile, rosemary, thyme, vetiver.

BLEND—Equal parts rosemary and Aroma Siez. Apply neat or mix with V-6 Mixing Oil and massage.

SUPPLEMENTS—ArthroTune, Coral Sea (highly bio-available calcium, contains 58 trace minerals), Essential Manna, Mineral Essence, Sulfurzyme, Super Cal.

DEVELOPMENT—Birch/wintergreen (with spruce), PanAway.

SUPPLEMENTS—Be-Fit, Coral Sea (highly bio-available calcium, contains 58 trace minerals), Power Meal, Super Cal, VitaGreen (stimulates and strengthens).

FATIGUE—<u>Aroma Siez</u>, cypress, Douglas fir, eucalyptus, grapefruit, Idaho balsam fir, **marjoram**, peppermint, ravensara, rosemary, thyme.

SUPPLEMENTS—ArthroTune, Coral Sea (highly bio-available calcium), Essential Manna (high in magnesium), Mineral Essence, Super Cal.

OVER-EXERCISED—Douglas fir, eucalyptus, **Idaho balsam fir**, ginger, lavender, thyme, White fir (with inflammation).

BATH—3 drops marjoram and 2 drops lemon in a tub of water. Soak.

BLEND—Equal parts of eucalyptus, peppermint, and ginger. Mix with V-6 Mixing Oil and massage.

RHEUMATISM (Muscular)—Rosemary, thyme.

SPRAINS—Black pepper, clove, eucalyptus, ginger, helichrysum, Idaho tansy, jasmine, lavender, lemongrass, **marjoram**, nutmeg, pine, rosemary, thyme, vetiver, White fir.

SPASMS—<u>Aroma Siez</u>, **basil**, Clary sage, cypress, lavender, jasmine, marjoram, <u>PanAway</u>, peppermint, Roman chamomile.

MASSAGE OILS—Cel-Lite Magic, Ortho Ease.

SUPPLEMENTS—ArthroTune, Coral Sea (highly bio-available calcium), Super Cal.

TINCTURES—Arthro Plus.

STIFFNESS—<u>Aroma Siez</u>, <u>PanAway</u>.

SUPPLEMENTS—ArthroTune.

SMOOTH MUSCLE—Bergamot, Black pepper, Clary sage, cypress, fennel, juniper, lavender, **marjoram**, melissa, neroli, peppermint, Roman chamomile, rosemary, sandalwood. Apply as a hot compress over the affected area.

****COMMENTS—Essential oils with high proportions of ester compounds are especially effective.*

TENSION (especially in shoulders and neck)—<u>Aroma Siez</u>, Douglas fir, helichrysum, juniper, lavender, **marjoram**, <u>Relieve It</u>, Roman chamomile, spruce.

BATH & SHOWER GELS—Evening Peace Bath & Shower Gel (relaxes tired, fatigued muscles and helps alleviate tension).

MASSAGE OILS—Ortho Ease and Ortho Sport.

TISSUE—

SUPPLEMENTS—Body Balance and Power Meal (contain a complete amino acid and vitamin profile and have a high level of predigested protein to maintain a good food supply for muscle tissue), AminoTech (contains amino acids which help increase formation of lean muscle tissue and prevent muscle from being broken down), Be-Fit (contains ingredients necessary to build muscle mass), UltraYoung/UltraYoung+ (increase production of growth hormone which increases formation of lean muscle tissue), WheyFit.

M

***COMMENTS—*Refer to the chapter entitled "How to Use - The Personal Usage Reference" in the Essential Oils Desk Reference under "Muscles" for some excellent blends to help improve circulation in the muscles and aid in the regeneration of muscle tissue.*

TONE—Basil, birch, Black pepper, cypress, ginger, grapefruit, juniper, lavender, lime, marjoram, orange, peppermint, petitgrain, pine, rosemary, thyme, wintergreen. Apply before exercise.

*SUPPLEMENTS—*Be-Fit (promotes formation of muscle tissue), Sulfurzyme, WheyFit.

***COMMENTS—*Poor muscle tone may indicate a sulfur deficiency.*

TORN MUSCLES—Helichrysum and spruce take pain away (use hot packs), ginger (circulation), **Lemongrass**.

*MASSAGE OILS—*Ortho Sport.

MUSCULAR DYSTROPHY: Aroma Siez, basil, eucalyptus, geranium, ginger, lavender, lemon, lemongrass, marjoram (combine with equal parts lemongrass), orange, pine, Relieve It, rosemary.

*MASSAGE OILS—*Ortho Ease, Ortho Sport.

*SUPPLEMENTS—*Megazyme, Mineral Essence, Power Meal, Sulfurzyme, Thyromin, Ultra Young, VitaGreen.

MYELIN SHEATH: ImmuneTune, ImmuPro, Radex, ImmuPower, and **cold** compresses using peppermint, juniper, and geranium *(remember, no heat!)*.

NAILS: Citrus Fresh, eucalyptus, frankincense, grapefruit, lavender, lemon (repeated use may help harden), lime, melaleuca, myrrh, oregano, patchouly, peppermint, ravensara, rosemary, thyme.

*BLEND—*Equal parts frankincense, lemon, and myrrh. Mix with a couple drops of Wheat Germ oil and apply 2-3 times per week.

*SUPPLEMENTS—*Coral Sea (highly bio-available calcium), Mineral Essence, Sulfurzyme (helps with growth and removal of ridges and cracks), Super Cal.

***COMMENTS—*A deficiency in sulfur can cause poor nail growth.*

NARCOLEPSY: Brain Power

*SUPPLEMENTS—*Mineral Essence, Thyromin, Ultra Young, VitaGreen.

***COMMENTS—* Establishing a routine*

Narcolepsy is a disorder that is characterized by sudden and uncontrollable drowsiness and attacks of sleep at unexpected and irregular intervals. It is frequently misdiagnosed as hypothyroidism (insufficient thyroid hormone), hypoglycemia (insufficient blood sugar), epilepsy, or multiple sclerosis. Proper diagnosis requires overnight monitoring with a device used to detect brain waves called an *electroencephalograph*.

of strict bedtimes and daytime naps may also help reduce the number of unexpected sleep attacks.

NASAL: See NOSE.

NAUSEA: Calamus, cardamom, clove, <u>Di-Tone</u> (over stomach and colon), ginger, juniper, ^Flavender, <u>M-Grain</u>, nutmeg, ^Fpeppermint (aromatic), rosewood, spearmint, tarragon. Apply behind ears and on Vita Flex points.
   BLEND—2 lavender, 2 spearmint, and 2 drops of another oil for your type of nausea. Mix together and put a little on a cotton ball and inhale three times a day or diffuse.

NECK: Basil, Clary sage, geranium, lemon, lemongrass, orange, helichrysum.
   CHRONIC PAIN—<u>PanAway</u>. Apply to base of big toe.

NEGATIVE IONS: When dispersed into the air through a cool-air nebulizing diffuser, the following oils ionize negatively: Bergamot, cedarwood, citronella, *Eucalyptus citriodora*, grapefruit, lavandin, lavender, lemon, lemongrass, mandarin, orange, patchouly, sandalwood.

> **Negative ions** are produced naturally by wind and rain. They help stimulate the parasympathetic nervous system which controls rest, relaxation, digestion, and sleep. However, if you live in an environment with an over-abundance of negative ions, such as in the country or by the ocean, you may benefit greatly by diffusing the oils listed under POSITIVE IONS. The production of more positive ions can help bring greater balance to the area and provide a more healthy environment.

M

N

NEGATIVITY: Sandalwood (removes negative programming from the cells).
   BREAKS UP—<u>Dream Catcher</u>, <u>Forgiveness</u>.
   DROWNING IN OWN—Grapefruit (aromatic).

NERVOUS SYSTEM: ^FBasil (stimulant and for nervous breakdown), bergamot, <u>Brain Power</u>, calamus, cedarwood (nervous tension), cinnamon bark, cumin (stimulant), <u>Di-Tone</u>, frankincense, geranium (regenerates nerves), ginger, Idaho balsam fir, jasmine (nervous exhaustion), juniper (better nerve function), lavender, lemon, lemongrass (for nerve damage; activates), marjoram (soothing), *Melaleuca ericifolia* (nervous tension), nutmeg (supports), orange, palmarosa (supports), <u>Peace & Calming</u>, pepper (stimulant), **peppermint** (soothes and strengthens; place on wrists or location of nerve damage), petitgrain (re-establishes nerve equilibrium), pine (stimulant), ravensara, Roman chamomile, rosemary, ^Fsage, sandalwood, spearmint, spruce (fatigue), valerian (central nervous system depressant), vetiver.

PERSONAL CARE—NeuroGen or Regenolone (both help nerve regeneration).

SUPPLEMENTS—Coral Sea (highly bio-available calcium, contains 58 trace minerals), Mineral Essence, Sulfurzyme, Super B.

TINCTURES—Nerv-Cal (supplies nerve tissues with calcium), Nerv-Us (helps heal nerve damage and relax nervous conditions). *Both tinctures are available through Creer Labs 801-465-5423.*

NERVOUSNESS—Cypress, goldenrod, orange, <u>Surrender</u>, tangerine.

PARASYMPATHETIC NERVES—See PARASYMPATHETIC NERVES. ᶠMarjoram (increases tone of).

VIRUS OF NERVES—Clove and frankincense.

NEURALGIA (severe pain along nerve): Cajeput, cedarwood, eucalyptus, helichrysum, juniper, lavender, ᶠmarjoram, nutmeg, pine, ᶠRoman chamomile.

NEURITIS: Cedarwood, clove, eucalyptus, juniper, lavender, ᶠRoman chamomile, yarrow.

NEUROLOGICAL PROBLEMS: Limit the use of oils with high *ketone* content.

***COMMENTS—*A 4 year old child was in a car accident where she suffered severe brain damage. The surgeon removed part of her brain which sent her into a coma. After being in a coma for two months, Dr. Friedmann was asked to help her. He used oils that are commonly used for neurological problems. He put <u>Valor</u> on the back of her neck, skull, and feet. He also used <u>Present Time</u> and <u>Awaken</u>. She came out of the coma and started doing physical therapy.*

NEUROMUSCULAR: Roman chamomile, tarragon.

NEUROPATHY: <u>Brain Power</u>, cedarwood, cypress, eucalyptus, geranium, helichrysum, juniper, <u>JuvaFlex</u>, lavender, lemongrass, peppermint, Roman chamomile, <u>Valor</u>.

PERSONAL CARE—NeuroGen, PD 80/20, Prenolone/Prenolone+, Regenolone.

SUPPLEMENTS—Body Balance, Essential Manna, Mineral Essence, Royal Essence, Sulfurzyme, Super B.

***COMMENTS—*Refer to the chapter entitled "How to Use - The Personal Usage Reference" in the <u>Essential Oils Desk Reference</u> under "Nerve Disorders" subcategory "Neuropathy" for some excellent blends.*

PAIN—<u>Relieve It</u>, helichrysum (best with cold compresses), <u>PanAway</u>. Massage with peppermint, juniper, and geranium and reapply cold compresses.

NEUROTONIC: Melaleuca, ᶠravensara, thyme.

NIGHT SWEATS: See HOT FLASHES and HORMONAL IMBALANCE. ^FSage.

NOSE: Melaleuca, rosemary.
> BLEEDING—Cypress, frankincense, lavender, lemon.
>> *BLEND*—2 cypress, 1 helichrysum, and 2 lemon in 8 oz. ice water. Soak cloth and apply to nose and back of neck.
>
> NASAL MUCUS MEMBRANE—Eucalyptus may help reduce inflammation.
> NASAL NASOPHARYNX—Eucalyptus.
> POLYPS—See POLYPS. Basil, citronella, frankincense, oregano, peppermint, <u>Purification</u>, <u>RC</u> (can be applied to inside of nose with cotton swab). Apply to exterior of nose (use caution because of close proximity to eyes) or breathe in diffused mist. A colon and liver cleanse may be helpful. Birch/wintergreen or <u>Valor</u> may also be applied to bridge of nose for possible structural realignment.
> ****COMMENTS—Nasal polyps are caused by an overproduction of fluid in the mucous membranes. They are seen with asthma, hay fever, chronic sinus infections, and cystic fibrosis. In fact, one source stated that one out of four people with cystic fibrosis have nasal polyps. They may also be a result of blockages in the brain or some trauma to the nose in which structural integrity has been compromised. Diet may also be a factor.*

NURSING: Clary sage (begins milk production), ^Ffennel or basil (increases milk production), geranium. Apply above breasts on lymph area and on spine at breast level.
> INCREASE MILK PRODUCTION—
>> *BLEND*—7 to 15 drops fennel and either 7 to 15 drops geranium or 5 to 10 drops Clary sage. Dilute 1-2 drops of blend in 2 Tbs. V-6 Mixing Oil.
>> *SUPPLEMENTS*—Body Balancing Trio Hers (Body Balance, Master Formula Hers, VitaGreen).
>
> DECREASE MILK PRODUCTION—Peppermint. Apply with cold compress over breasts. *Refer to Methods of Application under the Science and Application section the <u>Reference Guide for Essential Oils</u> for instructions on using cold compresses.*

OBESITY: See DIET, WEIGHT. Fennel, grapefruit, juniper, orange, rosemary, tangerine.
> *SUPPLEMENTS*—Power Meal (eat for breakfast as a meal replacement).
> REDUCE—Orange, tangerine.

OBSESSIVENESS: <u>Acceptance</u>, <u>Awaken</u>, Clary sage, cypress, <u>Forgiveness</u>, geranium, helichrysum, <u>Humility</u>, <u>Inner Child</u>, <u>Joy</u>, lavender, marjoram, <u>Motivation</u>, <u>Present Time</u>, rose, <u>Sacred Mountain</u>, sandalwood, <u>Valor</u>, ylang ylang.

ODORS: See DEODORANT. Bergamot, lavender, <u>Purification</u> (neutralizes and eliminates).
> BODY—<u>Purification</u> (obnoxious odors).

N
O

CONTROLLIING—Cedarwood.

OPENING (to receive): Fir (aromatic).

OPPOSITION: Valor.

ORAL INFECTIONS: ᶠRosewood.

OSTEOPOROSIS: See
          HORMONAL
          IMBALANCE. Aroma
          Siez, birch, chamomile
          (Roman and German),
          clove, cypress, fennel,
          fir (cortisone-like

> *Studies and clinical experience by Dr. John R. Lee indicate that bone mass can be reversed (regained) by as much as 41% with the use of Natural Progesterone. For information on Dr. Lee's book, see HORMONAL IMBALANCE.*

action), geranium, ginger, hyssop, lemon, nutmeg, oregano, PanAway, Peace &
          Calming, peppermint, pine, Relieve It, rosemary, spruce, thyme, wintergreen.
     SUPPLEMENTS—Arthro Plus, Coral Sea (highly bio-available calcium, contains 58
          trace minerals), PD 80/20, Prenolone/Prenolone+, Super Cal.

OVARIES: See HORMONAL IMBALANCE. Di-Tone, geranium, ᶠmyrtle, and/or
          ᶠrosemary (regulates).
     OVARIAN CYSTS—Basil.
          BLEND—5 frankincense and 5 Melrose. Mix and apply to lower back and abdomen.
          TINCTURES—Femalin has been reported to be very beneficial in getting rid of uterine
               and ovarian cysts. The following recipe has been used by some women who have
               had ovarian cysts:
          RECIPE #1—Douche with 3-4 droppers of Femalin in 6 oz. of water. Then, mix 2
               droppers of Femalin with 2 tsp. of olive oil. Before going to bed and while lying
               down, insert liquid blend into vagina and retain with a tampon throughout the
               night. In addition, flavor a glass of water with 2-3 droppers full of Femalin and
               drink. Do not put Femalin in juice as it may work negatively with the herbs. Feed
               the body with FemiGen.

OVERCOME AND RELEASE UNPLEASANT, DIFFICULT ISSUES IN LIFE:
          Acceptance, Release, Roman chamomile, SARA, Trauma Life.

OVEREATING: See EATING DISORDERS.

OVERWEIGHT: See OBESITY and WEIGHT.

OVERWHELMED: Acceptance, Hope, Release, Valor.

OXYGEN:

OXYGENATING—Fennel, fir, frankincense, oregano, sandalwood (increases oxygen around pineal and pituitary glands).

SUPPLEMENTS—Radex (increases oxygen).

PERSONAL CARE—Satin Facial Scrub - Mint or juniper (dispenses nutrients & oxygen).

> *All essential oils increase the ability of the body to take oxygen to the cells and to push toxins out. The oils pick up more oxygen and take it to the site of discomfort.*

OXYGEN EXCHANGE— Tsuga (increases by opening and dilating respiratory tract).

PAIN: See ACHES AND PAINS.

PAINTING: Add one 15 ml. bottle of your favorite essential oil (or oil blend) to any five gallon bucket of paint. Stir vigorously, mixing well, and then either spray paint or paint by hand. This should eliminate the paint fumes and after-smell.

PALPITATIONS: See HEART.

PANCREAS: Coriander, ᶠcypress (for insufficiencies), dill, fleabane, lemon, <u>Raven</u>, <u>RC</u>, rosemary, <u>Thieves</u>.

STIMULANT FOR—Fleabane, ᶠhelichrysum.

SUPPORT—Cinnamon bark, coriander, <u>EndoFlex</u>, fennel, geranium.

TINCTURE—Royal Essence.

SUPPLEMENTS—Megazyme, Stevia, Thyromin, VitaGreen.

PANCREATITIS:

WEAKNESS—Lemon, marjoram.

PANIC: <u>Awaken</u>, bergamot, birch, fir, frankincense, <u>Gathering</u>, <u>Harmony</u>, Idaho balsam fir, lavender, marjoram, myrrh, Roman chamomile, rosemary, sandalwood, spruce, thyme, <u>Valor</u>, <u>White Angelica</u>, wintergreen, ylang ylang.

PARALYSIS: <u>Awaken</u>, cypress, geranium, ginger, helichrysum, juniper, lemongrass, nutmeg, peppermint, <u>Purification</u>, <u>Valor</u>.

BLEND—Combine 6 cypress, 15 geranium, 10 helichrysum, 5 juniper, 2 peppermint and V-6 Mixing Oil. May rejuvenate nerve damage up to 60%. Put on location and on feet.

SUPPLEMENTS—Support the body with Body Balance, VitaGreen, Super B, Master Formula His/Hers. When it starts to reverse there will be pain, apply <u>PanAway</u> on location and on feet.

TINCTURES—Royal Essence (replaces mineral loss).

O

P

PARASITES: See ANTI-PARASITIC and INTESTINAL PROBLEMS. Anise, clove, <u>Di-Tone</u>, ^Ffennel, hyssop, melaleuca, Mountain savory, mugwort (blend with thyme), ^Foregano, tangerine, ^Ftarragon, ^Fthyme. Apply oil on stomach and feet to help pass parasites.

> *ParaFree was specifically designed to help the body rid itself of parasites. The essential oils contained in this supplement are: Black cumin, anise, fennel, laurel, vetiver, nutmeg, melaleuca alternifolia, Idaho tansy, clove, and thyme.*
>
> *Since this product is to be used orally and contraindications do exist, one would be well advised to review the book, <u>Essential Oil Safety—A Guide for Health Care Professionals</u> by Robert Tisserand and Tony Balacs or <u>Aromatherapy for Health Professionals</u> by Shirley and Len Price.*

ANTI-PARASITIC—^FNutmeg.

INTESTINAL—^FLemon, ravensara, ^FRoman chamomile.

   SUPPLEMENTS—Cleansing Trio (ComforTone, Megazyme, and ICP), ParaFree.

   ***COMMENTS—Individuals have passed parasites within 12 hours using Di-Tone on stomach.

PARASYMPATHETIC NERVOUS SYSTEM: ^FLemongrass (regulates), ^Fmarjoram (increases tone of), <u>Peace & Calming</u>, <u>Valor</u>.

   DIFFUSION—See NEGATIVE IONS for a list of oils that ionize negatively when diffused to help stimulate the parasympathetic

> *The Parasympathetic Nervous System is responsible for preparing us for feeding, digestion, and rest by slowing the heart, contracting the bronchi, dilating the arteries, and stimulating the digestive system.*

nervous system. *(See the Autonomic Nervous System chart in the Science and Application section of the <u>Reference Guide for Essential Oils</u>.)*

PARATHYROID: <u>EndoFlex</u>. Apply over the thyroid gland at the bottom of the throat or on the parathyroid Vita Flex point on feet.

> *The **parathyroid gland** is responsible for secreting a hormone necessary for the metabolism of calcium and phosphorus. It is located near or within the posterior surface of the thyroid gland.*

   PERSONAL CARE—EndoBalance.

PARKINSON'S DISEASE: See BRAIN, PINEAL GLAND, PITUITARY GLAND, and ALZHEIMER'S DISEASE. <u>Acceptance</u>, basil, bergamot, <u>Clarity</u> (brain function), cypress (circulation), frankincense, <u>Gathering</u> (high in sesquiterpenes and in frequency), geranium, helichrysum, juniper, lavender, lemon, marjoram, nutmeg, orange, <u>Peace & Calming</u>, peppermint, rosemary, sandalwood, thyme, <u>Valor</u>, vitex.

SUPPLEMENTS—
Cleansing Trio
(ComforTone,
Megazyme, and ICP),
JuvaTone, Power Meal
(contains Choline

> *Frankincense and sandalwood contain sesquiterpenes which have the ability to go beyond the blood-brain barrier. See PINEAL GLAND and PITUITARY GLAND.*

which is beneficial for Parkinson's disease), Sulfurzyme.

TINCTURES—Chelex.

The following recipe has been used by Dr. Terry Friedmann of Paradise Valley, Arizona:

RECIPE #1—Use the Cleansing Trio (ComforTone, Megazyme, and ICP) for one week, then add JuvaTone and 10 VitaGreen along with it. Drink 10 glasses of distilled water daily. Take one dropper full of Chelex tincture two times a day and diffuse the oil of helichrysum and frankincense together one hour at night.

TO PREVENT—Keep liver and blood clean with JuvaTone and the Cleansing Trio (ComforTone, Megazyme, and ICP). Massage with helichrysum and sandalwood to help chelate metallics out of the body.

PAST: <u>Present Time</u> (helps to bring you into the present so you can go forward).

PEACE: Juniper (aromatic), lavender (aromatic), marjoram, <u>Peace & Calming</u>, <u>Release</u>, <u>Trauma Life</u>, ylang ylang.
FINDING—Tangerine (aromatic).
PROMOTE—Roman chamomile.
SUPPLEMENTS—Cleansing Trio (ComforTone, Megazyme, and ICP) and JuvaTone.

PELVIC PAIN SYNDROME: Bergamot, clove, geranium, ginger, nutmeg, thyme.

PERIODONTAL DISEASE: See GUM DISEASE.

P

PERSONAL GROWTH:
ELIMINATING BLOCKED—Helichrysum, frankincense.
PERSONALITY (MULTIPLE)—<u>Inner Child</u>, <u>SARA</u>, and <u>Sensation</u>.

PERSPIRATION: Petitgrain, <u>Purification</u>.
SUPPLEMENTS—Cleansing Trio (ComforTone, Megazyme, and ICP).

PEST TROUBLES: See INSECT. Ravensara.

pH BALANCE: See ACIDOSIS and ALKALOSIS.
  SUPPLEMENTS—
    AlkaLime (combats yeast and fungus overgrowth and preserves the body's proper pH balance), ComforTone (to help clean out the colon), JuvaTone (to clean the liver), Megazyme and Mineral Essence (if body is too alkaline), VitaGreen (brings blood back to an alkaline pH).
  PERSONAL CARE—
    Genesis Hand & Body Lotion (balances pH on skin).

> *According to Dr. Robert O. Young in his book, <u>One Sickness, One Disease, One Treatment</u>, "disease is an expression of pH." He believes that there is only one disease which is "the constant over-acidification of the blood and tissues which disturbs the central regulation of the human body, all of which is mainly the result of an inverted way of living and eating." All sickness and disease that leads to death begins with an over-acidification of the blood and tissues and culminates with yeast and fungus. A normal healthy body should have a pH of about 7.2. (The use of saliva and urine test strips will show a much lower pH level due to the protein present in the solution. Saliva and urine tests from a healthy body should be about 6.6 to 6.8.) To maintain this pH, our diet should consist of 80% alkaline foods to 20% acid foods. "In the healing of disease, when the individual is acidic, the higher the ratio of alkaline elements in the diet, the faster will be the recovery."*

PHARYNGITIS: See also RHINOPHARYNGITIS. Goldenrod.

PHLEBITIS: Cypress, geranium, grapefruit, ᶠhelichrysum (prevents), ᶠlavender, Roman chamomile, or <u>Valor</u>. Massage toward heart and wear support hose until healed, possibly two to three months. Use <u>Aroma Life</u> every morning and night. Do the Raindrop Technique on leg.

PIMPLES: Clary sage, frankincense, <u>Gentle Baby</u>, <u>ImmuPower</u> (pimples in ears), lavender, lemongrass, melaleuca, <u>Melrose</u>, <u>Purification</u>, <u>Raven</u>, ravensara, <u>RC</u>.
  *PERSONAL CARE—*Rose Ointment (apply over top of other oil(s) used to enhance and extend their effectiveness).

PINEAL GLAND:
  OPENS AND INCREASES OXYGEN—
    <u>Acceptance</u>, <u>Brain Power</u>, Canadian Red cedar cedarwood, <u>Forgiveness</u>, frankincense,

> *The **pineal gland** synthesizes a hormone called melatonin in periods of darkness. The pineal gland and melatonin are being studied for their roles in aging, sleep, and reproduction.*
>
> *The pineal gland is also involved in the process of creativity and planning things to do. If the pineal gland is not open, negative emotions will be attracted back to the aura.*

<u>Gathering</u>, <u>Harmony</u>, <u>Inspiration</u>, <u>Into the Future</u>, <u>Release</u>, sandalwood (increases oxygen), spruce, <u>Trauma Life</u>, <u>3 Wise Men</u> (same frequency as pineal).
   ***COMMENTS— *Just smelling the essential oils will increase the oxygen production, particularly around the pineal and pituitary glands, and will help increase the secretion of anti-bodies, endorphins, and neuro-transmitters.*

PITUITARY: See ENDOCRINE SYSTEM.
   SUPPLEMENTS—Ultra Young (a spray neutriceutical which contains ingredients that are necessary for stimulating the pituitary gland into producing the human growth hormone (hGH) and allowing the body to utilize it).
   BALANCES—Geranium, ylang ylang. Apply to forehead, back of neck, and Vita Flex points on big toes.
   INCREASES OXYGEN— <u>3 Wise Men</u>, <u>Acceptance</u>, <u>Brain Power</u>, frankincense, <u>Forgiveness</u>, <u>Gathering</u>, <u>Harmony</u>, <u>Inspiration</u>, <u>Into the Future</u>, sandalwood, <u>Trauma Life</u>. Apply to the

> *The **pituitary gland** is located at the base of the brain and is considered to be the master gland because its secretions stimulate the other endocrine glands. The pituitary has an anterior and a posterior lobe. The anterior lobe secretes the human growth hormone (stimulates overall body growth), adrenocorticotropic hormone (controls steroid hormone secretion by the adrenal cortex), thyrotropic hormone (stimulates the activity of the thyroid gland), and three gonadotropic hormones (control growth and reproductive activity of the ovaries and testes). The posterior lobe secretes antidiuretic hormone and oxytocin. The antidiuretic hormone causes water retention by the kidneys. Oxytocin stimulates the mammary glands to release milk and also causes uterine contractions. An overactive pituitary during childhood can cause a child to be extremely tall while an underactive pituitary can result in the opposite.*
>
> ***Oils containing sesquiterpenes are especially effective in oxygenating the pineal and pituitary glands.*** *Frankincense and sandalwood are both high in sesquiterpenes. Blends containing both of these oils are: 3 Wise Men, Acceptance, Brain Power, Forgiveness, Gathering, Harmony, Inspiration, Into the Future, Trauma Life.*

forehead, back of neck, and Vita Flex points on big toes. Can also rub a couple drops of oil between hands, cup over nose and mouth, and breathe deeply (see COMMENT under PINEAL above).

PLAGUE: <u>Abundance</u>, ᶠclove, <u>Thieves</u> (annihilates bacteria).

PLEURISY: See LUNGS or ANTI-BACTERIAL. ᶠCypress, ᶠthyme.

PMS: See HORMONAL IMBALANCE. Angelica, anise, bergamot, ᶠClary sage, Exodus II, fennel, geranium, grapefruit, jasmine, lavender (aromatic), nutmeg, Peace & Calming, Roman chamomile, ᶠtarragon.

APATHETIC-TIRED-LISTLESS PMS—Bergamot, fennel, grapefruit, Roman chamomile.

> *BATH & SHOWER GELS*—Dragon Time Bath & Shower Gel.

> *BLEND*—10 drops Dragon Time and 4 drops basil. Rub blend around ankles, lower back, and lower stomach. Use before and during cycle.

IRRITABLE PMS—Bergamot, Clary sage, nutmeg, Roman chamomile.

> *MASSAGE OILS*—Before and during cycle, combine 10 drops Dragon Time with 4 basil and rub around ankles, lower back and lower stomach.

> *SUPPLEMENTS*—Essential Omegas, Exodus, PD 80/20, Prenolone/Prenolone+. Three times a day one week before cycle starts, take 2 droppers full of F.H.S. (available through Creer Labs 801-465-5423) in water. One week after the cycle, take Master Formula Hers four times a day and 6 VitaGreen a day. Also FemiGen (for PMS)—take 2 FemiGen three times a day before period, start again two days after cycle. Lady Love and Lady Flash (available through Creer Labs 801-465-5423).

VIOLENT AGGRESSIVE PMS—Bergamot, geranium, nutmeg.

> *SUPPLEMENTS*—Essential Omegas.

WEEPING-DEPRESSION PMS—Bergamot, Clary sage, geranium, nutmeg.

> *SUPPLEMENTS*—Essential Omegas.

PNEUMONIA: See RESPIRATORY SYSTEM (comments and recipe #1). Cajeput, eucalyptus, Exodus II, frankincense, ImmuPower (on spine), lavender, lemon, melaleuca, *Melaleuca ericifolia*, oregano, Raven (on back and feet), ravensara, Thieves (on feet) and thyme are good to use as compresses.

> *SUPPLEMENTS*—Exodus, Master Formula His/Hers, Ultra Young.
> One or more of the following can be used with great effect:
> 1. RC on chest.
> 2. Put 15 drops of RC in 2 cups of hot water in a bowl, wet towel, ring out, and put on chest with a dry towel on top.
> 3. Put 4 drops of RC or eucalyptus in ½ cup hot water, inhale steam deeply.
> 4. Raven in rectum, RC on chest and back (reverse each night).

> ***COMMENTS**—Refer to the chapter entitled "How to Use - The Personal Usage Reference" in the Essential Oils Desk Reference under "Pneumonia - Emphysema" for some excellent blend recipes and supplement recommendations.*

POISON OAK-IVY: Lavender, Melrose, Roman chamomile.

> *PERSONAL CARE*—Rose Ointment.

POLLUTION: See PURIFICATION. Purification.
   AIR—Lemon, peppermint, Purification.
   CIGARETTE SMOKE—Purification.
   WATER—Lemon, peppermint, Purification.
      SUPPLEMENTS—Radex.

POLYPS: See also NOSE:POLYPS. Di-Tone, Exodus II, peppermint, spikenard, and others
      with strong anti-bacterial properties (See ANTI-BACTERIAL).
      SUPPLEMENTS—ComforTone, Coral Sea (highly bio-available calcium, contains 58
         trace minerals), Exodus, Master Formula His/Hers, Megazyme, Super Cal.
   COMMENTS—*In two separate articles published in 1998, bacterial infection was
         found to exist when polyps were present. In the case of colorectal (intestinal)
         polyps, E. coli and similar bacteria were found to be adhering to the walls of
         the large intestine, and even partially penetrating the intestinal mucosa
         (Gastroenterology 1998; 115: 281-286). In the case of gastric polyps (small
         growths in the stomach lining), the Helicobacter pylori bacteria was found, and
         when eradicated, the polyps disappeared in 71% of the patients within a 12 to
         15 month period (Annals of Internal Medicine 1998; 129: 712-715).*

POSITIVE FEELINGS: Acceptance, Abundance, Envision, Forgiveness, Idaho tansy, Joy,
      Motivation, Live with Passion, 3 Wise Men (releases negative memory/trauma
      and reinforces positive feelings which creates greater spiritual awareness).

POSITIVE IONS: When
      dispersed into the air
      through a cool-air
      nebulizing diffuser, the
      following oils ionize
      positively: Cajeput,
      clove, cypress,
      eucalyptus,
      frankincense,
      helichrysum, juniper,

> *Positive ions are produced by electronic equipment and
> are typically found in man-made environments. They
> help stimulate the sympathetic nervous system, necessary
> for recovering, strengthening, and energizing. However,
> an over-abundance of positive ions can lead to stress
> and agitation. The diffusion of the oils listed under
> NEGATIVE IONS can help balance the ions and help
> produce a more stress free environment.*

P

   marjoram, *Melaleuca quinquenervia*, palmarosa, pine, ravensara, rosemary,
   thyme, ylang ylang.

POTASSIUM DEFICIENCY:
      SUPPLEMENTS—
         Essential Manna,
         Master Formula
         His/Hers, Mineral
         Essence, Thyromin.

> *Potassium is important for a healthy nervous system and
> a regular heart rhythm. It works with sodium to control
> the body's water balance and regulates the transfer of
> nutrients to the cells.*

POTENTIAL: <u>Acceptance</u>, <u>Awaken</u> (realize our highest potential), <u>Believe</u> (release our unlimited potential), <u>Gathering</u>, <u>White Angelica</u> (greater awareness of one's potential).

POWER: <u>Sacred Mountain</u>, <u>Surrender</u> (calming and relaxing to dominant personalities), <u>Valor</u>.

POWER SURGES: See HOT FLASHES.

PRAYER: Frankincense, <u>Inspiration</u>, <u>Sacred Mountain</u>.

PREGNANCY: Elemi, <u>Gentle Baby</u> (relieves stress during pregnancy; can also be used by fathers to relieve stress during delivery), geranium, grapefruit, jasmine, lavender, Roman chamomile, tangerine, ylang ylang.

    SUPPLEMENTS—PD 80/20, Prenolone/Prenolone+, ProMist, Thyromin (use before, during, and after).

    ANXIETY/TENSION—<u>Into the Future</u> (help let go of fear and trauma), <u>Present Time</u> (help mother focus on giving birth).

    BLEND—Add 10 drops lavender, 10 orange, 2 marjoram, 2 cedarwood, 1 Roman chamomile to 4 oz.

PREGNANCY SAFETY DATA

<u>Avoid During Pregnancy</u>

Single Oils: Basil, birch, calamus, cassia, cinnamon bark, hyssop, Idaho tansy, lavandin, rosemary, sage, tarragon.

Blends: Di-Tone, Dragon Time, Exodus II, Grounding, Mister.

Other: Estro, Exodus, FemiGen, Femalin, ParaFree, Protec,

<u>Use Cautiously During Pregnancy</u>

Single Oils: Angelica, cedarwood, chamomile (German/Blue), cistus, citronella, Clary sage, clove bud, cumin (Black), cypress, davana, fennel, laurel, marjoram, Mountain savory, myrrh, nutmeg, peppermint, rose, spearmint, vetiver, yarrow.

Blends: Aroma Siez, Clarity, Harmony, ImmuPower, Relieve It, Thieves.

Other: Prenolone/Prenolone+, ComforTone, Megazyme, ArthroTune, Dragon Time Massage Oil.

It was very difficult to compile a list of oils and products to be avoided during pregnancy. Each aromatologist has a different opinion. We feel that an oil that is unsafe is an oil that has been adulterated or one that is used improperly. Oils that are diluted, applied externally and in moderation should not create a problem. This list is a compilation of the safety data contained in aromatherapy books written by the following authors: Ann Berwick, Julia Lawless, Shirley & Len Price, Jeanne Rose, Robert Tisserand, and Tony Balacs.

sweet almond oil or V-6 Mixing Oil. Use as a massage oil or in bath water.
    SUPPLEMENTS—PD 80/20, Prenolone/Prenolone+, ProMist.
BABY (Newborn)—Frankincense (1 drop on crown for protection), myrrh (on remaining
    umbilical cord and around navel to protect from infection), <u>Valor</u> (1 drop - divide
    between both feet & 1-2 drops rubbed up spine to help ensure proper alignment).
BREASTS—Fennel (tone), Roman chamomile (sore nipples).
CONCEPTION—Do a proper cleansing for one year before. May want to start with the
    Master Cleanser (See CLEANSING for more information).
    SUPPLEMENTS— Cleansing Trio (especially ComforTone for the colon and ICP for
    the intestines), JuvaTone (cleanses liver).
CONSTIPATION— ComforTone can be taken during pregnancy as long as you don't get
    diarrhea. Diarrhea can cause cramping which could bring on labor.
    SUPPLEMENTS— JuvaTone (helps change genetics in the colon and purge the liver),
    Megazyme, Mint Condition.
DELIVERY—Clary sage, <u>Forgiveness</u>, <u>Gentle Baby</u>, <u>Harmony</u>, lavender (stimulates
    circulation, calming, antibiotic, anti-inflammatory, antiseptic), nutmeg (balances
    hormones, calms the central nervous system, alleviates anxiety, increases
    circulation, and good for blood supply), <u>Valor</u> (align mother's hips; apply along
    inside and bottom of each foot, then have someone hold feet–right palm to right
    foot and left palm to left foot–to balance energy flows; rub a couple drops along
    newborn's spine for alignment).
    ****CAUTION—Nutmeg is generally non-toxic, non-irritant, and non-sensitizing.
    However, large doses may cause nausea, stupor, and tachycardia. Use in
    moderation and with great care during pregnancy. See the safety data about
    nutmeg in the APPENDIX of this book.*
    AVOID EPISIOTOMY— <u>Gentle Baby</u> or geranium (neat or added to olive oil;
    massage perineum).
    BLEND—8 drops geranium, 5 drops lavender, 1 oz. V-6 Mixing Oil. Prepare three
    weeks before delivery and rub on perineum three times a day. One week before
    delivery, prepare same blend and add 5 drops fennel. Continue applying three
    times daily.
    DIFFUSE—<u>Hope</u>, <u>Joy</u>, <u>Motivation</u>, <u>Live with Passion</u>, <u>Peace & Calming</u>.
    UTERUS—Tone uterus with 1-3 drops of Clary sage around ankles (one woman
    dilated and had her baby in 1 ½ hours), <u>Dragon Time</u>, fennel, <u>Gathering</u>, sage.
    TRANSITION—Basil.
EARLY LABOR—Lavender (rub on tummy to stop).
ENERGY—Put equal portions of Roman chamomile, geranium, and lavender in V-6
    Mixing Oil.
HEMORRHAGING—Helichrysum and <u>Gentle Baby</u> together on lower back (prevent).
HIGH BLOOD PRESSURE—<u>Aroma Life</u> (heart). Avoid using hyssop, rosemary, sage,
    thyme, and possibly peppermint.
KEEP BABY IN BIRTH CANAL—<u>Gentle Baby</u>.

P

> ***COMMENTS***—*One mother would rub* <u>Gentle Baby</u> *on her little fingers and little toes when contracting. The she would squeeze the sides of her little fingers while someone else squeezed her little toes. This was repeated during contractions until the baby decided to stay in the birth canal.*

LABOR (during)—Clary sage (kick labor into gear; some have combined with fennel), <u>Gentle Baby</u> (apply to ankles and hands when labor starts), <u>Into the Future</u> (to help move past fear and trauma), jasmine (speed up contractions), <u>Present Time</u> (to help mother focus).

> *BLEND*—(**Use only when ready to deliver**). 2 oz. V-6 Mixing Oil, 8 drops Clary sage, 8 drops lavender, 8 drops jasmine. May be useful when trying to induce labor or augment a slow, lazy labor.
>
> PAIN—<u>PanAway</u> (apply to lower back and tummy area).
>
> ***COMMENTS***—*Refer to the chapter entitled "How to Use - The Personal Usage Reference" in the* <u>Essential Oils Desk Reference</u> *under "Pregnancy" for a wonderful blend to use during labor.*

LABOR (post)—Geranium, lavender.

> ***COMMENTS***—*Lavender is calming and has a slight analgesic effect. It also stimulates circulation, which is great for both mother and baby, and has anti-inflammatory and antiseptic properties. Geranium is one of the best oils to stimulate circulation, which in turn facilitates easy breathing. It has a contractive effect and helps pull together dilated tissues, so it is healing for the uterus and endometrium after the birth. Geranium is also an anti-depressant and is known for its uplifting effect* (<u>Alternative Medicine—A Definitive Guide</u>, *pp. 806-7).*

LACTATION—See MILK PRODUCTION.

MASTITIS (breast infection)—<u>Citrus Fresh</u> (with lavender), <u>Exodus II</u>, lavender, tangerine.

> *BLEND*—Equal amounts of lavender and tangerine. Dilute with some V-6 Mixing Oil and apply to breasts and under arms twice a day.
>
> *SUPPLEMENTS*—Exodus, ImmuGel.

MILK PRODUCTION—Clary sage (bring in milk), fennel or basil (increase), peppermint with cold compress (decrease). ***Caution: Fennel should not be used for more than 10 days as it will excessively increase flow through the urinary tract.***

> *SUPPLEMENTS*—Essential Manna, Power Meal, VitaGreen.

MISCARRIAGE (after)—Frankincense, geranium, grapefruit, lavender (may help prevent), Roman chamomile, spruce (2 drops on solar plexus).

> *SUPPLEMENTS*— JuvaTone, Cleansing Trio (ComforTone, Megazyme, and ICP).

MORNING SICKNESS— Calamus, <u>Di-Tone</u> (1-2 drops in water and sip or 1-2 drops around the navel), ginger, <u>M-Grain</u>, peppermint. Apply on or behind ears, down jaw bone, over stomach as a compress, on Vita Flex points on feet, on hands (rub together and smell), or put a drop on your pillow. Can also put 4 to 6 drops of

spearmint in a bowl of boiled and cooled water and place on floor beside the bed
overnight to keep stomach calm.

SUPPLEMENTS—
ComforTone,
Megazyme, Mint
Condition.

ON CHAKRAS—Awaken
(after pregnancy).

PLACENTA—Basil (has been

*Caution: Although Di-Tone is recommended for
morning sickness, it contains some oils which some
aromatologists strongly discourage using. It may have a
lot to do with purity. Use at your own risk. I did and it
worked for me!*

use to help retain), jasmine (helps expulsion).

POSTPARTUM DEPRESSION (Baby Blues)—See FEMALE PROBLEMS. Bergamot,
Clary sage, fennel, frankincense, geranium, Gentle Baby, grapefruit, Harmony,
Hope, jasmine, Joy, lavender, myrrh, nutmeg (use in moderation), orange, and
patchouly, Valor, vetiver, White Angelica.

SUPPLEMENTS—Essential Manna, Essential Omegas, ImmuPro.

SELF LOVE—Joy.

SKIN ELASTICITY—Aroma Life, Clarity, Dragon Time, Gentle Baby, Mister, M-Grain,
Relieve It. *Again, many of these blends contain oils that many aromatologists
feel should be avoided or used with caution during pregnancy.*

STRETCH MARKS—Gentle Baby (every day on tummy).

TOXEMIA (extremely high protein in urine)—Aroma Life.

PRIDE: Humility, peppermint (dispels).

PROCRASTINATION: Acceptance, Envision (emotional support), Magnify Your Purpose
(empowering and uplifting), Motivation (easier to take action, gets you out of the
mood of procrastination).

PROGESTERONE: EndoFlex, Grounding. *Progesterone is made from cholesterol and
helps to protect against cancer.*
PERSONAL CARE—PD 80/20, Prenolone/Prenolone+, ProMist.

PROSPERITY: Abundance, bergamot, cinnamon bark (aromatic), cypress.

PROSTATE: EndoFlex, helichrysum, juniper, Mister, yarrow.
PERSONAL CARE—EndoBalance, PD 80/20, Prenolone/Prenolone+, Protec
(designed to accompany the nightlong retention enema, it helps buffer the prostate
from inflammation, enlargement, and tumor activity).
SUPPLEMENTS—CortiStop (Men's), Master Formula HIS, ProGen (an herbal
support for the male glandular system; it may prevent prostate atrophy and
malfunction and protect men from prostate cancer).

DECONGESTANT—ᶠCypress, <u>Di-Tone</u>, <u>Dragon Time</u>, <u>Mister</u> (decongests prostate and
balances hormones), myrrh, ᶠmyrtle, sage, ᶠspruce, yarrow. Apply oils to inside
ankle and heel. <u>ImmuPower</u> on lower spine and in rectum.

   BLEND #1—Combine 15 frankincense and 5 <u>Mister</u> with 2 tsp. V-6 Mixing Oil.
   Insert blend into rectum with bulb syringe or pipet and retain throughout night.

   BLEND #2—Combine 10 frankincense and 10 lavender with 2 tsp. V-6 Mixing Oil.
   Insert blend into rectum with bulb syringe and retain throughout night.

   BLEND #3—Combine 10 frankincense, 5 myrrh, and 3 sage with 2 tsp. V-6 Mixing
   Oil. Insert blend into rectum with bulb syringe or pipet and retain through night.

ENLARGEMENT—Mix 10 drops of Mister with 1 Tbs. of V-6 Mixing oil and insert in
rectum and retain overnight. May also apply either sage, fennel, or yarrow to
posterior, scrotum, ankles, lower back, and bottom of feet.

INFLAMED—Cypress, lavender, thyme (<u>Alternative Medicine—A Definitive Guide</u>, p.
742).

STRENGTHEN—PD 80/20, Prenolone/Prenolone+, ProGen, Protec.

THOUGHT PATTERNS AND EMOTIONS—The prostate represents the masculine
principle. Men's PROSTATE problems have a lot to do with self-worth and also
believing that as they get older they become less of a man. Ideas may be in
conflict about sex, refusing to let go of the past, fear of aging, feeling like
throwing in the towel. May be feeling inadequate in sexual role, may be holding
onto unpleasant memories of previous relationships, or feeling unfulfilled in love.

PROSTATE CANCER: See
CANCER.

> *Prostate Cancer may be from repressed anger. Visualize
> the prostate healing, don't put energy into the cancer
> because it feeds the problem.*

PROTECTION: (from negative
influence) Clove
(aromatic), cypress,
fennel (protection from psychic attack), fir (aromatic), frankincense, <u>Harmony</u>,
<u>Joy</u>, <u>Sacred Mountain</u>, <u>Valor</u>, <u>White Angelica</u>.

PROTEIN: Carbonated water
prevents absorption of
protein. Protein
deficiency causes
Hypoglycemia.

> *A **protein deficiency**, either from the lack of protein
> intake or from the inability to digest it, creates an acidic
> pH in the blood. A high acidity level in the blood creates
> an environment for cell mutation and disease. See
> ACIDOSIS.*

   SUPPLEMENTS—Body
   Balance, Megazyme,
   Polyzyme (provides enzymes necessary for proper breakdown and digestion of
   protein), Power Meal (pre-digested protein), Sulfurzyme (helps digest protein),
   VitaGreen.

PSORIASIS: Bergamot, cajeput, cedarwood, ᶠhelichrysum, lavender, melaleuca, patchouly, Roman chamomile, ᶠthyme.

> *BLEND*—Combine 2-3 drops each of Roman chamomile and lavender for use as ointment for pH Balance.

> *PERSONAL CARE*—Rose Ointment (helps soften cracking skin), Lavender Volume Hair & Scalp Wash and Lavender Volume Nourishing Rinse for psoriasis.

PSYCHIC: Cinnamon bark (awareness), fennel (protect from attack), lemongrass. Diffuse.

> CENTERS—Elemi (balances, strengthens, fortifies).

PUBERTY: Fleabane (stimulates retarded puberty).

PULMONARY: See LUNGS.

PURGE: See CLEANSING.

PURIFICATION: <u>Abundance</u>, <u>Acceptance</u>, cedarwood, <u>En-R-Gee</u>, eucalyptus (aromatic), fennel (aromatic), lemon (aromatic), lemongrass (aromatic), melaleuca (aromatic), orange (aromatic), <u>Purification</u>, sage.

> AIR—Lemon (diffuse or add to spray bottle of water to deodorize and sterilize the air).

> CIGARETTE SMOKE—<u>Purification</u>.

> DISHES—2 drops of <u>Melrose</u> or lemon in the dish water for sparkling dishes and a great smelling kitchen.

> WATER—ᶠLemon, peppermint.

> CLOTHING—Adding oils to washer or dryer decreases bacteria, improves hygiene, and clothes have a fresh, clean smell.

> FURNITURE—A few drops of fir, lemon, or spruce oil on a dust cloth or 10 drops in a spray bottle work well for polishing, cleaning and disinfecting furniture, kitchens and bathrooms. You may also consider adding <u>Abundance</u> to increase your abundance. Lemon oil for dissolving gum and grease. <u>Purification</u> for mold and fungus. If you don't have a diffuser, you may want to add 10-12 drops of <u>Purification</u> to 8 oz of distilled water in a spray bottle and spray into the air.

PUS: See INFECTION and ANTI-INFECTIOUS. Melaleuca is useful in healing pus-filled wounds.

RADIATION: See CANCER. *Melaleuca quinquenervia*, <u>Melrose</u>, patchouly. May apply on location, bottom of feet, kidneys, thyroid, and diffuse.

> COMPUTER, T.V., MICROWAVE—Fill a wooden bowl half full of peat moss and half full of hazel nuts and 30 drops of <u>Melrose</u> then set on the appliance. Using an equipment diode may also help.

***COMMENTS—*Melrose* may help protect the body during radiation treatments if used 10 days before, during, and 10 days after. **Do not use on the day of radiation treatment**. According to Dr. Pénoël, massage with *Melaleuca quinquenervia* helps to prevent radiation side effects. Remember to keep all massage light and away from trauma area. Use with Radex.*

Valerie Woorwood suggests Recipe #1 below to be used at least two to three weeks before the radiation treatments begin. Don't use it during the treatment, but use it between treatments and for at least a month after your last treatment.

RECIPE #1—10 lavender, 5 German chamomile, 5 Roman chamomile, 5 tagetes, 5 yarrow, and 2 tsp. of vinca infused oil. Massage the entire torso, including the back and abdomen and the trauma area. This treatment will not conflict with the doctor's treatment. Note: Vinca is made from periwinkle which is known to contain alkaloids that in some cases can suppress the cancerous cells. (The Complete Book of Essential Oils & Aromatherapy, pp. 249-50).

RADIATION BURNS—Recipe #1 (in comment box above).

SIDE-EFFECTS–Recipe #2.

TREATMENTS—Radiation treatments can produce tremendous toxicity within the liver. Cut down on the use of oils with high *phenol* content to prevent increasing the liver toxicity.

The following Dr. Westlake formula utilizes Bach Flower Remedies to counteract the side-effects of cancer patients who have received radiation therapy.

RECIPE #2—"Mix 3.5 grams of sea salt with 100 mils of distilled water. Put into a 10 ml dropper bottle 2 drops of each of the following Bach Flower Remedies: Cherry Plum, Gentian, Rock Rose, Star of Bethlehem, Vine, Walnut and Wild Oat, and top up the bottle with the sea salt solution. Take 2 drops, three or four times a day, or add 10 to 15 drops to a bath. People who have been exposed to radiation sources, such as X-rays, cobalt therapy or other medical radiation therapies, or have been contaminated in an escape from a nuclear power station or who regularly use office or domestic equipment that gives out low-level radiation, such as color television sets, microwaves, and visual display units, would do well to use this formula in a bath once or twice a week." (Aromatherapy—An A to Z by Patricia Davis, p. 269)

CHEMOTHERAPY—Because of the greater amounts of toxicity produced, even greater care should be taken to limit the use of oils with high *phenol* content.

WEEPING WOUNDS FROM— Melaleuca, oregano, thyme.

SUPPLEMENTS—Radex (prevents build up). The apple pectin that is contained in ICP helps remove unwanted metals and toxins. It is also valuable in radiation therapy.

RASHES: Elemi (allergic), lavender, ʳmelaleuca, <u>Melrose</u>, palmarosa, <u>Release</u> (on Vita Flex points of feet), Roman chamomile. Red spots on body may indicate a Biotin deficiency; take Super C. *If the rash occurs from application of oils to the skin, it may be due to the oils reacting with accumulated synthetic chemicals (toxins) that are trapped in the fatty layers of the skin. Take the following steps: 1) Try diluting the oils first (1-3 drops of oil to ½ tsp. V-6 Mixing Oil), 2) reduce the number of oils used with each application (use oils one at a time), 3) reduce the amount of oils (number of drops) used, 4) reduce the frequency of application (more time between applications). Drinking pure (steam distilled) water helps promote the elimination of accumulated toxins from the body. Initiating programs to cleanse the bowels and blood will also help remove accumulated toxins and reduce the possible recurrences of the rash. If the rashes persist, discontinue use of the oils and consult your health care professional.*

PERSONAL CARE—KidScents Tender Tush, Rose Ointment.

***COMMENTS—*Dr. Friedmann had a patient who had a rash for three years on the side of the face and arms and the eyes were weeping. They had gone to five physicians for treatments and had no success. Dr. Friedmann did the following: 1) Did a culture of the eye and face and determined that the patient had staphylococcus. 2) Had the patient apply <u>Melrose</u> and lavender alternately morning and night. 3) Had the patient take Mineral Essence and Colloidal Essence (a colloidal silver product). After a short period of time, the patient's face and eyes totally cleared up and their arms were healing*

RAYNAUD'S DISEASE (feel cold; hands and feet turn blue): <u>Aroma Life</u>, clove, cypress, fennel, geranium, helichrysum, lavender, nutmeg, rosemary.

REFRESHING:

ESSENTIAL WATERS (HYDROSOLS)—Canadian Red Cedar (exhilarating), Peppermint, Spearmint. Spray into air or directly on face (don't spray directly in eyes or ears) diffuse using the Essential Mist Diffuser.

REGENERATING: Helichrysum, lavender, <u>Melrose</u>, or equal parts of <u>Thieves</u> and V-6 Mixing Oil.

SUPPLEMENTS—Body Balance, ImmuneTune, Power Meal.

REJECTION: <u>Acceptance</u>, <u>Joy</u>.

RELATIONSHIPS:

BATH & SHOWER GELS—Sensation Bath & Shower Gel contains oils used by Cleopatra to enhance love and increase the desire to be close to that someone special.

MASSAGE OILS—Sensation creates an exotic arousal; increases sexual desire. The fragrance creates a peaceful and harmonious feeling that is helpful in easing relationship stress.

PERSONAL CARE—Sensation Hand & Body Lotion.

ENHANCING—Ylang ylang.

ENDING RELATIONSHIPS—Basil.

RELAXATION: Citrus Fresh, Clary sage, frankincense, Gentle Baby, geranium, jasmine, lavender, Peace & Calming, Roman chamomile, sandalwood, Trauma Life (calming), ylang ylang.

BATH & SHOWER GELS—Evening Peace Bath & Shower Gel.

ESSENTIAL WATERS (HYDROSOLS)—Basil (relaxing to muscles), Lavender (soothing and calming), Melissa, Western Red Cedar. Spray into air or directly on face (don't spray directly in eyes or ears) or diffuse using the Essential Mist Diffuser.

DIFFUSION—See NEGATIVE IONS for oils that produce negative ions when diffused to help promote relaxation. Lavender, Peace & Calming.

MASSAGE OILS—Relaxation Massage Oil.

SENSE OF—Ylang ylang.

BLEND—1 bergamot, 2 lavender, 2 marjoram, and 4 rosewood.

RELEASE NEGATIVE TRAUMA: Inspiration, Release.

RESENTMENT: Forgiveness, Harmony, Humility, Idaho tansy, jasmine, Release, rose, White Angelica.

RESPIRATORY SYSTEM:

Abundance, anise, basil (restorative), bergamot (infections), cajeput (infections), Canadian Red cedar, Clary sage (strengthens), clove, Di-Tone, EndoFlex, ᶠeucalyptus (general stimulant and

> *Vita Flex points for the bronchial tubes are located between the bones on the tops of the feet. The sinuses are located at the base of the middle three toes on the bottom of the feet. One of the most effective ways of handling a respiratory problem is by doing rectal implants. There is a nerve that goes from the rectum to the lungs. The oils will travel in this manner in 3 seconds. The next best method is through inhalation.*

strengthens), *Eucalyptus radiata*, fennel (stimulant), ᶠfir (opens respiratory tract, increases oxygenation, decongests and balances), frankincense, goldenrod (discharges mucus), helichrysum (relieves), hyssop (opens respiratory system and discharges toxins and mucus), JuvaFlex, ledum (supports), lemon, marjoram (calming), melaleuca, *Melaleuca ericifolia*, Melrose, ᶠmyrtle, oregano (antiseptic), ᶠpeppermint (aid), pine (dilates and opens bronchial tract), RC, Raven (all respiratory problems), ravensara, rosemary verbenon, Sacred Mountain (soothing), ^Fspearmint, spruce, Thieves, tsuga (dilates and opens tract).

RECIPE #1—Dr. Young alternates the oils of Raven and RC in rectal implants. He uses 20 drops of the oil in 1 Tbs. of V-6 Mixing Oil and implants it rectally using a pipet (or glass dropper).

BLEND #1—3 birch/wintergreen, 8 eucalyptus, 6 fir, 6 frankincense, 1 peppermint, 10 ravensara and 1 oz. V-6 Mixing Oil.

BLEND #2—3 German chamomile, 10 fir, and 5 lemon.

ESSENTIAL WATERS (HYDROSOLS)—Canadian Red Cedar (supportive), Eucalyptus (soothing), Mountain Essence (enhanced respiratory action). Diffuse into air using the Essential Mist Diffuser.

SUPPLEMENTS—ImmuGel, Super C.

ACUTE—RC and Raven, Thieves.

BLEND #3—5 eucalyptus, 8 frankincense, 6 lemon, and 1 oz. V-6 Mixing Oil. Do a hot compress on chest and rub neat on bottom of feet under toes.

BLEND #4—3 tsp. *Eucalyptus radiata* (or any oil from the Myrtaceae botanical family), 1 tsp. Canadian Balsam fir (or any conifer oil). Apply to Vita Flex points on the feet, add to V-6 Mixing Oil and apply to chest area, or diffuse.

RESTLESSNESS: Acceptance, angelica, basil, bergamot, cedarwood, frankincense, Gathering, geranium, Harmony, Inspiration, Joy, lavender, orange, Peace & Calming, rose, rosewood, Sacred Mountain, spruce, Trauma Life, valerian, Valor, ylang ylang.

RHEUMATIC FEVER: Ginger, ^Ftarragon. Both help with pain.

RHEUMATISM: See ARTHRITIS.

RHINITIS: Basil.

> *Rhinitis is an inflammation of the nasal mucus membrane.*

RHINOPHARYNGITIS:
^FRavensara.

RINGWORM: See ANTI-FUNGAL. Geranium, lavender, melaleuca (Tea Tree), Melrose, myrrh, peppermint, Purification, RC, Raven, rosemary verbenon, thyme.

BLEND #1—2 lavender, 2 melaleuca, and 2 thyme, OR

BLEND #2—3 melaleuca, 2 peppermint, and 3 spearmint.

Apply 1-2 drops of blend (#'s 1 or 2 above) or Melrose on ringworm three times a day for ten days. Then mix 30 drops of melaleuca (Tea Tree) or Melrose with 2 Tbs. V-6 Mixing Oil and use daily until ringworm is gone.

MASSAGE OILS—Ortho Ease or Ortho Sport.

PERSONAL CARE—Rose Ointment.

ROMANTIC TOUCHES: Jasmine, patchouly, <u>Sensation</u>, ylang ylang; use these in small amounts.
   BATH & SHOWER GELS— Sensation Bath & Shower Gel.
   MASSAGE OILS—Sensation Massage Oil.
   PERSONAL CARE— Sensation Hand & Body Lotion.

ROSACEA (Acne Rosacea):
   Lavender. Dilute with V-6 Mixing Oil and apply daily after washing face with Orange Blossom Facial Wash and before applying Sandalwood Moisture Creme or Sandalwood Toner. Can also add extra lavender oil to Sandalwood Moisture Creme or Sandalwood Toner

> *Rosacea is a chronic, acne-like condition of the facial skin which typically first appears as a flushing or subtle redness on the cheeks, nose, chin or forehead that comes and goes. Left untreated, the condition progresses and the redness becomes more persistent, bumps and pimples appear, and small dilated blood vessels may become visible. In some cases the eyes may be affected, causing them to be irritated and bloodshot and, according to some doctors, can even cause blindness. In the more advanced cases, the nose becomes red and swollen from excess tissue. Currently, this condition can only be controlled.*

   PERSONAL CARE—Orange Blossom Facial Wash, Sandalwood Moisture Creme, Sandalwood Toner.

SACREDNESS: <u>Sacred Mountain</u> (sacred place of protection within self).

SADNESS: <u>Acceptance</u>, helichrysum, <u>Inspiration</u>, <u>Joy</u> (over heart), onycha (combine with rose in Massage Oil Base for calming/uplifting massage), orange (overcome), <u>3 Wise Men</u>, <u>Valor</u>. Wear as cologne or diffuse.

SAINT VITUS DANCE (Chorea):
   BLEND—5 <u>Aroma Siez</u>, 3 basil, 6 juniper, and 8 peppermint.

SANITATION: Citronella, lemongrass, <u>Purification</u>.

SCABIES: Bergamot, laurel, lavender and peppermint, pine, <u>Thieves</u> (needs to be diluted).

SCARRING: Frankincense (prevents), <u>Gentle Baby</u>, geranium, helichrysum (reduces), hyssop (prevents), ᶠlavender (burns), <u>Melrose</u>, rose (prevents), rosehip (reduces).
   PERSONAL CARE—Satin Body Lotion (moisturizes skin and promotes healing).
   BLEND #1—Equal parts helichrysum and lavender mixed with liquid lecithin.
   BLEND #2—3 rosemary, 15 rosewood, and 1 ¾ oz. Hazel Nut Oil.

> *BLEND #3*—6 lavender, 3 patchouly, 4 rosewood, and Vitamin E Oil.

PREVENT FORMATION—Frankincense, helichrysum, hyssop, myrrh, rose, rosehip seed
>   oil.

> *BLEND #4*—5 helichrysum, 2 patchouly, 4 lemongrass, 3 lavender in ¼ to ½ oz. V-6
>   Mixing Oil or Massage Oil Base.

> *BLEND #5*—Equal parts lavender, lemongrass, and geranium.

SCHMIDT'S SYNDROME: See
      ADDISON'S
      DISEASE. En-R-Gee,
      EndoFlex, Joy, nutmeg
      (increases energy;
      supports adrenal
      glands), sage (combine with nutmeg).

> *Schmidt's Syndrome is the same as Addison's Disease with the additional problem of low thyroid hormone production.*

> *SUPPLEMENTS*—ImmuPro, Master Formula His/Hers (3 times a day), Mineral
>   Essence (help supplement mineral loss), **Sulfurzyme** (shown to slow or reverse
>   autoimmune diseases), Super B (after each meal), Thyromin (first thing in
>   morning), VitaGreen.

> *TINCTURES*—Royal Essence (for energy).

SCIATICA: Aroma Life, cardamom, **cistus (followed by peppermint)**, fir, ᶠhelichrysum,
      Gentle Baby, hyssop, M-Grain, PanAway, peppermint, Relieve It, sandalwood,
      spruce (alleviates pain), ᶠtarragon, ᶠthyme, Valor. Apply a cold compress and
      lightly massage with Roman chamomile or lavender, and birch/wintergreen.
      Relief can also be obtained by applying Joy and lavender to the bottoms of the
      feet.

> *MASSAGE OIL*—Ortho Ease.

SCOLIOSIS: May be caused by a virus. DO THE RAINDROP TECHNIQUE!

> ***COMMENT*—The video, listed in the Bibliography, is highly recommended for a
>   professional visual presentation of this technique!*

> *BLEND*—8 basil, 12 birch/wintergreen, 5 cypress, 10 marjoram, and 2 peppermint.

CORRECT—Do the following (a variation of the Raindrop Technique) every seven to ten
>   days for a minimum of eight times to help get rid of SCOLIOSIS:

1. Rub Valor on feet.
2. Apply oregano and thyme using the Raindrop Technique up the spine.
3. Apply BLEND along the spine. Push or pull in the direction that the spine needs
    to be strengthened. Knead fingers clockwise three times. Then work two fingers
    up the spine with the other hand on top of the hand that is doing the kneading (do
    this three times).
4. Apply Aroma Siez and marjoram on the muscles on each side of the spine. Apply
    warm wet towel to back and have individual lay on their back.

5. Work the Vita Flex areas down the leg to the feet with basil, birch/wintergreen, cypress, and peppermint in V-6 Mixing Oil.
6. Work the spine Vita Flex areas on the feet then give feet a mild pull.
7. Put one hand under their chin and the other hand at the back of their neck. Have them breathe in and out as you gently rock and pull the neck in time with their breathing.
8. Take towel off. If the back gets too hot during massage apply more V-6 Mixing Oil.
9. Measure the spine to see how much it has changed.

SCRAPES: Lavender, ravensara.

SCURVY: ᶠGinger. Apply over kidneys and liver, and on corresponding Vita Flex points on the feet.
SUPPLEMENTS—Super C.

SECURITY: Christmas Spirit, Sacred Mountain.
CREATING—Acceptance, Roman chamomile.
FEELING OF—Cypress (aromatic).
IN THE HOME—Bergamot.
SELF SECURE—Oregano.

SEDATIVE: Among the most effective sedatives are: Bergamot, Citrus Fresh, lavender, neroli, and Peace & Calming. Other oils that may also help are: Angelica, cedarwood, Clary sage, coriander, cypress, elemi, frankincense, geranium, hyssop, jasmine, juniper, lavender, lemongrass, melissa, marjoram, onycha (benzoin), orange, patchouly, Roman chamomile, rose, sandalwood, tangerine, Trauma Life, valerian, vetiver (nervous system), ylang ylang. Use intuition as to which one may be best for the given situation. In addition, check the safety data for each of the oils in the APPENDIX of this book.

SEIZURE: See EPILEPSY.
GRAND MAL—Need to support the body. Aroma Siez (apply using the Raindrop Technique up the spine), Brain Power and Peace & Calming (diffuse and put around naval), Joy (over the heart), Sacred Mountain (back of neck and crown), and Valor (on feet).
SUPPLEMENTS—Cleansing Trio (ComforTone, Megazyme, and ICP), Essential Omegas.
****COMMENTS—Grand Mal seizures can sometimes be caused by zinc and copper imbalance. Mineral Essence provides zinc and copper in both ionic and colloidal form for optimal assimilation.*

S

SELF ADJUSTMENT: <u>Awaken</u>.

SELF ESTEEM: <u>Acceptance</u>, <u>Forgiveness</u>, <u>Joy</u>, <u>Valor</u>.
   BUILD—<u>Joy</u>, <u>Valor</u>.
   SELF LOVE—<u>Joy</u>, <u>Valor</u>.

SELF HYPNOSIS: Clary sage, geranium, patchouly.

SELF PITY: <u>Acceptance</u>, <u>Motivation</u>, <u>Valor</u>.

SENSORY SYSTEM (Senses): See AWARENESS. Birch/wintergreen.

SEXUAL ABUSE: <u>SARA</u> has a fragrance that when inhaled may enable one to relax into a
       mental state whereby one may be able to release and let go of the memory trauma
       of sexual and or ritual abuse.

SEX STIMULANT: ᶠCinnamon bark (general), ginger, goldenrod, rose, <u>Sensation</u>, ᶠylang
       ylang (sex drive problems).
       BATH & SHOWER GELS—Sensation Bath & Shower Gel contains oils used by
           Cleopatra to enhance love and increase the desire to be close to that someone
           special.
       MASSAGE OILS—Sensation creates an exotic arousal and increases sexual desire.
           The fragrance creates a peaceful and harmonious feeling that helps to ease
           relationship stress.
       PERSONAL CARE—PD 80/20, Prenolone/Prenolone+ (for both males and females),
           ProMist, Sensation Hand & Body Lotion.
       SUPPLEMENTS—Master Formula His/Hers, VitaGreen.
       TINCTURES—Royal Essence.
       OTHER—SE6 Tincture (available through Creer Labs 801-465-5423). Use 10-50
           drops of SE6 Tincture three times a day plus 2 droppers at bedtime for three to
           five days.
       AROUSING DESIRE—Clary sage.
       FRIGIDITY—See FRIGIDITY. Nutmeg (overcome).
       IMPOTENCE—Goldenrod (shows more potential than Viagra).
       INFLUENCES—Patchouly (aromatic).

SHINGLES: Bergamot, Blue cypress, eucalyptus, geranium, lavender, lemon, melaleuca
       (Tea Tree), ᶠravensara, Roman chamomile.
       BLEND—10 drops lavender, 10 melaleuca (Tea Tree), and 10 drops thyme mixed in
           Genesis Hand & Body Lotion. Rub on feet.
       MASSAGE OILS—Ortho Sport.
       PERSONAL CARE— PD 80/20, Prenolone/ Prenolone+.

SUPPLEMENTS—
    Cleansing Trio
    (ComforTone,
    Megazyme, and ICP),
    ImmuGel.
HERPES ZOSTER—
    Bergamot, *Eucalyptus radiata*, geranium, lavender, melaleuca (<u>Alternative Medicine—The Definitive Guide</u>, p. 972), Roman chamomile.

> *Shingles is an acute viral infection with inflammation of certain spinal or cranial nerves and the eruption of vesicles along the affected nerve path. It usually strikes only one side of the body and is often accompanied by severe neuralgia. Also called herpes zoster. Some say it is necessary to cleanse the liver.*
>
> *Dr. Schnaubelt says that his greatest success in helping individuals with shingles came from applying a blend of 50 percent Ravensara aromatica and 50 percent Calophyllum inophyllum (Tamanu). "Drastic improvements and complete remission occur within seven days." (<u>Alternative Medicine—The Definitive Guide</u>, p. 56).*

SHOCK: See FAINTING. <u>Aroma Life</u>, basil, <u>Clarity</u> (to keep from going into shock), <u>Gathering</u>, <u>Grounding</u>, helichrysum, <u>Inspiration</u>, <u>Joy</u>, melaleuca, melissa, myrrh, neroli, ᶠpeppermint, ᶠRoman chamomile, rosemary, <u>Valor</u>, ylang ylang.

SHOULDER (Frozen): Basil, birch/wintergreen, lemongrass, oregano, peppermint, White fir. Begin by applying White fir to shoulder Vita Flex point on foot (same side of body as frozen shoulder) to deal with any inflammation. Work it in with Vita Flex technique. Then check for improvement in pain reduction and/or range of motion (check after each oil to help determine what problem really was). In a similar manner apply lemongrass (for torn or pulled ligaments), basil (for muscle spasms), and birch/wintergreen (for bone problems) on the same Vita Flex point on the foot. After applying the oils to the foot and determining which oil(s) get the best results, apply same oil(s) on the shoulder and work it into the area with Vita Flex. Then apply peppermint (for nerves) and oregano (create thermal reaction to enhance elasticity of muscle and help it to stretch) on the shoulder and work each one into the area with Vita Flex. Finally, apply White fir to the other shoulder to create balance as the opposite shoulder will compensate for the sore one. Drink lots of water.
    PERSONAL CARE—Regenolone.
    SUPPLEMENTS—Sulfurzyme.

SINUS: Cedarwood, eucalyptus, ᶠhelichrysum, ᶠmyrtle, <u>PanAway</u>, <u>RC</u>, or <u>Thieves</u> on feet.
    COMMENTS— *Eucalyptus and other sinus oils work really well when rubbed on each side of the nose. It seems to clear the sinuses almost immediately.*

S

SINUSITIS: See RESPIRATORY SYSTEM. Cajeput, elemi, ᶠeucalyptus, *Eucalyptus radiata*, fir, ginger, *Melaleuca ericifolia*, myrtle, ᶠpine, ravensara, RC, ᶠrosemary. *SUPPLEMENTS*— ImmuneTune.

SKELETAL SYSTEM: See SCOLIOSIS. Valor ("chiropractor in a bottle"). Also try the RAINDROP TECHNIQUE.

SKIN: See ACNE, ALLERGIES, BRUISES, CUTS, DERMATITIS, ECZEMA, FACIAL OILS, PSORIASIS, WRINKLES. Acceptance, Aroma Life, cajeput, cedarwood, Roman and German chamomile (inflamed skin), Clarity, cypress, Dragon Time, frankincense, Gentle Baby (youthful skin), geranium, helichrysum, Inner Child, jasmine

> ***Contact-sensitization*** *is a type of allergic reaction which can occur when a substance comes into contact with the body. A few essential oils applied to the skin may cause sensitization, perhaps only after repeated application (the amount used is not significant). The skin reaction appears as redness, irritation, or vesiculation. A rule of thumb when applying oils to someone is that people with darker hair usually have less sensitive skin while those with blond or red hair are generally more sensitive.*
>
> ***Single oils:*** *Bergamot, cassia, cinnamon bark, citronella, clove, fennel, Laurus nobilis, ylang ylang.*
>
> *For a list of possible skin irritants, please see the APPENDIX of this book.*

(irritated skin), juniper, lavender, ledum (all types of problems), lemon, marjoram, ᶠmelaleuca (healing), Melrose, Mister, M-Grain, myrrh (chapped and cracked), ᶠmyrtle (antiseptic), orange, palmarosa (rashes, scaly, and flaky skin), patchouly (chapped; tightens loose skin and prevents wrinkles), ᶠpeppermint (itching skin), Relieve It, rosehip, rosemary, rosewood (elasticity and candida), sage, sandalwood (regenerates), Sensation, Valor, vetiver, Western Red cedar (nourishing), and ylang ylang.

AFTERSHAVE—Awaken can be used instead of aftershave lotion. Try adding Awaken to Sandalwood Moisture Creme, Satin Body Lotion, Sensation Hand & Body Lotion, or Genesis Hand & Body Lotion as an aftershave. KidScents Lotion makes a great aftershave as it soothes and rehydrates the skin (and smells good too).

BAR SOAPS—Lavender Moisturizing Soap, Lemon Sandalwood Cleansing Soap, Peppermint Cedarwood Moisturizing Soap, Sacred Mountain Moisturizing Soap for Oily Skin, Thieves Cleansing Soap.

BATH & SHOWER GELS—Dragon Time (for women who have lower back pain, stress and sleeping problems due to menstruation), Evening Peace (relaxes tired, fatigued muscles and helps to alleviate tension), Morning Start (dissolves oil and grease), and Sensation (aphrodisiac).

ESSENTIAL WATERS (HYDROSOLS)—Clary Sage, German Chamomile (soothes irritation and swelling), Eucalyptus (helps cleanse oily skin), Juniper (helps detoxify and cleanse), Lavender (soothing), Spearmint (helps cleanse blemished and oily skin). Spray directly onto the skin (don't spray directly into the eyes of ears).

PERSONAL CARE—Boswellia Wrinkle Creme, EndoBalance (helps moisturize dry, sun-damaged skin), Genesis Hand & Body Lotion (hydrates, heals, and nurtures the skin), Satin Facial Scrub - Mint or Juniper (eliminates layers of dead skin cells and slows down premature aging of the skin), NeuroGen (provide nutrients and moisturizers to deeper layers of the skin), Orange Blossom Facial Wash combined with Sandalwood Toner and Sandalwood Moisture Creme (cleans, tones, and moisturizes dry or prematurely aging skin), Prenolone, Regenolone (helps moisturize and regenerate tissues), Rose Ointment (for skin conditions and chapped skin), Satin Body Lotion (moisturizes skin leaving it feeling soft, silky, and smooth), Sensation Hand & Body Lotion (moisturizes, softens, and protects the skin from weather, chemicals, and household cleaners).

SUPPLEMENTS FOR SKIN—JuvaTone, Sulfurzyme, Ultra Young (helps firm and tighten skin by activating the production of skin proteins, collagen, and elastin).

TINCTURES—AD&E

AGING/WRINKLES—Carrot, frankincense, patchouly (prevents wrinkles), rose, rosehip (retards), rosewood (slows).

BATH & SHOWER GELS—Bath Gel Base (cleanses the pores of the skin) plus use your own choice of oils or blends to create the fragrance or therapeutic action you desire.

PERSONAL CARE—Boswellia Wrinkle Creme, EndoBalance, Genesis Hand & Body Lotion, Satin Facial Scrub - Mint or Juniper, PD 80/20, Prenolone/Prenolone+, Rose Ointment, Sandalwood Moisture Creme and Sandalwood Toner.

SUPPLEMENTS—Ultra Young (helps firm and tighten skin by activating the production of skin proteins, collagen, and elastin).

CHAPPED/CRACKED—Davana, elemi, myrrh, onycha (benzoin), patchouly.

BLEND #1—1 geranium, 1 patchouly, and 1 rosemary in Genesis Hand & Body Lotion or Satin Body Lotion.

BLEND #2—1-3 drops of both onycha (benzoin) and rose in Genesis Hand & Body Lotion, Satin Body Lotion (makes a wonderful hand cream), or Rose Ointment. May also add lemon and/or lavender for their additional healing properties.

PERSONAL CARE—Cinnamint Lip Balm.

DISEASE—Rose, Melrose.

DRY—Davana, Gentle Baby, geranium, jasmine, lavender, lemon, neroli, patchouly, Roman chamomile, ᶠrosewood, sandalwood.

S

ESSENTIAL WATERS (HYDROSOLS)—Clary Sage (supports cells). Spray directly onto the skin (don't spray directly into eyes or ears).

MASSAGE OILS—Sensation Massage Oil (silky and youthful skin).

PERSONAL CARE—EndoBalance, Genesis Hand & Body Lotion (hydrates, heals, and nurtures), NeuroGen, Orange Blossom Facial Wash (gently cleanses the skin), PD 80/20, Prenolone/ Prenolone+, Sandalwood Toner, Sandalwood Moisture Creme (hydrates), Satin Body Lotion (nourishes and moisturizes)

FACIAL MASK—Orange Blossom Facial Wash, Satin Facial Scrub - Mint or Juniper.

FEEDS SKIN AND SUPPLIES NUTRIENTS—All applicable Essential Oils, Boswellia Wrinkle Creme, EndoBalance, NeuroGen (deeper layers of the skin), Rose Ointment.

ITCHING—Peppermint.

PERSONAL CARE—Satin Body Lotion.

OILY (greasy) COMPLEXION—Bergamot, cajeput, Clary sage, cypress, jasmine, lavender, lemon, nutmeg, orange, ylang ylang.

ESSENTIAL WATERS (HYDROSOLS)—Eucalyptus (helps cleanse), Spearmint. Spray directly onto the skin (don't spray into eyes or ears).

SENSITIVE—Geranium, German chamomile, jasmine, lavender, neroli.

PERSONAL CARE—Satin Body Lotion.

SUNBURN—Add a little lavender or tamanu oil to some Satin Body Lotion.

PERSONAL CARE—LavaDerm Cooling Mist (use as often as necessary to keep skin cool and moist). May also use EndoBalance or Satin Body Lotion later to help maintain moisture.

SUNTAN—Sunsation Suntan Oil filters out the ultraviolet rays without blocking the absorption of vitamin D. It may also accelerate tanning.

TONES—Patchouly.

MASSAGE OILS—Cel-Lite Magic.

PERSONAL CARE—Satin Facial Scrub - Mint or Juniper, Sandalwood Toner with Sandalwood Moisture Creme.

SUPPLEMENTS—Ultra Young (helps firm and tighten skin by activating the production of skin proteins, collagen, and elastin).

SLEEP: Lavender (on spine), marjoram (aromatic), <u>Peace & Calming</u>, Roman chamomile (aromatic), valerian (disturbances).

DIFFUSION—See NEGATIVE IONS for oils that produce negative ions when diffused to help promote sleep. Lavender, <u>Peace & Calming</u>.

ESSENTIAL WATERS (HYDROSOLS)—Lavender (promotes). Spray into the air, on face (don't spray directly into eyes or ears) or diffuse using the Essential Mist diffuser.

SUPPLEMENTS—Ultra Young (restores deep sleep).

ANIMALS—Oils can be used on the paws of animals to help them relax and sleep when in pain. <u>Peace & Calming</u>, <u>Trauma Life</u>.

GOOD NIGHT SLEEP—1/4 cup bath salts, 10 drops geranium or lavender in bath and
    soak. Bath with Evening Peace Bath Gel.
RESTLESS—Lavender and <u>Gathering</u>.
SLEEPING SICKNESS—Geranium, juniper, <u>Peace & Calming</u> (on big toes, back of neck
    and navel), peppermint, or <u>Valor</u> (on feet).

SLIMMING AND TONING OILS: Basil, grapefruit, lavender, lemongrass, orange,
    rosemary, sage, thyme.

SLIVERS (SPLINTERS): Mix 10 drops <u>Thieves</u> with 4 Tbs. V-6 Mixing Oil and massage
    bottom of feet, arm pits, throat, and lower stomach. Put 30 drops of <u>Thieves</u> in
    Bath Gel Base and use in shower each day (this helps pull the slivers to gently
    massage them out) .

SMELL-LOSS OF: Basil (helps
    when loss of smell is
    due to chronic nasal
    catarrh), peppermint.
STIMULATE SENSORY
    CORTEX—<u>Brain
    Power</u>. Place under the
    tongue, behind the ears,
    and on the forehead.

> *Just smelling the oils helps stimulate the sense of smell.*
> ***To smell the oils,*** *first close the eyes, hold the left nostril
> closed, breathe in the smell of the oil through the right
> nostril, then breathe out through the mouth. Breathing
> in the fragrance of the oils in this manner stimulates
> every endocrine gland in the brain. Next hold the right
> nostril closed and repeat the process.*

    Can also place a couple drops of oil in the hands, rub them together in a clockwise
    motion, cup over nose and mouth, and breathe deeply.
    COMMENTS— *According to the* <u>Essential Oils Desk Reference</u>*, "Massage 1 or
    2 drops [of Brain Power] with a finger on the insides of cheeks in the mouth.
    Doing this 1 or 2 times a day will immediately improve the smell sensory
    cortex." (EDR-June 2002; Ch. 8; Brain Power; Application)*

SMOKING: <u>Purification</u>.
CIGARETTE—<u>Purification</u>.
STOP SMOKING—See ADDICTIONS. Clove (removes desire), <u>Present Time</u> (helps
    with insecurity), <u>Thieves</u> (on tongue before lighting up helps remove desire).
    SUPPLEMENTS—JuvaTone, Super C.
    COMMENTS— *One individual used JuvaTone to break a habit of smoking 2½
    packs of cigarettes a day for 20 years. Another individual who used JuvaTone
    went from smoking a pack a day to 1 cigarette in 1½ weeks.*

SOOTHING: <u>Gentle Baby</u>, myrrh, onycha (benzoin), <u>Release</u>, Roman chamomile, .

SORES: Melaleuca, pine, <u>Thieves</u>.

S

SORE THROAT: See THROAT.

SPACING OUT: <u>Grounding</u>, <u>Acceptance</u>, <u>Present Time</u>, <u>Sacred Mountain</u>.

SPASMS: See MUSCLES, ANTISPASMODIC. <u>Aroma Siez</u>, **basil**, calamus, ^Fcypress, jasmine (muscle), lavender (antispasmodic), marjoram (relieves), oregano, <u>Peace & Calming</u>, peppermint, Roman chamomile, spikenard, tarragon, and thyme.
    SPASTICITY—Cypress, ginger, juniper, lavender, lemon, rosemary, sandalwood.

SPINA BIFIDA: Work on the nervous system with eucalyptus, lavender, lemon, nutmeg, orange, Roman chamomile, rosemary, <u>3 Wise Men</u>.

> ***Spina Bifida*** *is a congenital defect of the back bone, usually the lower vertebrae varies from a small area of numbness to paralysis from the waist down. A mental handicap can occur.*

    Apply oil(s) to bottom of feet, along spine, forehead, back of neck, and diffuse. Do the Raindrop Technique.

SPINE: See BACK. Oils can be applied along the Vita Flex spine points on the feet as an alternative to working directly on the spine.
    CALCIFIED—Geranium, <u>PanAway</u> (on spine), rosemary.
      MASSAGE OILS—Ortho Ease for body massage.
      SUPPLEMENTS—Arthro Plus, ArthroTune, and Super C.
    DETERIORATING—<u>PanAway</u>.
      MASSAGE OILS—Ortho Ease.
      SUPPLEMENTS—ArthroTune, Super C.
      TINCTURES—Arthro Plus.
    PAIN—<u>Valor</u> and <u>PanAway</u> may relieve pain along the spine when applied to spine and Vita Flex points on feet.
      MASSAGE OILS—Ortho Sport.
    STIFFNESS—Marjoram, <u>Valor</u>. Do the Raindrop Technique.
      MASSAGE OILS—Ortho Sport.
    VIRUS—*Eucalyptus radiata*, <u>ImmuPower</u>, oregano, and Ortho Ease on Spine. Viruses tend to hibernate along the spine.

SPIRITUAL: <u>Awaken</u>, <u>Believe</u>, <u>Dream Catcher</u>, <u>Gathering</u>, <u>Gratitude</u>, <u>Humility</u>, <u>Inspiration</u>.
    AWARENESS—<u>Acceptance</u>, Canadian Red cedar, cedarwood, juniper, myrrh, <u>Sacred Mountain</u>, spruce, <u>White Angelica</u> (Aromatic), White lotus.
      BALANCING—<u>Joy</u>, <u>Into the Future</u>, spruce.
    INCREASE—<u>Believe</u>, cedarwood (enhances), frankincense (opening and enhancing spiritual receptivity; aromatic), <u>Gratitude</u>.
    INNER AWARENESS—<u>Believe</u>, <u>Gratitude</u>, <u>Inner Child</u>, <u>Inspiration</u>.

MEDITATION—Believe, Canadian Red cedar, frankincense, Inspiration, tsuga, White Angelica.
PRAYER—Gratitude, Inspiration, White Angelica.
PROTECTION—3 Wise Men (on crown and shoulders).
PURITY OF SPIRIT—Myrrh.
SPIRITUALLY UPLIFTING—Believe, Gratitude, Sacred Mountain.

SPLEEN: is a major receptor for infections. Laurel, marjoram.

SPORTS: See ACHES AND PAINS, BONES, INJURY, MUSCLES, TISSUE.
EXCEL IN—Clarity (on forehead), Peace & Calming (back of neck), PanAway (injuries), Valor (on feet for courage and confidence).
INJURIES—Helichrysum, lemongrass, Melrose, PanAway, Peace & Calming.
TRACK COMPETITION—
   BLEND—5 basil, 5 bergamot, and 2 tsp. V-6 Mixing Oil.
   MASSAGE OILS—Ortho Ease, Ortho Sport. Massage into the muscles to increase the oxygen and elasticity in the tissues to prevent the muscles and ligaments from tearing during strenuous exercise. It may also be used after to prevent the muscle from cramping.
   SUPPLEMENTS—VitaGreen.
   TINCTURES—Royal Essence.

SPRAINS: Aroma Siez, ginger, jasmine, lavender, ᶠmarjoram, PanAway, Peace & Calming, rose, sage. Make a cold compress with eucalyptus, lavender, Roman chamomile, or rosemary.

SPURS-BONE: See BONES. Lavender, RC (dissolves). Apply directly on location.

STAINS: Lemon (removes).

STAPH INFECTION: Black pepper or peppermint will make it more painful. Use oregano and hyssop; alternate with oregano and thyme to relieve the pain. Helichrysum, lavender, Purification.

STERILITY: Clary sage, ᶠgeranium, rose (wonderful for both men and women). Can also try jasmine, neroli, sandalwood, rosewood, and vetiver. Apply several together (or alternate individually) by massage or aromatic baths.
   PERSONAL CARE—EndoBalance, Prenolone/Prenolone+.
   SUPPLEMENTS—Body Balance, Power Meal.

STIMULATING: Basil, Black pepper, En-R-Gee, eucalyptus, fir, ginger, grapefruit, orange, patchouly, ᶠpeppermint, rose, rosemary, ᶠsage. Dilute with Massage Oil for stimulating massage. Adding a little Black pepper to an oil like rosemary can give it a little more power. Can also add a few drops of an oil or a couple oils to Bath Gel Base then add to bath water as the tub is filling.

ESSENTIAL WATERS (HYDROSOLS)—Basil, Juniper (to the nervous system), Thyme (to the scalp). Spray into air or directly on face (don't spray directly into eyes or ears) or diffuse using the Essential Mist Diffuser.

STINGS: See BITES.

STOMACH: ᶠBasil, calamus (supports), ginger, peppermint. Apply to stomach Vita Flex points on feet or use with a hot compress over the stomach area.

ACHE—<u>Di-Tone</u> (behind ears and down jaw bone), eucalyptus, geranium, lavender, peppermint, or rosemary.

ACID—Peppermint (put drop on finger and place on tongue). Put several drops of fresh lemon juice in warm water and sip slowly.

   SUPPLEMENTS—AlkaLime (acid-neutralizing mineral formula), Mint Condition.

BACTERIA or GERMS—Peppermint.

BLOATING—Fennel (1-2 drops in liquid as dietary supplement).

CRAMPS—Ginger, ᶠhelichrysum, lavender, onycha (benzoin), rosemary cineol, ᶠthyme (general tonic for), or flavor water with 5 drops of <u>Di-Tone</u> and drink for stomach pains.

TONIC—Tangerine.

UPSET—<u>Di-Tone</u>. Apply over stomach and colon, behind the ears, on Vita Flex points on the feet, and/or add 1 drop to 8 oz. rice or almond milk and drink. Can also place a couple of drops on the palms of the hands, rub together clockwise, then cup over nose and mouth and breathe deeply.

   SUPPLEMENTS—Mint Condition (taken before meals helps curb stomach upset).

STRENGTH: Cypress (aromatic), <u>Hope</u>, oregano, patchouly, ᶠpeppermint, <u>Raven</u>, Roman chamomile (strengthens positive imprinting in DNA), <u>Sacred Mountain</u>, <u>White Angelica</u>.

   SUPPLEMENTS—Be-Fit (enhances strength by promoting muscle formation), Power Meal, WheyFit (provides three high-quality sources of protein for enhanced strength), Wolfberry Bar.

STREP THROAT: See THROAT.

STRESS: <u>Aroma Life</u>, basil, <u>Believe</u>, ᶠbergamot, <u>Clarity</u>, Clary sage, cypress, elemi, <u>Evergreen Essence</u>, frankincense, geranium, grapefruit, <u>Harmony</u>, <u>Inspiration</u>, <u>Joy</u>, lavender (aromatic), <u>Lazarus</u> (available through Creer Labs 801-465-5423), marjoram, neroli, onycha (benzoin), <u>Peace & Calming</u>, pine, Roman chamomile (relieves stress), rosewood, <u>Sacred Mountain</u>, spruce, <u>Surrender</u>, tangerine, <u>3 Wise Men</u>, <u>Valor</u>, <u>White Angelica</u> and ylang ylang.

    BATH & SHOWER GELS—Evening Peace, Relaxation, or Sensation Shower Gel.

    MASSAGE OILS—Relaxation or Sensation Massage Oil.

    PERSONAL CARE—Sensation Hand & Body Lotion.

    SUPPLEMENTS—Coral Sea (highly bio-available, contains 58 trace minerals), ImmuPro, Master Formula His/Hers (Multi-Vitamin), Thyromin, Super B, and Super Cal.

    TINCTURES—Royal Essence.

CHEMICAL—Clary sage, geranium, grapefruit, lavender, lemon, patchouly, rosemary.

EMOTIONAL STRESS—Bergamot, Clary sage, <u>Evergreen Essence</u>, <u>Forgiveness</u>, <u>Gathering</u>, geranium, <u>Joy</u>, ravensara, sandalwood (layer on navel and chest), <u>Surrender</u>, <u>Trauma Life</u>.

ENVIRONMENTAL STRESS—Basil, bergamot, cedarwood, cypress, geranium, Roman chamomile.

MENTAL STRESS—Basil, bergamot, <u>Evergreen Essence</u>, geranium, grapefruit, lavender, patchouly, pine, sandalwood, <u>Surrender</u>.

PERFORMANCE STRESS—Bergamot, ginger, grapefruit, rosemary.

PHYSICAL STRESS—<u>Believe</u>, bergamot, fennel, <u>Gentle Baby</u>, geranium, <u>Harmony</u>, lavender, marjoram, <u>Peace & Calming</u>, Roman chamomile, rosemary, thyme, <u>Trauma Life</u> (calming).

    SUPPLEMENTS—ImmuPro.

RELATIONSHIP STRESS—See SEX STIMULANT.

    BATH & SHOWER GELS—Sensation Bath & Shower Gel.

    MASSAGE OILS—Sensation Massage Oil creates an exotic arousal, increasing sexual desire. The fragrance creates a peaceful and harmonious feeling that helps ease relationship stress. Relaxation Massage Oil also creates a peaceful and harmonious feeling. You may want to add jasmine and ylang ylang.

    PERSONAL CARE—Sensation Hand & Body Lotion.

STRESS THAT STARTS WITH TIREDNESS, IRRITABILITY, OR INSOMNIA—

    BLEND—15 Clary sage, 10 lemon, 5 lavender, and 1 oz. V-6 Mixing Oil.

    SUPPLEMENTS—ImmuPro, Super B.

STRETCH MARKS: <u>Gentle Baby</u>, ᶠlavender, mandarin, ᶠmyrrh, neroli.

    BLEND #1—3 rosemary, 15 rosewood, and 1 ¾ oz. Hazel Nut Oil.

    BLEND #2—6 lavender, 4 rosewood, 3 patchouly, and Vitamin E Oil.

    ***COMMENTS*—*Patricia Davis recommends adding mandarin and neroli to either rosehip seed oil or Almond oil to massage over tummy and hips.*

STROKE: See BLOOD: CLOTS and BROKEN BLOOD VESSELS. <u>Aroma Life</u>, calamus, cypress, helichrysum. Breathe deeply and apply to neck and forehead.

SUPPLEMENTS—Master Formula Hers/His, Power Meal, Sulfurzyme, Ultra Young, Wolfberry Power Bars.

HEAT—Lavender or peppermint (rub on neck and forehead).

MUSCULAR PARALYSIS—Lavender.

>   *BLEND*—Mix together equal parts of basil, lavender, and rosemary. Rub spinal column and paralyzed area (<u>Alternative Medicine—The Definitive Guide</u>, p. 978).

STRUCTURAL ALIGNMENT:

<u>Aroma Siez</u>, basil, birch, cypress, peppermint, Valor, wintergreen (apply on

> *<u>Valor</u> is considered a "chiropractor in a bottle." It may help to realign the spine and keep the body in balance.*

feet to reduce time and effort necessary for alignments and to increase amount of time the alignment remains effective). Do the Raindrop Technique.

MASSAGE OILS—Ortho Ease.

SUBCONSCIOUS: <u>Believe</u>, <u>Gratitude</u>, helichrysum (uplifts when diffused), Idaho balsam fir, Western Red cedar.

> *ESSENTIAL WATERS (HYDROSOLS)*—Western Red Cedar.

SUDORIFIC: Hyssop, juniper, lavender, Roman chamomile, rosemary, thyme.

> *A **sudorific** is an agent that causes sweating. It may be helpful in times of fever or when toxins need to be released through the skin.*

SUGAR:

> *SUPPLEMENTS*—Allerzyme (aids the digestion of sugars, starches, fats, and proteins).
>
> REMOVE ADDICTIONS TO SUGAR—Dill (on wrists).

> *Honey goes into the blood stream faster than sugar and can be harder on the system than sugar. Maple syrup is one of the most perfect sugars because it has equal proportions of positive and negative ions. It also has the same pH as the blood and it doesn't go into the blood as fast as honey or sugar. Diabetics and pre-diabetics should use black strap molasses instead of maple syrup.*

STOP EATING—<u>Peace & Calming</u>, <u>Purification</u>.

> *SUPPLEMENTS*—JuvaTone.

SUBSTITUTE—Stevia (liquid) or Stevia Select (powder). *Stevia Select can even be used on cereals and in other recipes as a sugar replacement. Experimentation may be necessary for proper amounts as Stevia Select tends to be more sweet than regular sugar.*

SUICIDE: See DEPRESSION and EMOTIONS.

SUNBURN: See BURNS.
> ᶠMelaleuca. Spray or
> rub with Roman
> chamomile and
> lavender. 5-6 drops of
> Roman chamomile
> added to lukewarm
> bath water helps reduce
> burning sensation.

*Dr. Alex Schauss, a prominent mineral researcher, has discovered that **burns** are painful because certain trace minerals are depleted from the skin and surrounding tissue. If the trace minerals are replenished to the affected area, then the pain will subside almost immediately. Many people have received instant pain relief when Mineral Essence was either taken internally or topically applied on the sunburn or burn.*

> *SUPPLEMENTS*—Mineral
> Essence (can apply directly on affected area).
> *PERSONAL CARE*—LavaDerm Cooling Mist (use as often as needed to keep skin
> cool and moist), Satin Body Lotion.
> PREVENT BLISTERING—Apply 2-3 drops of lavender with Satin Body Lotion.

SUN SCREEN: ᶠHelichrysum.
> *PERSONAL CARE*—Sunsation Suntan Oil helps filter out the ultraviolet rays without
> blocking the absorption of vitamin D, which is important to skin and bone
> development. It also ACCELERATES TANNING.

SUPPORTIVE: Myrrh.

SWELLING: See EDEMA (for swelling from water retention). Helichrysum, lemongrass,
tangerine.

**SYMPATHETIC NERVOUS
SYSTEM:** Black
pepper, Brain Power,
Clarity, *Eucalyptus
radiata*, ginger,
peppermint.

The Sympathetic Nervous System is responsible for preparing our bodies for action by stimulating the heart, dilating the bronchi, contracting the arteries, and inhibiting the digestive system.

> Stimulation of certain areas of the Sympathetic Nervous System can be achieved
> by application of any of the above oils at the appropriate places along the spinal
> column (*refer to the Autonomic Nervous System chart in the Science and
> Application section of the Reference Guide for Essential Oils*).
> *SUPPLEMENTS*—Coral Sea (highly bio-available, contains 58 trace minerals),
> Mineral Essence, Power Meal, Sulfurzyme, Super Cal, Ultra Young.

SYMPATHY: Acceptance, Awaken, Present Time.

TACHYCARDIA (Rapid Heartbeat): See ANXIETY, HEART, SHOCK, or STRESS.
Aroma Life (combine with ylang ylang), goldenrod, Idaho tansy, lavender, neroli, orange, PanAway, Relieve It, Roman chamomile, rose, ᶠrosemary, ᶠylang ylang (smell on tissue or straight from bottle in emergency). Apply over heart and to heart Vita Flex points on the left hand and elbow (see illustration under HEART) and on the left foot. Add oils to V-6 Mixing Oil or Massage Oil for massage, or add them to Bath Gel Base for an aromatic bath. Continue to use regularly to help prevent recurrence.
TINCTURES—HRT.
SUPPLEMENTS—CardiaCare, Sulfurzyme.

TALKATIVE: Cypress (for over talkative).

TASTE: Helichrysum (1 drop on tongue), peppermint (for impaired taste).
SUPPLEMENTS—Mineral Essence, Super B, Super C (enhances flavor).

TEETH: See DENTAL INFECTION.
CAVITIES—Brush teeth with Thieves. *Put a drop on your toothpaste if you can't handle it straight.*
PERSONAL CARE—Dentarome/Dentarome Plus Toothpaste (contains Thieves), Fresh Essence Mouthwash (contains Thieves), KidScents Toothpaste (for children).
***COMMENTS—*People have had regeneration of their teeth in as little as four months by brushing their teeth with Thieves.*
FILLINGS—(to help eliminate toxins from mercury in the system) Idaho balsam fir (22 drops in a capsule, once in morning, once at night). Can also combine Idaho balsam fir with helichrysum and/or frankincense.
SUPPLEMENTS—Radex and Super C, Cleansing Trio (ComforTone, Megazyme, and ICP), Detoxzyme (5 in morning and 5 at night until body says stop! Then back off to 1 or 2 per day).
GUM SURGERY—Helichrysum every 15 minutes for the pain.
TEETHING PAIN—German chamomile, Thieves.
TOOTHACHE—Cajeput, ᶠclove, melaleuca, Purification (anti-bacterial), Roman chamomile. Apply on location (on gums) and along jawbone.
PERSONAL CARE—Dentarome/Dentarome Plus Toothpaste (contains Thieves), Fresh Essence Mouthwash (contains Thieves).
TOOTHPASTE—Thieves.
***COMMENTS—*You may want to put 10-12 drops of Thieves in 2 oz. of water in a small spray bottle. Mist in mouth or on toothbrush and brush.*
RECIPE—Combine 4 tsp. green or White clay, 1 tsp. salt, 1 to 2 drops peppermint, 1 to 2 drops lemon, mix clockwise.

PERSONAL CARE—Dentarome/Dentarome Plus Toothpaste (contains <u>Thieves</u>), Fresh Essence Mouthwash (contains <u>Thieves</u>), KidScents Toothpaste (for children).

NERVE PAIN—Melaleuca (put 1 drop in small amount of water and hold in mouth for one to two minutes to help calm nerves).

TEMPERATURE: See FEVER or THYROID.

SUPPLEMENTS—Thyromin (balances the temperature in the body).

LOWER—Bergamot, eucalyptus, lavender, melissa, peppermint. Cypress and rosemary induce sweating to lower temperature indirectly. Use oils in baths or mix with cool water and sponge over body or area.

ESSENTIAL WATERS (HYDROSOLS)—Lavender, Melissa, Peppermint. Spray directly on body or diffuse with Essential Mist Diffuser.

RAISE—Marjoram, onycha (benzoin), thyme. Add to V-6 Mixing Oil or Massage Oil for brisk massage. Locally warming (rubefacient) oils like Black pepper, juniper, and rosemary help raise temperature in cold extremities.

TENDONITIS: Basil, ᶠbirch, cypress, lavender, ginger, <u>PanAway</u>, peppermint, <u>Relieve It</u>, rosemary, wintergreen. Apply oils in Raindrop fashion on location and ice pack.

PAIN RELIEF—Birch/wintergreen and peppermint. If pain and inflammation is a result of torn or infected ligaments or tendons, then lemongrass and helichrysum can be helpful when added to any of these oils.

TENNIS ELBOW: Birch, eucalyptus, helichrysum, <u>PanAway</u>, peppermint, rosemary, wintergreen.

> ***Tennis Elbow** is the painful inflammation of the tendon on the outer side of the elbow that usually results from excessive strain on and twisting of the forearm.*

BLEND #1—10 eucalyptus, 10 peppermint, 10 rosemary, and 1 Tbs. V-6 Mixing Oil. Mix and apply, then ice pack. Can also try alternating cold and hot packs.

BLEND #2—Equal parts lemongrass, helichrysum, marjoram, and peppermint. Mix and apply, then ice pack.

TENSION: Basil (nervous), bergamot (nervous), ᶠcedarwood, frankincense, <u>Harmony</u>, lavender, *Melaleuca ericifolia* (nervous), <u>Peace & Calming</u>, <u>Trauma Life</u> (balances and calms), valerian, ylang ylang. Apply on hands, cup over nose and mouth and breathe deeply or diffuse. Mix a few drops of oil, or oils of choice, in ½ cup Epsom salts and add to bath water.

AQUA ESSENCE BATH PACKS—Finally, some of the most popular essential oil blends have been combines with the latest hydro-diffusion technology to create the perfect solution for adding oils to your bath water. Place a packet in the tub while

T

adding hot water and the oils are perfectly dispersed into the water. The packets contain 10 ml of oil and are reusable. Try either <u>Valor</u> or <u>Peace & Calming</u>.
RELIEVE—Grapefruit, Roman chamomile.
  MASSAGE OILS—Ortho Ease, Relaxation.
  PERSONAL CARE—Prenolone/Prenolone+.

TESTICLES: ᶠRosemary.
  REGULATION—<u>Aroma Siez</u> (combine with <u>Mister</u>), Clary sage, geranium, sandalwood, yarrow.
    PERSONAL CARE—Prenolone+.
    SUPPLEMENTS—Mineral Essence, ProGen, Ultra Young+.

THOUGHTS: <u>Inspiration</u> (relieves negative), ravensara (lifts emotions).

THROAT: Calamus (helps remove phlegm), ᶠcypress, oregano. Myrrh and peppermint are also very effective for removing phlegm and mucus from the throat area.
  DRY—Grapefruit, lemon.
  INFECTION IN—Clary sage, ᶠlemon, oregano, ᶠpeppermint.
  LARYNGITIS—See LARYNGITIS.
  SORE—Rub one of the following on the throat: Bergamot, cajeput, geranium, ginger, <u>ImmuPower</u>, ᶠmelaleuca, myrrh, oregano, <u>RC</u>, sandalwood, <u>Thieves</u>, or put 1 drop of <u>Thieves</u> in 32 oz. water and drink. Inhalations with Clary sage, eucalyptus, lavender, sandalwood, thyme.
    TINCTURES—Gargle with Royal Essence.
  STREP—Geranium, ginger, or <u>Thieves</u> (rub on throat every time it feels sore; dilute well!). Also hyssop, laurel, melaleuca (combine with <u>Thieves</u> and dilute), oregano, ravensara (combine with <u>Melrose</u>).
    SUPPLEMENTS—ImmuneTune, ImmuPro, Super C.
    TINCTURES—Royal Essence (gargle every hour).

THRUSH: Bergamot, eucalyptus, ᶠlavender, marjoram, rose, thyme.
  VAGINAL—Geranium, ᶠmelaleuca, ᶠmyrrh, patchouly, rosemary.

THYMUS: Elemi, <u>ImmuPower</u> (apply on throat and chest), ravensara, <u>Thieves</u> (dilute with V-6 Mixing Oil and apply over thymus or apply neat on bottom of feet).
  STIMULATES—<u>ImmuPower</u>, ᶠspruce.
    SUPPLEMENTS—Ultra Young (reverses aging of the thymus gland).

THYROID:

DYSFUNCTION—Clove.

NORMALIZES HORMONAL
IMBALANCE
OF—Myrtle.

HYPERTHYROIDISM—<u>Endo</u>
<u>Flex</u>, ᶠmyrrh, myrtle,
ᶠspruce.

> *The **thyroid gland** is situated in the neck and regulates the body's metabolic rate.*
>
> *To determine whether or not the thyroid needs help, you must monitor your basal cell temperature. Place a thermometer under your arm pit before getting out of bed in the morning and rest quietly for 10 minutes. A temperature below 97.6° F (36.5° C) may indicate hypothyroidism (low thyroid function) and a temperature above 98° F (36.7° C) may indicate hyperthyroidism.*

   SUPPLEMENTS—
   Sulfurzyme.

   BLEND #1—Equal parts
   lemongrass and myrrh.
   Can apply undiluted on
   thyroid and parathyroid Vita Flex points under big toes or dilute with small
   amount of V-6 Mixing Oil and apply on throat just under the Adam's apple.

   BLEND #2—Equal parts myrrh and spruce. Apply as directed in Blend #1 above.

HYPOTHYROIDISM—Clove, <u>EndoFlex</u> (apply on top of big toes), ᶠmyrtle, peppermint,
   spearmint. Combine lemongrass with any or all of these oils and apply as directed
   in BLEND #1 above.

   SUPPLEMENTS—Thyromin (regulates metabolism, balances body temperature,
   prevents fatigue; *follow directions for use as specified in the Supplements
   section under Thyromin*).

   ****COMMENTS*—*One of the signs of thyroid deficiency is rough, dry skin on the
   bottoms of the feet.*

REGULATION—Ledum.

SUPPORTS—<u>EndoFlex</u>, myrrh (rub on hands and feet), myrtle.

   SUPPLEMENTS—Cleansing Trio (ComforTone, Megazyme, and ICP), Power Meal,
   VitaGreen (enhances effect of Thyromin), Thyromin (regulates metabolism,
   balances body temperature, prevents fatigue; *follow directions for use as
   specified in the Supplements section of the <u>Reference Guide for Essential Oils</u>
   under Thyromin*).

TINNITUS: (Ringing in the ears.) See EAR. Juniper, helichrysum. Apply to mastoid bone
   behind ear.

TIRED: See ENERGY, EXHAUSTION, and FATIGUE.

TISSUE: Basil, elemi (rejuvenates), helichrysum, lavender, lemongrass, lime (tightens
   connective tissue), marjoram, <u>Melrose</u>, Roman chamomile, sandalwood.
   SUPPLEMENTS—Be-Fit (builds muscle tissue), Body Balance (for elasticity in
   tissues), AminoTech (builds lean muscle tissue), Power Meal (pre-digested

protein), WheyFit. Biotin (found in Body Balance) is important for damaged tissue.

ANTI-INFLAMMATORY—Myrrh.

BONE AND JOINT REGENERATION—

    BLEND—5 drops birch/wintergreen, 2 German chamomile, 1 Blue tansy, 7 fir, 5 helichrysum, 5 hyssop, 4 lemongrass, 8 sandalwood, 8 spruce, and 1 oz. V-6 Mixing Oil.

CLEANSES TOXINS FROM—Fennel.

CONNECTIVE TISSUE, WEAK—<u>Aroma Siez</u>, helichrysum, lavender, lemongrass, patchouly.

    MASSAGE OILS—Ortho Ease.

DEEP TISSUE PAIN—Helichrysum, <u>PanAway</u>, <u>Relieve It</u>.

    MASSAGE OILS—Ortho Ease and Ortho Sport.

REPAIR—Elemi (builds), helichrysum (scar tissue and reduces tissue pain), hyssop (scars), lemongrass (repairs connective tissue), orange, rosewood, sage (firms tissue), <u>Relieve It</u> (deep tissue damage).

    PERSONAL CARE—Rose Ointment (to help maintain, protect, and keep the scab soft), Satin Body Lotion (to moisturize and promote healing).

REGENERATE—Geranium, helichrysum, lemongrass, <u>Melrose</u>, ᶠpatchouly, rosehip.

    ****COMMENTS*—Use helichrysum and <u>Melrose</u> together for traumatized tissue (cuts, wounds, and abrasions).*

TMJ (Temporomandibular Joint Disorder or TMD): <u>3 Wise Men</u>. Apply on temple and side of face, in front of ear and down to the jaw. Cover with ice packs for 10 minutes at a time, 3-4 times a day. May be best to seek advise from a healthcare professional, especially a dentist.

TONIC:

DIGESTIVE—ᶠGerman chamomile, *Melaleuca quinquenervia*.

GENERAL—Angelica, basil, cajeput, cardamom, cinnamon bark, cistus, Clary sage, cumin, galbanum, geranium, ginger, grapefruit, juniper, lemon, lemongrass, lime, mandarin, marjoram, melissa, Mixta chamomile, Mountain savory, myrrh, neroli, nutmeg, orange, palmarosa, patchouly, sandalwood, spruce, ylang ylang. Best way to restore tone in a body that is run-down is to apply oils by massage when possible. Baths are next in effectiveness to massage is not possible or between massages.

HEART—Lavender, thyme.

NERVE—Carrot, Clary sage, melaleuca, ᶠravensara, thyme.

SKIN—lemon, lime, spearmint, spikenard.

STOMACH—Tangerine.

UTERINE—Jasmine, thyme.

TONSILLITIS: (Inflamed tonsils, most often due to streptococcal infection.) See STREP
    THROAT. Bergamot, clove, goldenrod, ᶠginger, lavender, lemon (gargle),
    ᶠmelaleuca, Roman chamomile, Thieves. Apply on throat, lungs, and Vita Flex
    points.
    DIFFUSE—Bergamot, clove, geranium, lavender, lemon, melaleuca (Tea Tree),
    onycha (benzoin), Thieves, thyme. Breathe deeply through mouth.
    PERSONAL CARE—Fresh Essence Mouthwash.
    ***COMMENTS—*Use caution when considering surgery (tonsillectomy) for recurring
    tonsillitis as doctors have discovered that the only area of the body that can
    synthesize the antibody to poliomyelitis (polio) is the tonsils.*

TOOTHACHE: See TEETH.

TOXEMIA: Aroma Life, cypress.
    SUPPLEMENTS—
    Essential Manna,
    Exodus.
    TINCTURES—Rehemogen.

> **Toxemia**—*poisoned condition of the blood caused by
> the presence of toxic materials, usually bacterial but
> occasionally chemical or hormonal in nature. When
> bacteria themselves find entrance into the bloodstream,
> the condition is known as bacteremia. The term toxemia
> is also sometimes applied to preeclampsia, a condition
> that occasionally occurs in late pregnancy and is
> characterized by high blood pressure and kidney
> malfunction.*
> *(Microsoft® Encarta® Online Encyclopedia 2000)*

TOXINS: Fennel, fir, hyssop
    (opens respiratory
    system and discharges
    toxins and mucus),
    lemongrass (helps
    increase lymphatic
    circulation for enhanced toxin removal), patchouly (digests toxic wastes).
    SUPPLEMENTS—Cleansing Trio (ComforTone, Megazyme, and ICP). These
    cleansing products may help remove toxic by-products from the body.
    ***COMMENTS—*Another way to help remove toxins through the skin is to add 2 cups
    of Apple Cider Vinegar to warm bath water and soak for 25 minutes.*

TRANSITION IN LIFE: Acceptance, Awaken (into achieving success), basil, cypress. May
    also want to concentrate on the emotional blends of Valor, Motivation,
    Grounding, Release, Hope, and Joy (*refer to the pages on "Auricular Emotional
    Therapy" and "Emotional Release" in the Science and Application section of
    the Reference Guide for Essential Oils*).

TRAUMA: See SHOCK. Release (feet and liver), Joy (heart), 3 Wise Men (crown); use all
    three blends in succession. May also diffuse. Envision, Forgiveness, Hope, and
    Release can also aid in releasing emotional trauma (*Refer to each blend
    separately in the Blends section of the Reference Guide for Essential Oils for*

possible applications). <u>Trauma Life</u> is an excellent blend for helping to cope with shock or emotional trauma. Apply on forehead and on palms then rub palms together, cup over nose and mouth, and inhale deeply. Others that may help are <u>Valor</u> (on the feet), <u>SARA</u> (on temples), <u>Peace & Calming</u> (on palms; place hands together over heart in prayer position).

****COMMENTS—Concentrate on relaxing to help release the trauma. Also, if after an emotional or physical trauma you find you don't like the smell of a particular oil, it may be the one you need most to help unlock the trauma. Try exposing yourself to it a little at a time until the healing is finished.*

SUPPLEMENTS—ImmuPro, Mineral Essence, Super C.

TRAVEL SICKNESS: See MOTION SICKNESS.

TUBERCULOSIS (T.B.): Cajeput, ᶠcedarwood, ᶠcypress, ᶠ*Eucalyptus radiata*, lemon, ᶠmyrtle, peppermint, rosemary verbenon, sandalwood, or ᶠthyme linalol. <u>Exodus II</u> (on spine and Raven on back with a hot compress), <u>ImmuPower</u> (on spine daily), <u>Raven</u> (1-2 drops in V-6 Mixing Oil as a rectal implant), <u>RC</u> (on chest and back– reverse each night with Raven), rose, rosemary, <u>Thieves</u> (on feet). A hot compress can be used when applying oils to the chest or back. DO THE RAINDROP TECHNIQUE.

SUPPLEMENTS—Exodus, ImmuGel, ImmuneTune, ImmuPro, Radex, Royal Essence, Super C, VitaGreen. Do a colon and liver cleanse with the Cleansing Trio (ComforTone, Megazyme, and ICP), and JuvaTone.

TINCTURES—Rehemogen.

BLEND—1-2 drops each of Eucalyptus radiata, myrtle, Mountain savory, and ravensara in 1 Tbsp. V-6 Mixing Oil. Apply as a rectal implant.

****COMMENTS—Refer to the chapter entitled "How to Use - The Personal Usage Reference" in the Essential Oils Desk Reference under "Tuberculosis" for a specific regimen using the blends and supplements.*

AIRBORNE BACTERIA—<u>Purification</u>, <u>Raven</u>, <u>RC</u>, <u>Sacred Mountain</u>, <u>Thieves</u>. Alternate diffusing different oils to help control spread of bacteria like *Mycobacterium tuberculosis*.

BLEND—Equal amounts of cypress and <u>Sacred Mountain</u>. Diffuse.

PULMONARY—Cypress, eucalyptus, <u>Inspiration</u>, ᶠoregano, ravensara.

BLEND—Equal amounts of frankincense and <u>ImmuPower</u>. Diffuse or dilute with V-6 Mixing Oil and massage on chest or back. Can also apply to Vita Flex lung points on hands and feet.

TUMORS: See CANCER.

ANTI-TUMORAL—Clove, ᶠfrankincense, ledum (may be more powerful than frankincense). Apply directly on tumor.

LIPOMA–Frankincense and clove, grapefruit, ginger, ledum.

PERSONAL CARE—Prenolone/Prenolone+.
***COMMENTS—Avoid the use of elemi as the oxidation of d-limonene (a principle
constituent of elemi) has been known to cause tumor growth!

TYPHOID: (Fever from contamination of the Salmonella typhosa bacteria) See ANTI-
BACTERIAL. ᶠCinnamon bark, lemon, <u>Melrose</u>, Mountain savory, peppermint,
<u>Purification</u>, <u>Raven</u>, ravensara, <u>RC</u>. Diffuse or dilute with V-6 Mixing Oil or
Massage Oil Base and apply over intestines and on intestine Vita Flex points on
the feet.

ULCERS: Bergamot, cinnamon bark, clove, elemi, ᶠfrankincense, geranium, ᶠGerman
chamomile, lemon, ᶠmyrrh, oregano, rose, thyme, vetiver. Add one drop of oil to
rice or almond milk and take as dietary supplement. May also be applied over
stomach by hot compress.

SUPPLEMENTS—Use
ComforTone to help
destroy the bacteria,
then use Megazyme (if
aggravation occurs,
take Mint Condition
first), Master Formula
His/Hers, and Mint
Condition (may help
soothe the ulcers; take with ComforTone).

> While some sources claim that sixty percent of all **ulcers**
> are caused by bacteria, F. Batmanghelidj, M.D.
> maintains that the majority of ulcers are only
> dehydration of the stomach lining. In his book, <u>Your
> Body's Many Cries for Water</u>, Dr. Batmanghelidj shows
> that rehydration is the simplest cure for this and many
> other adverse health conditions.

DUODENAL—(Damaged mucous membrane in a portion of the small intestine). Same
oils as listed above.
SUPPLEMENTS—AlkaLime.
GASTRIC—See GASTRITIS. ᶠGeranium.
LEG—(From lack of circulation in lower extremities and possible bacterial, fungal, or
viral infection). <u>Gentle Baby</u>, geranium, German chamomile, lavender, <u>Melrose</u>,
patchouly, <u>Purification</u>, Roman chamomile, rosewood, <u>Sensation</u>.
***COMMENTS—Dilute oils with V-6 Mixing Oil or Massage Oil Base and
massage lower extremities to stimulate circulation. Thyromin may be needed
to help with overall circulation.
MASSAGE OILS—Sensation.
PERSONAL CARE—Rose Ointment.
BLEND—Equal drops of lavender and either <u>Melrose</u> or <u>Purification</u> applied to
location. Can cover with Rose Ointment.
MOUTH—See CANKERS. Basil (mouthwash), myrrh, orange.
BLEND #1—1 drop each of sage and clove and 1-3 drops lavender. Apply directly on
location.
PEPTIC—Flavor a quart of water with 1 drop of cinnamon bark oil and sip all day.

SUPPLEMENTS—AlkaLime.

STOMACH—Bergamot, frankincense, geranium, orange, peppermint. Use as food flavoring, apply to stomach, and Vita Flex points.

SUPPLEMENTS—AlkaLime, Cleansing Trio (ComforTone, Megazyme, and ICP), Master Formula His/Hers, Royaldophilus (can help coat stomach and protect sensitive tissues while rebuilding).

ULCERATIONS—Cleanse liver and colon (See CLEANSING). Lavender, <u>Melrose</u>, rose.

PERSONAL CARE—Rose Ointment.

VARICOSE ULCERS—See VARICOSE ULCERS.

ULTRAVIOLET RAYS: Sunsation Suntan Oil blocks ultraviolet rays without blocking the absorption of Vitamin D.

UNWIND: See MASSAGE. Lavender, <u>Peace & Calming</u>. Diffuse, rub between hands and inhale deeply, or combine with V-6 Mixing Oil or Massage Oil for massage.

MASSAGE OILS—Relaxation.

BATH & SHOWER GELS—Evening Peace.

UPLIFTING: <u>Believe</u>, bergamot, birch, <u>Brain Power</u>, fir (emotionally uplifting), grapefruit, helichrysum, Idaho balsam fir, Idaho tansy, jasmine, lavender, myrrh, orange, <u>Live with Passion</u>, ravensara, <u>Sacred Mountain</u>, <u>Sensation</u>, spruce, <u>3 Wise Men</u>, tsuga, wintergreen. Diffuse or wear as perfume or cologne.

BLEND—3 birch/wintergreen, 3 lavender, 3 orange, 3 spruce and 1 oz. V-6 Mixing Oil. Wear a few drops of this blend as a perfume or cologne or apply over the heart, on the chest, neck, and/or shoulders, and behind the ears. Can also apply a few drops on both hands, rub together, cup over nose and mouth and breathe deeply.

BATH & SHOWER GELS—Morning Start, Sensation.

ESSENTIAL WATERS (HYDROSOLS)—Basil, Melissa, Mountain Essence, Peppermint, Idaho Tansy (mentally). Spray into air directly on face (don't spray directly into eyes or ears) or diffuse using the Essential Mist Diffuser.

URETER:

INFECTIONS IN—See BLADDER: INFECTION or KIDNEYS:

> *The **ureter** is the duct that carries the urine away from the kidneys to the bladder.*

INFECTION. ᶠLemon, ᶠmyrtle. Apply as specified below in Urinary Tract Infection.

URINARY TRACT: Bergamot, <u>ImmuPower</u>, lavender, ledum, melaleuca (Tea Tree), pine (antiseptic), ᶠsage, ᶠsandalwood, rosemary, tarragon, ᶠthyme (infection).

GENERAL—Bergamot, ᶠeucalyptus (general stimulant).

INFECTION—See BLADDER INFECTION. Bergamot, cajeput, ᶠcedarwood, <u>Di-Tone</u>, <u>EndoFlex</u>, geranium, hyssop, <u>ImmuPower</u>, <u>Inspiration</u> (effective by itself), juniper, lemongrass, <u>Melrose</u>, onycha, <u>Purification</u> (effective by itself), tarragon. Apply 2-3 drops of oil directly over bladder. May also apply a hot compress.

BLEND #1—Equal parts sage and <u>Purification</u>.

BLEND #2—Equal parts thyme and <u>Melrose</u>.

BLEND #3—Equal parts oregano and <u>Thieves</u>.

BLEND #4—Equal parts juniper and <u>EndoFlex</u>.

***COMMENTS—With any of the above blends, dilute with V-6 Mixing Oil and massage over lower back and pubic area or apply with hot compress.

SUPPLEMENTS—AlkaLime.

TINCTURES—K&B.

RECIPE #1—Add 1 drop Mountain savory to 3 droppers of K&B tincture in distilled water and drink every few hours.

***COMMENTS—Refer to the chapter entitled "How to Use - The Personal Usage Reference" in the <u>Essential Oils Desk Reference</u> under "Urinary Tract/Bladder Infection" for a unique blend of 14 different oils to specifically help with infection.

STONES IN—ᶠFennel, ᶠgeranium. Apply oils over pubic area and lower back with hot compress. *See Master Cleanser under CLEANSING.*

SUPPORT—Cypress, geranium, goldenrod, juniper, laurel, melaleuca.

TINCTURES—K&B.

UTERUS: Cedarwood, frankincense, geranium, jasmine, lemon, myrrh.

INFLAMMATION—Elemi.

REGENERATION OF TISSUE—Frankincense, sage, tarragon. Add 1-3 drops of each to 1 tsp. V-6 Mixing Oil, insert into vagina, and retain overnight.

PERSONAL CARE—PD 80/20, Prenolone/Prenolone +.

SUPPLEMENTS—Body Balance, FemiGen.

TINCTURES—Femalin (take internally and as a douche with 12 drops in 6 oz. distilled water morning and evening before retention implant).

UTEROTONIC—Thyme.

UTERINE CANCER—See CANCER. Cedarwood, frankincense, geranium, <u>ImmuPower</u>, lemon, myrrh. Oils can be applied to the reproductive Vita Flex points on the feet, mostly around the front of the ankle, on either side of the ankle under the ankle bone, and up the Achilles tendon. The most effective application of oils is by vaginal retention implant. Add 2-5 drops of any of these single oils or a combination of any of them to 1 tsp. V-6 Mixing Oil, insert into vagina and retain overnight. A tampon may be used if necessary to help retain the oil.

U
V

TINCTURES—Femalin (take internally and as a douche with 12 drops in 6 oz. distilled water morning and evening before retention implant).

UTERINE CYSTS—Femalin has been reported to be very beneficial in getting rid of uterine and ovarian cysts. See HORMONAL IMBALANCE.

BLEND #4—1 dropper of Femalin tincture mixed with 5 frankincense and 4 clove. Douche twice a day, retain for 20 minutes. Do for 90 days and rest for one month and repeat.

VAGINAL:

APPLICATION METHODS—Mix desired oil(s) with water and either use in a douche or sitz bath. After a douche, a capsule of Royaldophilus can be inserted in the vagina to help repopulate friendly bacteria and flora. Desired oil(s) may also be mixed with V-6 Mixing Oil and either applied directly or by soaking a tampon in mixture, inserting, and leaving in all day or night.

CANDIDA (thrush)—ᶠBergamot, lavender, laurel, ᶠmelaleuca, ᶠmyrrh, rosemary, spikenard, ᶠthyme. *See Application Methods above.*

SUPPLEMENTS—AlkaLime, Royaldophilus, and/or Stevia Select with FOS (important to re-establish the intestinal flora). Yogurt or Royaldophilus mixed with a little bit of water may be applied directly to relieve the pain associated with candida.

***COMMENTS—Focus on the underlying problem of system-wide yeast infection. See CANDIDA. Also, refer to the chapter entitled "How to Use - The Personal Usage Reference" in the Essential Oils Desk Reference under "Fungal Infections" for some excellent blend recipes for dealing with vaginal yeast infections.

INFECTION—ᶠCinnamon bark (be extremely careful; dilute well), Clary sage, cypress, eucalyptus, hyssop, juniper, lavender, laurel, melaleuca, <u>Melrose</u>, myrrh, Mountain savory, oregano, ᶠrosemary, ᶠrosewood, sage, <u>3 Wise Men</u>, thyme. Apply oregano and thyme along the spine using the Raindrop Technique. *See also Application Methods above.*

BLEND #1—Equal parts oregano, thyme, and <u>Melrose</u>. Dilute with V-6 Mixing Oil or Massage Oil and apply as described in Application Methods above.

BLEND #2—3 drops rosemary, 2 drops *Melaleuca quinquenervia*, 2 drops oregano, and 1 drop thyme. Dilute with V-6 Mixing Oil or Massage Oil and apply as described in Application Methods above. Can also apply as hot compress over lower abdominal area.

BLEND #3—5 drops <u>Melrose</u>, 2 drops oregano, and 1 drop thyme in 1 Tbsp. V-6 Mixing Oil or Massage Oil. Use as douche or vaginal retention implant as described in Application Methods above.

INFLAMMATION OF VAGINA—Eucalyptus, lavender, melaleuca, yarrow.

RETENTION IMPLANT—Used to cleanse and nourish the female reproductive system or as a support when taking products like the FemiGen supplement or the Femalin tincture. Best when done after a colon and liver cleanse using the Cleansing Trio (ComforTone, ICP, Megazyme).

BLEND #4—Dilute 2 drops *Melaleuca quinquenervia*, 1 drop lavender, and 1 drop bergamot in 1 Tbsp. V-6 Mixing Oil. Insert and retain overnight.

BLEND #5—Dilute 2 drops frankincense and 7 drops Purification in 1 Tbsp. V-6 Mixing Oil. Insert and retain overnight.

VAGINITIS—ᶠCinnamon bark (be extremely careful; dilute well), *Eucalyptus radiata*, ᶠrosemary, ᶠrosewood. Valerie Woorwood suggests the following douche recipe that should be used daily for three days a week only.

RECIPE #1—1 lavender, 1 melaleuca (Tea Tree), 1 tsp. of vinegar, ½ tsp. lemon juice, and 2 ½ cups of warm water. Mix thoroughly.

VARICOSE ULCERS: Eucalyptus, geranium, lavender, melaleuca (Tea Tree), thyme, yarrow.

VARICOSE VEINS: <u>Aroma Life</u>, <u>Aroma Siez</u>, basil, bergamot, <u>Citrus Fresh</u>, ᶠcypress (as bath oil), geranium, helichrysum (especially during pregnancy), Idaho tansy (helps weak veins), juniper, lavender, ᶠlemon (tonic for circulatory system), ᶠlemongrass, orange, ᶠpeppermint, rosemary, spikenard, tangerine, yarrow.

MASSAGE OILS—Cel-Lite Magic (strengthens vascular walls).

SUPPLEMENTS—Super B, Thyromin, VitaGreen.

TINCTURES—Rehemogen, Royal Essence.

BLEND #1—1-3 drops each of lemongrass and <u>Aroma Life</u> with Cel-Lite Magic.

BLEND #2—1-3 drops each of basil and <u>Aroma Siez</u>. Massage above the affected vein toward the heart.

***COMMENTS—*Refer to the chapter entitled "How to Use - The Personal Usage Reference" in the <u>Essential Oils Desk Reference</u> under*

Varicose veins are abnormal swelling of the veins in the legs. It is most often a symptom of poor circulation and a loss of elasticity of the vascular walls and particularly their valves. If the valves do not work properly, blood accumulates in the veins instead of flowing back to the heart. This accumulation of blood causes the vein to become swollen and twisted. *Hemorrhoids* are varicose veins of the anus or rectum usually resulting from constipation. Cleanse the colon.

Helichrysum dissolves the coagulated blood inside and outside of the veins. Cypress strengthens the veins. Massage *above* the affected vein toward the heart with helichrysum and cypress every morning and night; wear support hose until healed; it may take from three months to a year to heal completely. It is important to vary the essential oils being used. Try using lavender, juniper or rosemary instead of cypress and helichrysum. See DIET, CIRCULATORY SYSTEM.

Caution: Do not rub below the affected area as it may increase the pressure on the vein

"Varicose Veins" for more specific blend recipes and instructions regarding treatment.

VASCULAR SYSTEM: <u>Aroma Life</u>, cypress, frankincense, helichrysum, ᶠlemongrass (strengthens vascular walls). Apply as a full body massage, over heart, and on bottom of the feet.

> *MASSAGE OILS*—Cel-Lite Magic (strengthens vascular walls).

> *The **vascular system** refers to the vessels or veins that carry and circulate fluids (blood and lymph) throughout the body.*

CLEANSING—See CHELATION and METALS.

SUPPLEMENTS— JuvaTone, VitaGreen, and Radex work very well together. Other supplements include AD&E, ImmuGel, ImmuneTune, Megazyme, and Super C.

TINCTURES—HRT, K&B, Rehemogen, Royal Essence.

BLEND—1-3 drops each of helichrysum and <u>Aroma Life</u> with Cel-Lite Magic Massage Oil. Massage on the body to help dilate the blood vessels and enhance the chelation of metallics.

VASODILATOR: See BLOOD. Lemongrass, marjoram.

VEINS: See VASCULAR SYSTEM above.
CIRCULATION IN VASCULAR WALLS OF VEINS—<u>Aroma Life</u>, cypress, lemon.
BLOOD CLOT IN VEIN—Cypress and helichrysum (rub neat on location to dissolve).

VERTIGO: See EARS, EQUILIBRIUM and DIZZINESS. Ginger.

VIRAL DISEASE: Cinnamon bark.
SUPPLEMENTS—ParaFree, Super C, ImmuneTune, ImmuPro, ImmuGel.
ANTI-VIRAL—Oregano.
INFECTION—Cajeput, melaleuca, oregano, ravensara, thyme. Apply along spine, bottom of feet, and diffuse.
BLEND—Mix one drop each of lavender, orange, and spruce and apply to chest. Then put 10 drops of frankincense in a cap full of Evening Peace Bath Gel and add to bath as a bubble bath and soak.

VIRUSES: (often hibernate along the spine) Massage <u>ImmuPower</u> and oregano along the spine. Also use bergamot, cypress, *Eucalyptus radiata*, lavender, *Melaleuca quinquenervia* (viral and fungal infection), ravensara (viral infection), ᶠrosemary, <u>Thieves</u>. DO THE RAINDROP TECHNIQUE!
SUPPLEMENTS—ImmuPro, Royaldophilus (up to 4 a day, 30 minutes before eating).

AIRBORNE VIRUSES—<u>ImmuPower</u> on throat and chest, <u>Thieves</u> on feet. Diffuse.

ASTHMA—See ASTHMA.

EBOLA VIRUS—This virus cannot live in the presence of cinnamon bark or oregano.

EPSTEIN BARR VIRUS—See EPSTEIN BARR. Strengthen immune system, ensure proper thyroid function, and work on hypoglycemia. <u>ImmuPower</u>, <u>Thieves</u>.
> *SUPPLEMENTS*—Exodus, ImmuneTune, ImmuGel, ImmuPro, Wolfberry Bars.

RESPIRATORY—*Eucalyptus radiata*.

SPINE—5 oregano and 5 thyme. Put on bottom of the feet and up the spine using the Raindrop Technique.

VISUALIZATION: <u>Awaken</u>, <u>Dream Catcher</u>, helichrysum, <u>PanAway</u>. Diffuse or wear as perfume or cologne.

VITAL CENTERS: Oregano and sage may strengthen the vital centers of the body.

VITAMINS: *See the SUPPLEMENT section of the <u>Reference Guide for Essential Oils</u>.*
> *SUPPLEMENTS*—Body Balance, Coral Sea (highly bio-available, contains 58 trace minerals), Power Meal, Sulfurzyme (sulfur necessary for proper assimilation of Vitamin C), Super B, Super C, Super Cal.
>
> *TINCTURES*—AD&E.

CHILDREN—
> *SUPPLEMENTS*—Mighty Mist (vitamin spray), Mighty Vites (chewable vitamin tablets).

VITILIGO: Frankincense, <u>Melrose</u>, myrrh, <u>Purification</u>, sage, sandalwood, vetiver. Apply behind ears and to back of neck. Then rub hands together, cup over nose and mouth, and breathe deeply. Can also be applied to Vita Flex points

> *Vitiligo* is a disease in which the skin pigmentation is absent in certain areas of the body. It looks as if patches of skin have been bleached white. This may be due to a malfunction of the pineal gland and possibly the pituitary gland as well. *See PINEAL and PITUITARY for oils and products that can help oxygenate these glands. Another possible remedy includes daily exposure of the eyes to full-spectrum light without contacts or eyeglasses.*

relating to the pineal and pituitary glands on the feet and hands.

VOICE (hoarse): Bergamot, jasmine.
> *BLEND*—Add one drop each of <u>Melrose</u> and lemon to 1 tsp. honey. Swish around in mouth for a couple of minutes to liquify then swallow.

VOID: <u>3 Wise Men</u> (replaces the void; place on crown).

VOMITING: See NAUSEA. ᶠFennel, nutmeg, ᶠpeppermint (aromatic).
  MASSAGE OR COMPRESS (over stomach)—Black pepper, fennel, lavender,
    peppermint, Roman chamomile, rose.

WARMING: Cinnamon bark, onycha (benzoin), oregano, thyme.

WARTS: Cinnamon bark, colloidal silver, clove, cypress, frankincense (excellent for more
    stubborn warts), jasmine, lavender, lemon (may dilute in 2 tsp. apple cider
    vinegar), Melrose, oregano, Thieves. Dilute 1 to 2 drops of oil in a few drops of
    V-6 Mixing Oil and apply on location.
  BLEND—5 cypress, 10
    lemon, 2 Tbs. apple
    cider vinegar, AD&E
    tincture. Apply twice
    daily and bandage.
    Keep a bandage on it
    until wart is gone.
  TINCTURES—AD&E.
  GENITAL—Frankincense
    (excellent for more
    stubborn warts), hyssop, melaleuca, oregano, Thieves, thyme. Dilute 1-2 drops of
    oil in a few drops of V-6 Mixing Oil and apply on location.
  PLANTER—Oregano.

> *Stanley Burroughs touts clove oil as being wonderful for
> corns, skin cancer, and warts. He suggests using your
> finger to apply a small amount of clove oil directly on
> warts or corns. After a short time, use an emery stick to
> scrape off the top of the wart or corn and apply the oil
> again. Repeat several times daily until wart or corn
> disappears. The same technique can be used for skin
> cancer. (Healing for the Age of Enlightenment, p. 104.)*

WASTE: *Refer to Chapter 20 in the Essential Oils Desk Reference for lots of information
    on Cleansing and Digestion using essential oils and supplements.*
  ELIMINATING—ᶠLavender (through lymphatic system).
    SUPPLEMENTS—Cleansing Trio (ComforTone, Megazyme, and ICP). These
    cleansing products help eliminate toxic waste from the body.

WATER DISTILLATION: Add 3-5 drops of your favorite oil to the post-filter on your
    distiller. The oils will help increase the oxygen and frequency of the water. Try
    lemon, and peppermint.

WATER PURIFICATION: ᶠLemon, orange. H2Oils packets are wonderful for purifying
    and flavoring drinking water at the same time. Packets can be left in a container
    of water overnight to allow the oils to be effectively dispersed throughout the
    water. Try lemon, lemon/grapefruit, or lemon/orange.
  REMOVE NITRATES—Peppermint.

WATER RETENTION: See EDEMA, DIURETIC, and HORMONAL IMBALANCE.

WEAKNESS:
> AFTER ILLNESS—Thyme (physical).

WEALTH: <u>Abundance</u>, bergamot.
> ATTRACTS—Cinnamon bark (aromatic).
> MONEY—Ginger, patchouly.

WEIGHT: See HORMONAL IMBALANCE and pH BALANCE. **Proper exercise** is
> absolutely important! *Refer to the Supplement section of the <u>Reference Guide</u>*
> *<u>for Essential Oils</u> for instructions on how to use Body Balance, ThermaBurn,*
> *and ThermaMist for different weight problems.*
>> SUPPLEMENTS—Enzyme
>> products: Allerzyme
>> (aids the digestion of
>> sugars, starches, fats,
>> and proteins),
>> Carbozyme (aids the
>> digestion of

> ***Weight gain*** *is often attributed to slow metabolism, lack of exercise, low fiber, poor diet, stress, enzyme deficiency, hormonal imbalance, low thyroid function, and poor digestion and assimilation. It can also result from too much insulin being produced by the body.*

>> carbohydrates), Detoxzyme (helps maintain and support a healthy intestinal
>> environment), Fiberzyme (aids the digestion of fiber and enhances the absorption
>> of nutrients), Polyzyme (aids the digestion of protein and helps reduce swelling
>> and discomfort), and Lipozyme (aids the digestion of fats). Body Balancing Trio
>> (BodyBalance Mater Formula His/Her, VitaGreen), Cleansing Trio
>> (ComforTone, Megazyme, and ICP).
> CONTROL—<u>EndoFlex</u> (while taking Thyromin, a drop of <u>EndoFlex</u> under the tongue two
> or three times a day can help).
>> SUPPLEMENTS—Thyromin.
> EMOTIONS—Excessive weight may be due to unresolved childhood emotions. Any or
> all of the following may help: <u>Acceptance</u>, <u>Forgiveness</u>, <u>Inner Child</u>, <u>SARA</u> (*Refer*
> *to the "Emotional Release" part of the Science and Application section or to*
> *the Blend section of the <u>Reference Guide for Essential Oils</u> for more*
> *information on each of these blends*).
> WEIGHT LOSS—<u>EndoFlex</u> (on throat, under big toes), <u>Joy</u>, and <u>Motivation</u>.
>> BLEND #1—Put 5 lemon and 5 grapefruit in 1 gallon of water and drink during the
>> day. Add more grapefruit to dissolve fat faster. This same thing can now be done
>> easier and more effectively by using the H2Oils packet with lemon/grapefruit.
>> Just leave the packet in a gallon of purified drinking water overnight and the oils
>> will disperse throughout the water.
>> BLEND #2—4 lavender, 4 basil, 3 juniper, 8 grapefruit, 5 cypress. Mix and apply to
>> feet, on location, as a body massage, or use in bath. Blend is used to emulsify fat.
>> MASSAGE OILS—Massage whole body with Cel-Lite Magic after showering.

PERSONAL CARE—If the weight problem is related to a hormonal imbalance, Prenolone/Prenolone+ or ProMist combined with Thyromin and <u>EndoFlex</u> may help.

SUPPLEMENTS—Use Body Balance (helps to be at ideal weight) to replace breakfast and dinner, ComforTone, ICP, and Megazyme to promote proper elimination of waste material from the bowels, ThermaBurn or ThermaMist to naturally suppress the appetite and regulate the metabolism, and Thyromin to ensure proper thyroid function. Eat a normal meal at lunch, but watch fat intake. Other products that may help are AlkaLime (improves digestion), Power Meal, Sulfurzyme, Ultra Young (may help improve fat-to-lean ratios), and WheyFit (high quality, lactose-free proteins from three different sources). Master Formula His/Hers is also important to use.

UNDERWEIGHT—Drink Body Balance with meals. Feed cells with Mineral Essence.

WELL BEING: <u>Citrus Fresh</u>, Idaho tansy, <u>Release</u> (emotional), rose.
FEELING OF—<u>Harmony</u>, spearmint.
PROMOTES—Eucalyptus, geranium, lavender, lemon, lime.
   SUPPLEMENTS—Cleansing Trio (ComforTone, Megazyme, and ICP).

WHIPLASH: See TRAUMA or SHOCK. <u>Aroma Siez</u>, basil, birch (bones), helichrysum (bruising), hyssop (inflammation), juniper, lemongrass (strained ligaments), marjoram (muscles), PanAway, <u>Relieve It</u>, Roman chamomile, spruce, wintergreen (bones).
   SUPPLEMENTS—ArthroTune, Sulfurzyme, Super C.
   TINCTURES—Arthro Plus.
   ***COMMENTS—*Remember to think through every physical aspect of the injury (ie. muscle damage, nerve damage, inflammation, ligament strain, bone injury, fever, and emotions). Select oils for each area of concern.*

WHOLENESS: Ones own spirituality and oneness with the Creator. Apply each of the following blends, one right after the other: <u>Awaken</u> over the heart and on the forehead, <u>Sacred Mountain</u> on the crown of the head and over the thymus, and <u>White Angelica</u> on the shoulders. Then rub hands together, cup over nose and mouth, and breathe deeply to inhale the aroma of all three blends together.

WHOOPING COUGH: See CHILDHOOD DISEASES. Cinnamon bark, Clary cage, cypress, grapefruit, hyssop, lavender, Foregano. Apply on chest, throat, and Vita Flex points. Use a hot compress for deeper penetration.
   DIFFUSE—Basil, eucalyptus, lavender, melaleuca, peppermint, Roman chamomile, rose, thyme.

WITHDRAWAL: See ADDICTIONS.

WORKAHOLIC: Basil, geranium, lavender, marjoram. Rub a couple drops between hands, cup over nose and mouth and breathe deeply. Can also be diffused.

WORMS: See RINGWORM or PARASITES. Bergamot, Di-Tone (helps expel intestinal worms), lavender, melaleuca, peppermint, Roman chamomile, rosemary verbenon, thyme. For intestinal worms, apply a few drops over abdomen with a hot compress or add to V-6 Mixing Oil (½ to 1 oz.) and use as a retention enema for 15 minutes or more. Can also apply on intestine and colon Vita Flex points on the feet.

    BLEND—Mix 6 drops Roman chamomile, 6 eucalyptus, 6 lavender, and 6 lemon with 2 Tbs. V-6 Mixing Oil. Apply 10-15 drops of blend over abdomen with a hot compress and on intestine and colon Vita Flex points on the feet.

    SUPPLEMENTS—Cleansing Trio (ComforTone, Megazyme, and ICP), ParaFree.

WORRY: Bergamot. Diffuse.

WOUNDS: Bergamot, cajeput, Fclove (infected wounds), cypress, elemi (infected), eucalyptus, frankincense, galbanum, geranium, juniper, lavender (combine with any of these other oils), melaleuca (Tea Tree), myrrh, onycha (benzoin), peppermint (when wound has closed, will soothe, cool, and reduce inflammation), Roman chamomile (add to Rose Ointment for an excellent first aid salve), rose, rosemary, rosewood, thyme, tsuga.

    BLEND #1—Lavender with Purification or Melrose.

    RECIPE #1—First, 1-3 drops of helichrysum on the fresh wound will help stop the bleeding and a drop of clove will help with pain. Once bleeding is stopped, a drop of lavender (to help start the healing),

> *Dr. Marcy Foley maintains that "Each person will have a unique picture which created their healing challenges, and will require that each of these areas be addressed for a complete healing to take place." This is especially true for surface **wounds** where each aspect of the trauma must be considered. For example, there may also be damage to muscles, nerves, ligaments, or bones; there may be infection or inflammation; and there may be an emotion or even fever to deal with. Oils should be considered for each of these different areas as well.*

a drop of Melrose (to help fight infection), and a drop of lemongrass (for possible ligament damage) can be applied. Other oils such birch/wintergreen, thyme, or sage may also be applied depending on the extent of the injury. Rose Ointment can then be applied to help seal the wound and extend the effectiveness of the applied oils, and then cover it all with a bandage. When changing the bandage, myrrh, onycha, or patchouly can be applied to help promote further healing.

    Thieves or Purification may be necessary to help fight any occurrence of infection.

    PERSONAL CARE—Rose Ointment (seals and protects).

W
Y
Z

SUPPLEMENTS—Stevia extract (apply on closed wound to help reduce scarring).
CHILDREN (and INFANTS)—Lavender and/or Roman chamomile. Helichrysum and peppermint are best diluted with lavender or Rose Ointment first to help minimize stinging effect on open wounds.

    BLEND #2—(for Bruises or Wounds) 1-3 drops each of helichrysum and lavender diluted in 1/8 oz. V-6 Mixing Oil or Massage Oil Base.

BLEEDING—Rose, helichrysum, lemon.

    BLEND #3—Equal amounts of Roman chamomile, geranium, and lemon. Can alternate with cypress, hyssop, palmarosa, and rose. Apply directly with a compress 2-3 times a day for 3-4 days then reduce to once a day until healed.

DISINFECT—Hyssop, Idaho tansy, lavender, melaleuca, Mountain savory, thyme (thymol and linalol). Apply 1-2 drops directly on wound.

HEALING—See SCARRING. Helichrysum, Idaho tansy, lavender, melaleuca (pus-filled wounds), myrrh, neroli, onycha (benzoin), patchouly, ravensara, sandalwood, tsuga, yarrow. Apply directly on wound followed by Rose Ointment.

INFLAMMATION—German chamomile (helps reduce).

SURGICAL—Melrose, peppermint (cooling and soothing), <u>Purification</u>, <u>Thieves</u>.

    BLEND #4—3 helichrysum, 3 frankincense, 4 lavender in 2 tsp. V-6 Mixing Oil. Reapply a few drops of blend when changing bandages.

WEEPING—Juniper, myrrh, patchouly, tarragon.

    BLEND #5—5 drops Roman chamomile, 10 lavender, 3 tarragon, and 2 oz. V-6 Mixing Oil. Apply as a hot compress.

WRINKLES: Carrot, cistus, Clary sage, cypress, elemi, fennel, frankincense, galbanum, geranium, helichrysum, lavender, lemon, myrrh, neroli,

> *Wrinkles occur as we mature and as we lose oxygen to the tissues. Essential oils oxygenate the tissues and thereby slow down the premature aging of the skin.*

orange, oregano, patchouly, rose, rosemary, rosewood, sandalwood, spikenard, thyme, ylang ylang.

    AFTERSHAVE—<u>Awaken</u> can be used instead of aftershave lotion. KidScents Lotion works well to rehydrate the skin after shaving.

    BLEND #1—3 lavender, 4 geranium, 2 patchouly, 6 rosewood, and 1 oz. V-6 Mixing Oil. Rub on wrinkles in an upward, lifting motion.

    BLEND #2—1 frankincense, 1 lavender, and 1 lemon. It's like magic for wrinkles. Rub on morning and night around the eyes.

    BLEND #3—5-10 drops frankincense added to Sandalwood Moisture Creme.

    BLEND #4—Equal amounts of sandalwood, helichrysum, geranium, lavender, and frankincense. Combine with either Genesis Hand & Body Lotion or Satin Body Lotion and apply.

    PERSONAL CARE—Rose Ointment, Sandalwood Moisture Creme, Satin Body Lotion.

    SUPPLEMENTS—Megazyme, PD 80/20, Prenolone/Prenolone+, Thyromin (thyroid function affects the skin), Ultra Young.

PREVENT—<u>Gentle Baby</u> and patchouly (prevents and retards).

    PERSONAL CARE—Boswellia Wrinkle Creme (collagen builder), Satin Facial Scrub - Mint or Juniper, NeuroGen (helps moisturize deep tissues), Wolfberry Eye Creme. The following three items can be used together to help tone the skin and prevent wrinkles: Orange Blossom Facial Wash, Sandalwood Toner, Sandalwood Moisture Creme.

SMOOTH—Add 2 drops frankincense to a little Genesis Hand & Body Lotion or Satin Body Lotion and apply.

    PERSONAL CARE—Boswellia Wrinkle Creme (collagen builder).

YEAST: See CANDIDA.

YIN and YANG: Ylang ylang (balances)

YOGA: Cedarwood, sandalwood, spruce, tsuga.

ZEST (for life): <u>En-R-Gee</u>, <u>Motivation</u>, nutmeg, <u>Legacy</u>, <u>Live with Passion</u>. Diffuse.

NOTES

Appendix

Single Oil Summary Information

The following chart displays summary information about each of the single oils, including: botanical name, safety data, and the products (blends, personal care products, bath and shower gels, tinctures, massage oils, and supplements) that contain the single oil. The safety data includes possible skin reactions and conditions during which use of that particular oil should be limited or completely avoided (refer to the legend following this chart). **Note:** This safety data is provided for **EXTERNAL USE ONLY! Essential oils should never be taken internally** unless specifically instructed by a healthcare professional.

Single Oil Name	Botanical Name	Safety Data	Products containing Single Oil
Angelica	*Angelica archangelica* (Umbelliferae)	(GRAS), D, P, PH	Awaken, Forgiveness, Grounding, Harmony, Legacy, Live with Passion, Surrender
Anise	*Pimpinella anisum* (Umbelliferae)	(GRAS), CS	Awaken, Di-Tone, Dream Catcher, Allerzyme, Carbozyme, ComforTone, Detoxzyme, Fiberzyme, ICP, Lipozyme, Megazyme, ParaFree, Polyzyme, Power Meal
Basil	*Ocimum basilicum* (Labiatae)	(GRAS), E*, P*, SI	Aroma Siez, Clarity, Legacy, M-Grain, ArthroTune
Bergamot	*Citrus bergamia* (Rutaceae)	(GRAS), CS*, PH*	Awaken, Clarity, Dream Catcher, Forgiveness, Gentle Baby, Harmony, Joy, Joy Aqua Essence, Legacy, White Angelica, EndoBalance, Genesis Hand and Body Lotion, Prenolone, Prenolone+, Rosewood Moisturizing Hair & Scalp Wash, Rosewood Moisturizing Nourishing Rinse, Sandalwood Moisture Creme, Sandalwood Toner, Dragon Time Bath Gel, Evening Peace Bath Gel, Femalin Tincture
Birch	*Betula alleghaniensis* (Betulaceae)	E*, P*	
Black Cumin	*Nigella sativa*		ParaFree
Blue Cypress	*Callitris intratropica*		Brain Power
Buplevere	*Bupleurum fruticosum*		Legacy

Single Oil Name	Botanical Name	Safety Data	Products containing Single Oil
Cajeput	*Melaleuca leucadendra* (Myrtaceae)	(FA/FL), SI	Legacy
Calamus	*Acorus calamus (Araceae)*		Exodus II
Cardamom	*Elettaria cardamomum* (Zingiberaceae)	(GRAS)	Clarity, Legacy
Carrot	*Daucus carota* (Umbelliferae)	(GRAS)	Legacy, Rose Ointment
Cassia	*Cinnamomum cassia* (Lauraceae)	(GRAS), CS*, SI*	Exodus II
Cedar	*Cedrus canadensis* (Cupressaceae)		Evergreen Essence
Cedar, Canadian Red	*Thuja plicata* (Cupressaceae)	CS	Legacy
Cedar, Western Red	*Thuja plicata* (Cupressaceae)		Red Cedar Essential Water, KidScents Lotion
Cedar Leaf	*Thuja occidentalis* (Cupressaceae)		Legacy
Cedarwood	*Cedrus atlantica* (Pinaceae)	P	Brain Power, Grounding, Inspiration, Into the Future, Legacy, Live with Passion, Sacred Mountain, SARA, KidScents Bath Gel, KidScents Lotion, Sacred Mountain Aqua Essence, Sacred Mountain Bar Soap, Peppermint Cedarwood Bar Soap, Cel-Lite Magic Massage Oil
Chamomile (German/Blue)	*Matricaria chamomilla/recutita* (Compositae)	(GRAS), P, SI	EndoFlex, Legacy, Surrender, K&B Tincture, JuvaTone, ComforTone
Chamomile (Mixta)	*Chamaemelum mixtum* (Compositae)		Radex
Chamomile (Roman)	*Chamaemelum nobile* (Compositae)	(GRAS), SI	Clarity, Forgiveness, Gentle Baby, Harmony, Joy, Joy Aqua Essence, JuvaFlex, Legacy, M-Grain, Motivation, Surrender, Genesis Hand and Body Lotion, KidScents Tender Tush, Lemon Sage Clarifying Hair & Scalp Wash, Lemon Sage Clarifying Nourishing Rinse, Sandalwood Toner, Satin Body Lotion, Wolfberry Eye Creme, Dragon Time Bath Gel, Evening Peace Bath Gel, Chelex Tincture, K&B Tincture, Rehemogen Tincture

Single Oil Name	Botanical Name	Safety Data	Products containing Single Oil
Cinnamon Bark	*Cinnamomum verum* (Lauraceae)	CS*, P*, SI*	Christmas Spirit, Exodus II, Gathering, Legacy, Magnify Your Purpose, Thieves, Cinnamint Lip Balm, Thieves Bar Soap, ImmuGel, Mineral Essence, Wolfberry Bar
Cistus	*Cistus ladanifer* (Cistaceae)	(FA/FL), P	ImmuPower, Legacy, ImmuneTune, KidScents Tender Tush
Citronella	*Cymbopogon nardus* (Gramineae)	(GRAS), CS*, P, SI	Legacy, Purification, Sunsation Suntan Oil
Clary Sage	*Salvia sclarea* (Labiatae)	(GRAS), A, P	Dragon Time, Into the Future, Legacy, Live with Passion, EndoBalance, Lavender Volume Hair & Scalp Wash, Lavender Volume Nourishing Rinse, Prenolone, Prenolone+, Rosewood Moisturizing Hair & Scalp Wash, Rosewood Moisturizing Nourishing Rinse, Dragon Time Bath Gel, Evening Peace Bath Gel, Estro Tincture, Femalin Tincture, Cel-Lite Magic Massage Oil, Dragon Time Massage Oil, CortiStop (Women's), FemiGen
Clove	*Syzygium aromaticum* (Myrtaceae)	(GRAS), CS*, P, SI	Abundance, En-R-Gee, ImmuPower, Legacy, Longevity, Melrose, PanAway, Thieves, Dentarome Plus Toothpaste, KidScents Toothpaste, Thieves Bar Soap, K&B Tincture, Royal Essence Tincture, Essential Omegas, ImmuGel, Longevity Capsules, Megazyme, ParaFree, Radex
Coriander	*Coriandrum sativum* L. (Umbelliferae)	(GRAS), ST	Legacy
Cumin	*Cuminus cyminum* (Umbelliferae)	(GRAS), P, PH*	ImmuPower, Legacy, Detoxzyme, Protec, Radex
Cypress	*Cupressus sempervirens* (Cupressaceae)	P	Aroma Life, Aroma Siez, Legacy, RC, Arthro Plus Tincture, H-R-T Tincture, Cel-Lite Magic Massage Oil, ArthroTune, Body Balance, Power Meal, Super Cal
Davana	*Artemisia pallens* (Compositae)	(FA/FL), P	Trauma Life
Dill	*Anethum graveolens* (Umbelliferae)	(GRAS), E	Legacy
Elemi	*Canarium luzonicum* (Burseraceae)	(FA/FL)	Legacy, Ortho Sport Massage Oil
Eucalyptus	*Eucalyptus globulus* (Myrtaceae)	(FA/FL)	Legacy, RC, Fresh Essence Mouthwash, Chelex Tincture, Ortho Sport Massage Oil
Eucalyptus Citriodora	*Eucalyptus citriodora* (Myrtaceae)	CS	Legacy, RC

Single Oil Name	Botanical Name	Safety Data	Products containing Single Oil
Eucalyptus Dives	*Eucalyptus dives* (Myrtaceae)		Legacy
Eucalyptus Polybractea	*Eucalyptus polybractea* (Myrtaceae)		Legacy
Eucalyptus Radiata	*Eucalyptus radiata* (Myrtaceae)		Legacy, Raven, RC, Thieves, Thieves Bar Soap
Fennel	*Foeniculum vulgare* (Umbelliferae)	(GRAS), CS, E, P	Di-Tone, Dragon Time, JuvaFlex, Legacy, Mister, Allerzyme, Carbozyme, Detoxzyme, EndoBalance, Fiberzyme, Lipozyme, Prenolone, Prenolone+, Dragon Time Bath Gel, Estro Tincture, Femalin Tincture, K&B Tincture, Dragon Time Massage Oil, CortiStop (Women's), FemiGen, ICP, Megazyme, ParaFree, Power Meal, ProGen
Fir	*Abies alba* (Pinaceae)	(FA/FL), SI	En-R-Gee, Grounding, Into the Future, Legacy, Sacred Mountain, Sacred Mountain Aqua Essence, Sacred Mountain Bar Soap, ArthroTune, ImmuneTune
Fir, Balsam	*Abies balsamea* (Pinaceae)	(FA/FL), SI	Legacy
Fir, Douglas	*Pseudotsuga menziesii* (Pinaceae)	SI	Legacy, Regenolone
Fir, Idaho Balsam	*Abies grandis* (Pinaceae)	SI, PH	Believe, Gratitude
Fir, Red	*Abies magnifica* (Pinaceae)	SI	Evergreen Essence
Fir, White	*Abies grandis* (Pinaceae)	SI	Evergreen Essence, Legacy, Mountain Essence Essential Water
Fleabane	*Conyza canadensis* (Compositae)		Legacy, CortiStop (Men's and Women's), ProMist, ThermaBurn, Ultra Young, Ultra Young Plus
Frankincense	*Boswellia carteri* (Burseraceae)	(FA/FL)	Abundance, Acceptance, Believe, Brain Power, Exodus II, Forgiveness, Gathering, Gratitude, Harmony, Humility, ImmuPower, Inspiration, Into the Future, Legacy, Longevity, 3 Wise Men, Trauma Life, Valor, Boswellia Wrinkle Creme, KidScents Tender Tush, Protec, Wolfberry Eye Creme, Valor Bar Soap, Valor Aqua Essence, CortiStop (Men's and Women's), Exodus, ThermaBurn
Galbanum	*Ferula gummosa* (Umbelliferae)	(FA/FL)	Exodus II, Gathering, Gratitude, Legacy

Single Oil Name	Botanical Name	Safety Data	Products containing Single Oil
Geranium	*Pelargonium graveolens* (Geraniaceae)	(GRAS), CS	Acceptance, Clarity, EndoFlex, Envision, Forgiveness, Gathering, Gentle Baby, Harmony, Humility, Joy, Joy Aqua Essence, JuvaFlex, Legacy, Release, SARA, Trauma Life, White Angelica, Boswellia Wrinkle Creme, EndoBalance, Genesis Hand and Body Lotion, Lemon Sage Clarifying Hair & Scalp Wash, Lemon Sage Clarifying Nourishing Rinse, Prenolone, Prenolone+, Rosewood Moisturizing Hair & Scalp Wash, Rosewood Moisturizing Nourishing Rinse, Satin Body Lotion, Wolfberry Eye Creme, Dragon Time Bath Gel, Evening Peace Bath Gel, KidScents Bath Gel, KidScents Lotion, Melaleuca Geranium Bar Soap, K&B Tincture, JuvaTone
Ginger	*Zingiber officinale* (Zingiberaceae)	(GRAS), CS, PH	Abundance, Di-Tone, Legacy, Live with Passion, Magnify Your Purpose, Allerzyme, Carbozyme, ComforTone, Fiberzyme, ICP, Lipozyme, Mint Condition
Goldenrod	*Solidago canadensis* (Asteraceae)		Legacy
Grapefruit	*Citrus x paradisi* (Rutaceae)	(GRAS)	Citrus Fresh, Legacy, Cel-Lite Magic Massage Oil, Body Balance, Power Meal, ProMist, Super C, ThermaMist
Helichrysum	*Helichrysum italicum* (Compositae)		Aroma Life, Brain Power, Forgiveness, JuvaFlex, Legacy, Live with Passion, M-Grain, PanAway, Trauma Life, Chelex Tincture, ArthroTune, CardiaCare
Hyssop	*Hyssopus officinalis* (Labiatae)	(GRAS), E*, HBP*, P*	Exodus II, Harmony, ImmuPower, Legacy, Relieve It, White Angelica, Exodus
Jasmine	*Jasminum officinale* (Oleaceae)	(GRAS)	Clarity, Dragon Time, Forgiveness, Gentle Baby, Harmony, Inner Child, Into the Future, Joy, Joy Aqua Essence, Legacy, Live with Passion, Sensation, Genesis Hand & Body Lotion, Lavender Volume Hair & Scalp Wash, Lavender Volume Nourishing Rinse, Satin Body Lotion, Sensation Hand & Body Lotion, Dragon Time Bath Gel, Evening Peace Bath Gel, Sensation Bath Gel, Dragon Time Massage Oil, Sensation Massage Oil
Juniper	*Juniperus osteosperma* and/or *J. scopulorum* (Cupressaceae)		Di-Tone, Dream Catcher, En-R-Gee, Grounding, Hope, Into the Future, Legacy, 3 Wise Men, Allerzyme, Carbozyme, Fiberzyme, Juniper Satin Facial Scrub, Lipozyme, NeuroGen, Morning Start Bath Gel, Morning Start Bar Soap, Arthro Plus Tincture, K&B Tincture, Cel-Lite Magic Massage Oil, Ortho Ease Massage Oil, ArthroTune

Single Oil Name	Botanical Name	Safety Data	Products containing Single Oil
Laurel	*Laurus nobilis* (Lauraceae)	(GRAS), CS, P*	Legacy, Exodus, ParaFree
Lavandin	*Lavandula x hybrida* (Labiatae)	(GRAS), E, P*	Purification, Release
Lavender	*Lavandula angustifolia* CT linalol (Labiatae)		Aroma Siez, Brain Power, Dragon Time, Envision, Forgiveness, Gathering, Gentle Baby, Harmony, Legacy, M-Grain, Mister, Motivation, RC, SARA, Surrender, Trauma Life, LavaDerm Cooling Mist, Lavender Essential Water, Lavender Volume Hair & Scalp Wash, Lavender Volume Nourishing Rinse, KidScents Tender Tush, Orange Blossom Facial Wash, Sandalwood Moisture Creme, Sunsation Suntan Oil, Wolfberry Eye Creme, Dragon Time Bath Gel, Lavender Bar Soap, Estro Tincture, Dragon Time Massage Oil, Relaxation Massage Oil, ProGen
Ledum	*Ledum groenlandicum* (Ericaceae)		Legacy
Lemon	*Citrus limon* (Rutaceae)	(GRAS), PH*, SI*	Citrus Fresh, Clarity, Forgiveness, Gentle Baby, Harmony, Joy, Joy Aqua Essence, Legacy, Raven, Surrender, Thieves, Genesis Hand and Body Lotion, KidScents Detangler, KidScents Shampoo, Lavender Volume Hair & Scalp Wash, Lavender Volume Nourishing Rinse, Lemon Sage Clarifying Hair & Scalp Wash, Lemon Sage Clarifying Nourishing Rinse, Orange Blossom Facial Wash, Dragon Time Bath Gel, Evening Peace Bath Gel, Thieves Bar Soap, Lemon Sandalwood Bar Soap, H-R-T Tincture, AlkaLime, AminoTech, Berry Young Delights, Berry Young Juice, Body Balance, CardiaCare, ImmuGel, ImmuneTune, JuvaTone, Mineral Essence, Power Meal, Super C, VitaGreen, WheyFit
Lemongrass	*Cymbopogon flexuosus* (Gramineae)	(GRAS), SI*	Di-Tone, En-R-Gee, Inner Child, Legacy, Purification, Allerzyme, Carbozyme, Fiberzyme, Lipozyme, NeuroGen, Sunsation Suntan Oil, Morning Start Bath Gel, Morning Start Bar Soap, Ortho Ease Massage Oil, Ortho Sport Massage Oil, Be-Fit, Body Balance, ICP, VitaGreen
Lime	*Citrus aurantifolia* (Rutaceae)	(GRAS), PH*	Legacy, Lemon Sage Clarifying Hair & Scalp Wash, Lemon Sage Clarifying Nourishing Rinse, AlkaLime, AminoTech, Mighty Vites, Super C
Mandarin	*Citrus reticulata* (Rutaceae)	(GRAS), PH	Citrus Fresh, Joy, Joy Aqua Essence, Legacy, Dragon Time Bath Gel, Mighty Vites, Super C

Single Oil Name	Botanical Name	Safety Data	Products containing Single Oil
Marjoram	*Origanum majorana* (Labiatae)	(GRAS), P	Aroma Life, Aroma Siez, Dragon Time, Legacy, M-Grain, RC, Dragon Time Bath Gel, Arthro Plus Tincture, Ortho Ease Massage Oil, Ortho Sport Massage Oil, ArthroTune, CardiaCare, Super Cal
Melaleuca (Tea Tree)	*Melaleuca alternifolia* (Myrtaceae)	(FA/FL), CS	Legacy, Melrose, Purification, Rose Ointment, Sunsation Suntan Oil, Melaleuca Geranium Bar Soap, Femalin Tincture, Rehemogen Tincture, Royal Essence Tincture, ParaFree, Radex
Melaleuca ericifolia (formerly Rosalina)	*Melaleuca ericifolia* (Myrtaceae)	(FA/FL)	Legacy, Melaleuca Geranium Bar Soap
Melaleuca quinquenervia	*Melaleuca quinquenervia* (Myrtaceae)	(FA/FL), CS	Melrose, Radex
Melissa	*Melissa officinalis* (Labiatae)	(GRAS)	Brain Power, Forgiveness, Hope, Humility, Legacy, Live with Passion, Melissa Essential Water, White Angelica, VitaGreen
Mountain Savory	*Satureja montana* (Labiatae)	(GRAS), P*, SI*	ImmuPower, Legacy, Surrender
Mugwort	*Artemisia vulgaris* (Asteraceae)	P*	
Myrrh	*Commiphora myrrha* (Burseraceae)	(FA/FL), P	Abundance, Exodus II, Gratitude, Hope, Humility, Legacy, 3 Wise Men, White Angelica, Boswellia Wrinkle Creme, Protec, Rose Ointment, Sandalwood Moisture Creme, Sandalwood Toner, Thyromin
Myrtle	*Myrtus communis* (Myrtaceae)		EndoFlex, Inspiration, Legacy, Mister, Purification, RC, JuvaTone, ProGen, ThermaBurn, Thyromin
Neroli	*Citrus aurantium bigaradia* (Rutaceae)	(GRAS)	Acceptance, Humility, Inner Child, Legacy, Live with Passion, Present Time
Nutmeg	*Myristica fragrans* (Myristicaceae)	(GRAS), E*, P	EndoFlex, En-R-Gee, Legacy, Magnify Your Purpose, Royal Essence Tincture, Be-Fit, ParaFree, Power Meal, ThermaBurn
Onycha	*Styrax benzoin* (Styracaceae)	(FA/FL)	
Orange	*Citrus sinensis* (Rutaceae)	(GRAS), PH*	Abundance, Christmas Spirit, Citrus Fresh, Envision, Harmony, Inner Child, Legacy, Longevity, Peace & Calming, Peace & Calming Aqua Essence, SARA, Berry Young Juice, Body Balance, Essential Omegas, ImmuneTune, ImmuPro, Longevity Capsules, Mighty Vites, Power Meal, Super C, Wolfberry Bar

Single Oil Name	Botanical Name	Safety Data	Products containing Single Oil
Oregano	*Origanum compactum* (Labiatae)	(GRAS), SI*	ImmuPower, Legacy, Regenolone, Ortho Sport Massage Oil, ImmuGel
Palmarosa	*Cymbopogon martinii* (Gramineae)	(GRAS)	Clarity, Forgiveness, Gentle Baby, Harmony, Joy, Joy Aqua Essence, Legacy, Genesis Hand & Body Lotion, Rose Ointment, Dragon Time Bath Gel, Evening Peace Bath Gel
Patchouly	*Pogostemon cablin* (Labiatae)	(FA/FL)	Abundance, Di-Tone, Legacy, Live with Passion, Magnify Your Purpose, Peace & Calming, Allerzyme, Carbozyme, Fiberzyme, Lipozyme, Peace & Calming Aqua Essence, Orange Blossom Facial Wash, Rose Ointment
Pepper (Black)	*Piper nigrum* (Piperaceae)	(GRAS), SI*	Dream Catcher, En-R-Gee, Legacy, Relieve It, Royal Essence Tincture, Cel-Lite Magic Massage Oil, ArthroTune
Peppermint	*Mentha piperita* (Labiatae)	(GRAS), CS, HBP, P	Aroma Siez, Clarity, Di-Tone, Legacy, M-Grain, Mister, PanAway, Raven, RC, Relieve It, Allerzyme, Carbozyme, Cinnamint Lip Balm, Dentarome/ Dentarome Plus Toothpaste, Fiberzyme, Fresh Essence Mouthwash, Fresh Essence Plus Mouthwash, Lipozyme, Mint Satin Facial Scrub, NeuroGen, Polyzyme, Regenolone, Satin Body Lotion, Morning Start Bath Gel, Peppermint Cedarwood Bar Soap, Peppermint Essential Water, Morning Start Bar Soap, Ortho Ease Massage Oil, Ortho Sport Massage Oil, Relaxation Massage Oil, ComforTone, CortiStop (Men's and Women's), Essential Manna (Carob Mint Flavor), Megazyme, Mineral Essence, Mint Condition, ProGen, ProMist, ThermaMist, Thyromin
Petitgrain	*Citrus aurantium* (Rutaceae)	(GRAS)	Legacy
Pine	*Pinus sylvestris* (Pinaceae)	(FA/FL), SI	Evergreen Essence, Grounding, Legacy, RC, Lemon Sage Clarifying Hair & Scalp Wash, Lemon Sage Clarifying Nourishing Rinse, ImmuneTune
Pine, Black	*Pinus nigra* (Pinaceae)	SI	Evergreen Essence
Pine, Lodge Pole	*Pinus contorta* (Pinaceae)	SI	Evergreen Essence
Pine, Piñon	*Pinus edulis* (Pinaceae)	SI	Evergreen Essence
Pine, Ponderosa	*Pinus ponderosa* (Pinaceae)	SI	Evergreen Essence

Single Oil Name	Botanical Name	Safety Data	Products containing Single Oil
Ravensara	*Ravensara aromatica* (Lauraceae)		ImmuPower, Legacy, Raven, ImmuneTune
Rosalina (Australian)	See Melaleuca ericifolia		
Rose (Bulgarian)	*Rosa damascena* (Rosaceae)	(GRAS), P	Envision, Forgiveness, Gathering, Gentle Baby, Harmony, Humility, Joy, Joy Aqua Essence, Legacy, SARA, Trauma Life, White Angelica, Rose Ointment
Rosehip	*Rosa canina* (Rosaceae)	(GRAS)	Legacy, Rose Ointment, Sandalwood Moisture Creme, Wolfberry Eye Creme
Rosemary cineol	*Rosmarinus officinalis* CT 1,8 cineol (Labiatae)	(GRAS), E*, HBP*, P*	Clarity, En-R-Gee, JuvaFlex, Legacy, Melrose, Purification Thieves, Morning Start Bath Gel, Thieves Bar Soap, Morning Start Bar Soap, Chelex Tincture, Femalin Tincture, Rehemogen Tincture, Royal Essence Tincture, Be-Fit, ComforTone, ICP, ImmuGel, JuvaTone, Polyzyme, VitaGreen
Rosemary verbenon	*Rosmarinus officinalis* CT verbenon (Labiatae)	(GRAS), E*, HBP, P	Legacy, Orange Blossom Facial Wash, Sandalwood Moisture Creme
Rosewood	*Aniba rosaeodora* (Lauraceae)		Acceptance, Believe, Clarity, Forgiveness, Gentle Baby, Gratitude, Harmony, Humility, Inspiration, Joy, Joy Aqua Essence, Legacy, Magnify Your Purpose, Sensation, Valor, Valor Aqua Essence White Angelica, Genesis Hand & Body Lotion, KidScents Lotion, KidScents Tender Tush, Rose Ointment, Rosewood Moisturizing Hair & Scalp Wash, Rosewood Moisturizing Nourishing Rinse, Sandalwood Moisture Cream, Sandalwood Toner, Satin Body Lotion, Sensation Hand & Body Lotion, Wolfberry Eye Creme, Dragon Time Bath Gel, Evening Peace Bath Gel, Sensation Bath Gel, Lavender Bar Soap, Valor Bar Soap, H-R-T Tincture, Relaxation Massage Oil, Sensation Massage Oil
Sage	*Salvia officinalis* (Labiatae)	(GRAS), E*, HBP*, P*	EndoFlex, Envision, Legacy, Magnify Your Purpose, Mister, Protec, Lemon Sage Clarifying Hair & Scalp Wash, Lemon Sage Clarifying Nourishing Rinse, Dragon Time Bath Gel, K&B Tincture, Dragon Time Massage Oil, FemiGen, ProGen
Sage, Spanish	*Salvia lavandulifolia*	(GRAS)	Harmony

Single Oil Name	Botanical Name	Safety Data	Products containing Single Oil
Sandalwood	*Santalum album* (Santalaceae)	(FA/FL)	Acceptance, Brain Power, Dream Catcher, Forgiveness, Gathering, Harmony, Inner Child, Inspiration, Legacy, Live with Passion, Magnify Your Purpose, Release, 3 Wise Men, Trauma Life, White Angelica, Boswellia Wrinkle Creme, KidScents Tender Tush, Rosewood Moisturizing Hair & Scalp Wash, Rosewood Moisturizing Nourishing Rinse, Sandalwood Moisture Creme, Sandalwood Toner, Satin Body Lotion, Evening Peace Bath Gel, Lemon Sandalwood Bar Soap, Ultra Young, Ultra Young Plus
Spearmint	*Mentha spicata* (Labiatae)	(GRAS), P	Citrus Fresh, EndoFlex, Legacy, Cinnamint Lip Balm, Fresh Essence Plus Mouthwash, Relaxation Massage Oil, Mint Condition, ProMist, ThermaBurn, ThermaMist, Thyromin
Spikenard	*Nardostachys jatamansi* (Valerianaceae)		Exodus II, Humility, Legacy, Exodus
Spruce	*Picea mariana* (Pinaceae)	(FA/FL)	Abundance, Christmas Spirit, Envision, Gathering, Grounding, Harmony, Hope, Inner Child, Inspiration, Legacy, Motivation, Present Time, RC, Relieve It, Sacred Mountain, Sacred Mountain Aqua Essence, Surrender, 3 Wise Men, Trauma Life, Valor, Valor Aqua Essence, White Angelica, Sacred Mountain Bar Soap, Valor Bar Soap, ArthroTune
Spruce, Colorado Blue	*Picea pungens* (Pinaceae)		Evergreen Essence
Tamanu	*Calophyllum inophyllum* (Bintangor)		
Tangerine	*Citrus nobilis* (Rutaceae)	(GRAS)	Citrus Fresh, Dream Catcher, Inner Child, Legacy, Peace & Calming, KidScents Detangler, KidScents Shampoo, Peace & Calming Aqua Essence, Relaxation Massage Oil, ComforTone
Tansy, Blue	*Tanacetum annum* (Compositae)		Acceptance, Dream Catcher, JuvaFlex, Legacy, Peace & Calming, Release, SARA, Valor, KidScents Detangler, KidScents Shampoo, KidScents Tender Tush, Peace & Calming Aqua Essence, Valor Aqua Essence, Dragon Time Bath Gel, Evening Peace Bath Gel, Valor Bar Soap, JuvaTone
Tansy, Idaho	*Tanacetum vulgare* (Compositae)		ImmuPower, Into the Future, Legacy, ParaFree
Tarragon	*Artemisia dracunculus* (Compositae)	(GRAS), E*, P*	Di-Tone, Legacy, Allerzyme, Carbozyme, ComforTone, Fiberzyme, ICP, Lipozyme, Megazyme, Mint Condition

Single Oil Name	Botanical Name	Safety Data	Products containing Single Oil
Thyme	*Thymus vulgaris* (Labiatae)	(GRAS), HBP	Legacy, Longevity, Dentarome Plus Toothpaste, Fresh Essence Mouthwash, KidScents Toothpaste, Rehemogen, ImmuGel, Longevity Capsules, ParaFree, Radex
Thyme linalol	*Thymus vulgaris* CT Linalol (Labiatae)	(GRAS)	Legacy
Thyme, Red	*Thymus serpyllum* (Labiatae)	(GRAS)	Ortho Ease
Tsuga	*Tsuga canadensis* (Pinaceae)	(FA/FL), SI*	Grounding, Legacy
Valerian	*Valeriana officinalis* (Valerianaceae)	(FA/FL), CS	Legacy, Trauma Life
Vetiver	*Vetiveria zizanoides* (Gramineae)	P	Legacy, Fresh Essence Plus Mouthwash, Melaleuca Geranium Bar Soap, Ortho Ease Massage Oil, Ortho Sport Massage Oil, ParaFree
Vitex	*Vitex negundo* (Labiatae)		Legacy
White Lotus	*Nymphaea lotus* (Nymphaeaceae)		
Wintergreen	*Gaultheria procumbens* (Ericaceae)	E*, P*	Legacy, PanAway, Raven, Dentarome/ Dentarome Plus Toothpaste, Fresh Essence Mouthwash, Regenolone, Rosewood Moisturizing Hair & Scalp Wash, Rosewood Moisturizing Nourishing Rinse, Arthro Plus Tincture, Ortho Ease Massage Oil, Ortho Sport Massage Oil, ArthroTune, Be-Fit, Super Cal
Yarrow	*Achillea millefolium* (Compositae)	CS, P	Dragon Time, Legacy, Mister, Prenolone/ Prenolone+, Dragon Time Massage Oil, ProGen

Single Oil Name	Botanical Name	Safety Data	Products containing Single Oil
Ylang Ylang	*Cananga odorata* (Annonaceae)	(GRAS), CS	Aroma Life, Clarity, Dream Catcher, Forgiveness, Gathering, Gentle Baby, Gratitude, Grounding, Harmony, Humility, Inner Child, Joy, Joy Aqua Essence, Legacy, Motivation, Peace & Calming, Peace & Calming Aqua Essence, Present Time, Release, Sacred Mountain, Sacred Mountain Aqua Essence, SARA, Sensation, White Angelica, Boswellia Wrinkle Creme, EndoBalance, Genesis Hand & Body Lotion, Lemon Sage Clarifying Hair & Scalp Wash, Lemon Sage Clarifying Nourishing Rinse, Prenolone/ Prenolone+, Satin Body Lotion, Sensation Hand & Body Lotion, Dragon Time Bath Gel, Evening Peace Bath Gel, Sensation Bath Gel, Sacred Mountain Bar Soap, H-R-T Tincture, Dragon Time Massage Oil, Relaxation Massage Oil, Sensation Massage Oil, CardiaCare, FemiGen

Safety Data Legend:

A	**Avoid** during and after consumption of **alcohol**
CS	Could possibly result in **contact sensitization** (redness or irritation of the skin due to repeated application of a substance) (rotate or use different oils)
CS*	Repeated use can result in **extreme contact sensitization** (rotate between different oils)
D	**Avoid** if **diabetic**
E	Use with **caution** if susceptible to **epilepsy** (small amounts or in dilution)
E*	**Avoid** if susceptible to **epilepsy** (can trigger a seizure)
HBP	Use with **caution** if dealing with **high blood pressure** (small amounts)
HBP*	**Avoid** if dealing with **high blood pressure**
P	Use with **caution** during **pregnancy** (small amounts or in dilution)
P*	**Avoid** during **pregnancy**
PH	**Photosensitivity**–direct exposure to sunlight after use could cause dermatitis (test first)
PH*	**Extreme Photosensitivity**–direct exposure to sunlight after use can cause severe dermatitis (avoid exposing affected area of skin to direct sunlight for 12 hours)
SI	Could possibly result in **skin irritation** (dilution may be necessary)
SI*	Can cause **extreme skin irritation** (dilution highly recommended)
ST	Can cause **stupification** in high doses (use only small amounts or in dilution)

Blend Summary Information

The following chart displays summary information about each of the oil blends, including: single oils contained in the blend, possible uses or areas of application, and safety data. The safety data includes possible skin reactions and conditions during which use of that particular blend should be limited or completely avoided (refer to the legend following the chart).
Note: This safety data is provided for **EXTERNAL USE ONLY! Essential oils should never be taken internally** unless specifically instructed by a healthcare professional.

Blend Name	Single Oil Contents	Uses/Application Areas	Safety Data
Abundance	Myrrh, cassia, frankincense, patchouly, orange, clove, ginger, spruce	Diffuse; Wrists, ears, neck, face; Wallet/Purse; Painting; Perfume	CS*, SI
Acceptance	Geranium, Blue tansy, frankincense, sandalwood, neroli, rosewood (Carrier: Almond oil)	Diffuse; *Liver*, heart, *chest*, face, ears, neck, thymus, wrists; Sacral chakra; Perfume	
Aroma Life	Cypress, marjoram, helichrysum, ylang ylang (Carrier: Sesame seed oil)	Heart; Vita Flex heart points—under left ring finger, under left ring toe, above left elbow, arteries on neck; Spine	
Aroma Siez	Basil, marjoram, lavender, peppermint, cypress	Muscles; Neck; Heart; Vita Flex points; Full body massage; Bath	
Awaken	Oil Blends of Joy, Forgiveness, Dream Catcher, Present Time, Harmony	Diffuse; Chest, heart, *forehead*, neck, temples, wrists; Perfume; Full body massage; Bath	
Believe	Idaho balsam fir, rosewood, frankincense	Diffuse; *Heart, forehead, temples*; Perfume	
Brain Power	Cedarwood, sandalwood, frankincense, melissa, Australian Blue cypress, lavender, helichrysum	Diffuse; Neck, throat, nose; Inside of cheeks; Perfume	
Christmas Spirit	Orange, cinnamon bark, spruce	Diffuse; Crown; Perfume; Place on pine boughs or fireplace logs; Add to potpourri	CS*, SI*
Citrus Fresh	Orange, tangerine, mandarin, grapefruit, lemon, spearmint	Diffuse; Ears, heart wrists; Perfume; Full body massage; Bath; Purify drinking water	SI*, PH*
Clarity	Basil, cardamom, rosemary cineol, peppermint, rosewood, geranium, lemon, palmarosa, ylang ylang, bergamot, Roman chamomile, jasmine	Diffuse; Forehead, neck, temples, wrists; Perfume; Bath	SI, P, PH*

Blend Name	Single Oil Contents	Uses/Application Areas	Safety Data
Di-Tone	Tarragon, ginger, peppermint, juniper, anise, fennel, lemongrass, patchouly	Vita Flex points—feet and ankles; stomach; abdomen, bottom of throat; Compress	P, E
Dragon Time	Clary sage, fennel, lavender, jasmine, yarrow, marjoram	Vita Flex points; Diffuse; Abdomen, lower back, location	P
Dream Catcher	Sandalwood, bergamot, ylang ylang, juniper, Blue tansy, tangerine, Black pepper, anise	Diffuse; Forehead, eye brows, *temples*, ears, throat chakra; Perfume; Pillow; Bath or sauna	PH
EndoFlex	Spearmint, sage, geranium, myrtle, nutmeg, German chamomile (Carrier: Sesame seed oil)	Thyroid, kidneys, liver, pancreas, glands; Vita Flex points	SI, E
En-R-Gee	Rosemary cineol, juniper, nutmeg, fir, Black pepper, lemongrass, clove	Diffuse; Wrists, ears, neck, temples, feet; Full body massage; Perfume	SI*, E
Envision	Spruce, sage, rose, geranium, orange, lavender	Vita Flex points; Diffuse; Wrists, *temples*; Bath; Massage	HBP, E, P
Evergreen Essence	Colorado Blue spruce (*Picea pungens*), Ponderosa pine (*Pinus ponderosa*), pine, Red fir (*Abies magnifica*), cedar (*Cedrus canadensis*), White fir, Black pine (*Pinus nigra*), Piñon pine (*Pinus edulis*), Lodge Pole pine (*Pinus contorta*)	*Diffuse*; Hands, bottoms of feet	CS, SI
Exodus II	Cinnamon bark, cassia, calamus, myrrh, hyssop, frankincense, spikenard, galbanum (Carrier: Olive oil)	Vita Flex points; Spine (dilute well)	CS*, SI*, P*
Forgiveness	Frankincense, sandalwood, lavender, melissa, angelica, helichrysum, rose, rosewood, geranium, lemon, palmarosa, ylang ylang, bergamot, Roman chamomile, jasmine (Carrier: Sesame seed oil)	Diffuse; *Navel*, heart, ears, wrists; Perfume	
Gathering	Galbanum, frankincense, sandalwood, lavender, cinnamon bark, rose, spruce, geranium, ylang ylang	Diffuse; *Forehead, heart, temples*, neck, thymus, face, chest; Perfume	
Gentle Baby	Geranium, rosewood, palmarosa, lavender, Roman chamomile, ylang ylang, rose, lemon, bergamot, jasmine	Diffuse; Ankles, lower back, abdomen, feet, face, neck; Massage; Perfume; Bath	
Gratitude	Idaho balsam fir, frankincense, rosewood, myrrh, galbanum, ylang ylang	Diffuse; *Heart, forehead, temples*; Perfume	

Blend Name	Single Oil Contents	Uses/Application Areas	Safety Data
Grounding	Juniper, angelica, ylang ylang, cedarwood, pine, spruce, fir, tsuga	Diffuse; *Brain stem, back of neck, sternum*, temples	SI
Harmony	Hyssop, spruce, lavender, frankincense, geranium, ylang ylang, orange, sandalwood, angelica, Spanish sage (*Salvia lavandulifolia*), rose, rosewood, lemon, palmarosa, bergamot, Roman chamomile, jasmine	Diffuse; Each chakra; Ears, feet, heart; *Energy meridians*, crown; Perfume	P, E*, HBP, PH
Hope	Melissa, myrrh, juniper, spruce (Carrier: Almond oil)	Diffuse; *Ears*; Chest, heart, temples, solar plexus, neck, feet, wrists; Perfume	
Humility	Geranium, ylang ylang, frankincense, spikenard, myrrh, rose, rosewood, melissa, neroli (Carrier: Sesame seed oil)	Diffuse; *Heart, neck, temples*	
ImmuPower	Cistus, frankincense, hyssop, ravensara, Mountain savory, oregano, clove, cumin, Idaho tansy	Diffuse; Throat, chest, spine, feet; Thymus; Veins in neck, under arm pits	SI, P, E
Inner Child	Orange, tangerine, jasmine, ylang ylang, spruce, sandalwood, lemongrass, neroli	Diffuse; *Navel, chest, temples, nose*	PH*, SI
Inspiration	Cedarwood, spruce, rosewood, sandalwood, frankincense, myrtle, mugwort	Diffuse; *Horns*, crown, shoulders, back of neck	
Into the Future	Frankincense, jasmine, Clary sage, juniper, Idaho tansy, fir (Carrier: Almond oil)	Diffuse; Bath; Heart, wrists, neck; Compress; Full body massage	
Joy	Lemon, mandarin, bergamot, ylang ylang, rose, rosewood, geranium, palmarosa, Roman chamomile, jasmine	Diffuse; *Heart*, ears, neck, thymus, temples, forehead, wrists; Bath; Compress; Massage; Perfume	PH*
JuvaFlex	Fennel, geranium, rosemary cineol, Roman chamomile, Blue tansy, helichrysum (Carrier: Sesame seed oil)	Vita Flex points; Feet, spine, LIVER; Full body massage	SI
Legacy	(See LEGACY in Blend section for complete list of 91 single oils)	Diffuse; Forehead, wrists, sternum, feet; Perfume	CS, SI
Live with Passion	Melissa, helichrysum, Clary sage, cedarwood, angelica, ginger, neroli, sandalwood, patchouly, jasmine	Wrists, *temples, chest, forehead*; Bath; Perfume or cologne	

Blend Name	Single Oil Contents	Uses/Application Areas	Safety Data
M-Grain	Basil, marjoram, lavender, peppermint, Roman chamomile, helichrysum	DIFFUSE; Forehead, crown, shoulders, neck, temples; Vita Flex points; Massage	
Magnify Your Purpose	Sandalwood, nutmeg, patchouly, rosewood, cinnamon bark, ginger, sage	Vita Flex points; Feet, wrists, *temples*; Diffuse; Bath; Massage	E, P, CS, SI
Melrose	Melaleuca (*alternifolia* & *quinquenervia*), rosemary cineol, clove	Diffuse; Forehead, liver; Topically on location	CS, SI
Mister	Sage, fennel, lavender, myrtle, yarrow, peppermint (Carrier: Sesame seed oil)	Vita Flex points; Ankles, lower pelvis, prostate (dilute); Compress	P*, E
Motivation	Roman chamomile, ylang ylang, spruce, lavender	Diffuse; Chest, neck; *Solar plexus*, sternum, feet, navel, ears; wrists, palms; Perfume	
PanAway	Wintergreen, helichrysum, clove, peppermint	Compress on spine; Vita Flex on feet; Topically on location	
Peace & Calming	Tangerine, orange, ylang ylang, patchouly, Blue tansy	Diffuse; Navel, nose, neck, feet; Bath; Perfume	PH
Present Time	Neroli, spruce, ylang ylang (Carrier: Almond oil)	*Thymus*; Neck, forehead	
Purification	Citronella, lemongrass, rosemary cineol, melaleuca, lavandin, myrtle	Diffuse; Vita Flex points; Ears, feet, temples; Topically on location	CS, SI
Raven	Ravensara, *Eucalyptus radiata*, peppermint, wintergreen, lemon	Diffuse; Vita Flex points; Lungs, throat; Pillow; Suppository (diluted)	SI
RC	4 eucalyptuses (E. globulus, E. radiata, E. australiana, E. citriodora), myrtle, marjoram, pine, cypress, lavender, spruce, peppermint	DIFFUSE; Chest, back, feet; Sinuses, nasal passages; Ears, neck, throat; Compress; Massage	
Release	Ylang ylang, lavandin, geranium, sandalwood, Blue tansy (Carrier: Olive oil)	*Compress on liver*; Ears, feet, Vita Flex points; Perfume	
Relieve It	Spruce, Black pepper, hyssop, peppermint	Apply on location of pain	SI, P, E, HBP
Sacred Mountain	Spruce, ylang ylang, fir, cedarwood	Diffuse; *Solar plexus, brain stem*, crown, neck, ears, thymus, wrists; Perfume	SI
SARA	Blue tansy, rose, lavender, geranium, orange, cedarwood, ylang ylang (Carrier: Almond oil)	*Energy centers*; Vita Flex points; *Temples, nose*; Places of abuse	

Blend Name	Single Oil Contents	Uses/Application Areas	Safety Data
Sensation	Rosewood, ylang ylang, jasmine	Diffuse; Apply on location; Massage; Bath	
Surrender	Lavender, Roman chamomile, German chamomile, angelica, Mountain savory, lemon, spruce	*Forehead, rim of ears, nape of neck, chest, solar plexus*; Bath	P, SI
Thieves	Clove, lemon, cinnamon bark, *Eucalyptus radiata*, rosemary cineol	Diffuse; Feet, throat, stomach, intestines; Thymus, arm pits (Dilute well for topical uses!)	CS*, SI*, P
3 Wise Men	Sandalwood, juniper, frankincense, spruce, myrrh (Carrier: Almond oil)	Diffuse; *Crown of head*; Neck, forehead, solar plexus, thymus; Perfume	
Trauma Life	*Citrus hystrix* (Leech Lime), davana, geranium, spruce, helichrysum, rose, sandalwood, frankincense, lavender, valerian	Diffuse; Spine; Feet, chest, ears, neck, forehead	
Valor	Spruce, rosewood, Blue tansy, frankincense (Carrier: Almond oil)	*FEET*; Diffuse; Heart, wrists, solar plexus, neck to thymus, spine; Perfume	
White Angelica	Geranium, spruce, myrrh, ylang ylang, hyssop, bergamot, melissa, sandalwood, rose, rosewood (Carrier: Almond oil)	Diffuse; *Shoulders*, crown, chest, ears, neck, forehead, wrists; Bath; Perfume	PH

Note: Italicized application areas represent the most effective areas for **emotional applications**.

Safety Data Legend:

A	**Avoid** during and after consumption of **alcohol**
CS	Could possibly result in **contact sensitization** (redness or irritation of the skin due to repeated application of a substance) (rotate or use different oils)
CS*	Repeated use can result in **extreme contact sensitization** (rotate between different oils)
D	**Avoid** if **diabetic**
E	Use with **caution** if susceptible to **epilepsy** (small amounts or in dilution)
E*	**Avoid** if susceptible to **epilepsy** (can trigger a seizure)
HBP	Use with **caution** if dealing with **high blood pressure** (small amounts)
HBP*	**Avoid** if dealing with **high blood pressure**
P	Use with **caution** during **pregnancy** (small amounts or in dilution)
P*	**Avoid** during **pregnancy**
PH	**Photosensitivity**–direct exposure to sunlight after use could cause dermatitis (test first)
PH*	**Extreme Photosensitivity**–direct exposure to sunlight after use can cause severe dermatitis (avoid exposing affected area of skin to direct sunlight for 12 hours)
SI	Could possibly result in **skin irritation** (dilution may be necessary)
SI*	Can cause **extreme skin irritation** (dilution highly recommended)
ST	Can cause **stupification** in high doses (use only small amounts or in dilution)

Bibliography

D'Adamo, Dr. Peter J., *4 Blood Types, 4 Diets, Eat Right For Your Type*. New York, NY: G.P. Putnam's Sons, 1996.

Balch, M.D., James, and Phyllis Balch, C.N.C. *Prescription for Nutritional Healing*. Garden City Park, NY: Avery Publishing Group, 1990.

Becker, M.D., Robert O. *The Body Electric*. New York, NY: Wm. Morrow, 1985.

Burroughs, Stanley. *Healing for the Age of Enlightenment*. Auburn, CA: Burroughs Books, 1993.

Burton Goldberg Group, The. *Alternative Medicine: The Definitive Guide*. Fife, WA: Future Medicine Publishing, Inc., 1994.

DeVita, Sabina M. *Electromagnetic Pollution. A Hidden Stress to Your System*. Marble Hill, MO: Stewart Publishing Company, 2000.

---------------. *Essential Oils Desk Reference*. Essential Science Publishing, Third Printing May 2000.

Fischer-Rizzi, Suzanne. *Complete Aromatherapy Handbook*. New York, NY: Sterling Publishing, 1990.

Foley, Marcy. *Embraced by the Essence! Your Journey into Wellness Using Pure Quality Essential Oils*. Boulder, Colorado: Holistic Wellness Foundation I, April 2000.

Gattefosse, Ph.D., Rene-Maurice. *Gattefosse's Aromatherapy*. Essex, England: The C.W. Daniel Company Ltd., 1937 English translation.

---------------. *Integrated Aromatic Medicine*. Proceedings from the First International Symposium, Grasse, France. Essential Science Publishing, March 2000.

Lawless, Julia. *The Encyclopaedia of Essential Oils*. Rockport, MA: Element, Inc., 1992.

Lee, M.D., John R. *Natural Progesterone: The Multiple Roles of a Remarkable Hormone.* Sebastopol, CA: BLL Publishing, 1995.

Maury, Marguerite. *Marguerite Maury's Guide to Aromatherapy.* C.W. Daniel, 1989.

Pènoël, M.D., Daniel and Pierre Franchomme. L'aromatherapie exactement. Limoges, France: Jollois, 1990.

Price, Shirley, and Len Price. *Aromatherapy for Health Professionals.* New York, NY: Churchill Livingstone Inc., 1995.

Price, Shirley, and Penny Price Parr. *Aromatherapy for Babies and Children.* San Francisco, CA: Thorsons, 1996.

Rose, Jeanne. *The Aromatherapy Book: Applications and Inhalations.* Berkeley, CA: North Atlantic Books, 1992.

Ryman, Danièle. *Aromatherapy: The Complete Guide to Plant & Flower Essences for Health and Beauty.* New York: Bantam Books, 1993.

Tisserand, Maggie. *Aromatherapy for Women: a Practical Guide to Essential Oils for Health and Beauty.* Rochester, VT: Healing Arts Press, 1996.

Tisserand, Robert. *Aromatherapy: to Heal and Tend the Body.* Wilmot, WI: Lotus Press, 1988.

Tisserand, Robert. *The Art of Aromatherapy.* Rochester, VT: Healing Arts Press, 1977.

Tisserand, Robert, and Tony Balacs. *Essential Oil Safety: A Guide for Health Care Professionals.* New York, NY: Churchill Livingstone, 1995.

Valnet, M.D., Jean. *The Practice of Aromatherapy: a Classic Compendium of Plant Medicines and their Healing Properties.* Rochester, VT: Healing Arts Press, 1980.

Watson, Franzesca. *Aromatherapy Blends & Remedies.* San Francisco, CA: Thorsons, 1995.

Wilson, Roberta. *Aromatherapy for Vibrant Health and Beauty: a practical A-to-Z reference to aromatherapy treatments for health, skin, and hair problems.* Honesdale, PA: Paragon Press, 1995.

Worwood, Valerie Ann. *The Complete Book of Essential Oils & Aromatherapy.* San Rafael, CA: New World Library, 1991.

Young, N.D., D. Gary. *An Introduction to Young Living Essential Oils.* Payson, UT: Young Living Essential Oils, 2000.

Young, N.D., D. Gary. *Aromatherapy: The Essential Beginning.* Salt Lake City, UT: Essential Press Publishing, 1995.

Young, Ph.D., Robert O. *One Sickness, One Disease, One Treatment.* Alpine, UT: Self-published, 1995.

Video Listing

---------------. *Essential Tips for Happy, Healthy Pets.* The Vision Firm, LLC, 2000.

Eaton, Cathy. *Raindrop Therapy.* Health is Your Wealth Enterprises, 1997.

Woloshyn, Tom. *Vita Flex Instruction.* Vita-Gem Enterprises, 1998.

Young, ND, D. Gary. *Raindrop Technique.* Young Living Essential Oils, 2000.

Index

This is an index of only the oil blends, personal care products, bath & shower gels, tinctures, massage oils, and supplements that appear in the Personal Guide section of this book. This index does not include any single oils as they have numerous entries in the "Personal Guide" section and would tend to make this index somewhat unusable. Also, possible uses for each single oil are already listed in the "Single Oil" section of the <u>Reference Guide for Essential Oils</u>. For summary information on each single oil, refer to the "Single Oil Summary Information" chart in the Appendix of this book.

Products Available from Abundant Health

Code	Wt‡	Product Description	Price
HEALTH RELATED BOOKS			
1000	46	**COIL BOUND - REFERENCE GUIDE BUNDLE** (1001 & 1002)	$30.00
1001	34	**COIL BOUND - Reference Guide for Essential Oils**	24.00
1002	12	**COIL BOUND - Quick Reference Guide for Using Essential Oils**	10.00
9049	80	**Essential Oils Desk Reference/Pocket Reference Bundle**	47.95
9048	64	**Essential Oils Desk Reference** (Second Edition)	38.00
9047	16	**Essential Oils Pocket Reference**	12.50
9065	18	**Integrated Aromatic Medicine - Grasse Symposium**	29.95
9026	6	**The Truth Behind Growth Hormone: Its Promise and Peril**	3.75
9027	6	**Longevity Secrets**	4.75
9011	3	**A New Route to Robust Health**	2.50
9016	4	**Pregnenolone**	3.50
9052	12	**Electromagnetic Pollution**	8.50
9020	16	**What Your Doctor May Not Tell You About Menopause**	13.00
9021	16	**What Your Doctor May Not Tell You About Premenopause**	13.00
9023	17	**The Miracle of MSM: The Natural Solution for Pain**	19.00
9024	13	**Your Body's Many Cries for Water**	14.00
9025	13	**Grow Young with HGH**	13.00
9030	20	**Feelings Buried Alive Never Die...**	14.00
9031	17	**Healing Feelings... From Your Heart**	14.00
9035	12	**Releasing Emotional Patterns with Essential Oils**	14.00
9050	31	**Essential Oil Safety**	47.00
9057	23	**The Essential Oil Cookbook** (180 recipes using 25 essential oils)	22.00
9045	48	**Embraced by the Essence**	33.00
9019	17	**Healing with Aromatherapy**	12.00
9060	33	**Aromatherapy for Health Professionals**	32.00
9070	16	**Aromatherapy for Babies and Children**	14.00
9075	8	**Veterinary Aromatherapy**	14.00
9080	85	**Alternative Medicine–A Definitive Guide**	29.00
9081	60	**An Alternative Medicine Guide to CANCER**	39.00
MASSAGE TABLES (Stock Colors Available: Teal or Raspberry)			
9610	640	**Avalon 30" Massage Table w/ Standard Crescent Face Rest**	352.00
9620	688	**Avalon 30" Massage Table w/ Standard Crescent Face Rest and Carrying Case**	410.00

| 9630 | 688 | **Spirit 30" Massage Table w/ Standard Crescent Face Rest** | 412.00 |
| 9640 | 736 | **Spirit 30" Massage Table w/ Standard Crescent Face Rest and Carrying Case** | 467.00 |

VIDEOS & VITA FLEX PRODUCTS (Volume Discounts Available)

9202	11	**VIDEO: Raindrop Technique** *by D. Gary Young*	$15.50
9227	11	**VIDEO: Essential Tips for Happy, Healthy Pets**	14.75
9302	11	**VIDEO: Vita Flex Instruction**	25.00
9301	20	**Vita Flex Roller** (Also known as **"Relax-a-Roller"**)	20.00
9040	11	**Healing for the Age of Enlightenment** (book)	11.00

GLASS and PLASTIC PRODUCTS (Others available - Call or see website)

9100	3	**5/8 Dram Amber Glass Vials** (w/orifice reducers) - 1 doz.	3.75
9135	104	**5/8 Dram Amber Glass Vials** (w/orifice reducers) - 38 doz.	114.00
9115	2	**5/8 Dram Blue Glass Vials** (w/orifice reducers) - ½ doz.	4.00
9116	2	**5/8 Dram Green Glass Vials** (w/orifice reducers) - ½ doz.	4.00
9140	3	**Pipettes** (Glass Droppers) - 1 doz.	3.50
9150	2	**1/6 Dram Clear Sample Vials** (w/dabber cap or clip) - 1 doz.	2.00
9160	4	**2 Dram (7.4 ml) Amber Glass Vials** w/dropper cap) - ½ doz.	3.75
9170	6	**4 Dram (14.7 ml) Amber Glass Vials** w/dropper cap) - ½ doz.	4.00
9180	12	**1 oz. Amber Glass Vials** w/dropper cap) - ½ doz.	4.00
9123	.5	**Spray Top for 1 oz. Amber Glass Vial**	.40
9120	3	**2 oz. Amber Glass Vial** (w/spray top)	.85
9125	3	**2 oz. Blue Glass Vial** (w/spray top)	1.10
9190	4	**2 oz. Plastic Bottles** w/snap top cap - ½ doz.	2.00

DIFFUSERS (Volume Discounts Available)

9310	13	**Battery Operated Diffuser w/ Power Adapter & 5 Pads**	35.00
9309		**Refill Pads for Battery Operated Diffuser**	.20
9320	17	**Economy Model Diffuser**	32.00
9330	18	**Silent Model Diffuser**	62.00
9340	35	**Professional Model Diffuser**	70.00
9345	45	**Deluxe Serenity Model Diffuser**	90.00
9360	12	**Diffuser Timer** with on/off switch and 96 possible settings (programmable in 15 minute increments over a 24 hour period!)	12.00

VIAL CARRYING CASES and OIL STORAGE/DISPLAY RACKS

9550	6	**Essential Bags**–Carrying Case for 30 - 15 ml vials (Disc. Avail)	31.95
9560	4	**Essential Bags**–Carrying Case for 16 - 5/8 dram vials (Disc.)	13.95
9535	18	**Essential Portfolios**–Professional Presentation Case for 32 vials	29.65
9545	8	**Essential Portfolios**–Professional Presentation Case for 8 vials	13.45

9573	288	**PREMIUM 3-Shelf Solid Oak Storage/Display Rack** (Holds 144 vials) It is 15" high x 21.75" wide x 8.5" deep; has two removable shelves with routed holes to keep your oils in place.	119.95
ELECTROMAGNETIC FIELD (EMF) PROTECTION			
9700	1	**Cellular Phone Diode** provides excellent protection against EMF from cellular or cordless phones, blow dryers, or any appliance.	19.95

‡ Weight is all shown in ounces.   Prices subject to change without notice!

Call for Wholesale Prices & Volume Discounts!!!

Abundant Health
478 S. Geneva Rd.
Orem, UT 84058

Orders: 1-888-718-3068 / 801-705-4832
Fax: 1-877-568-1988 / 801-705-4830
E-Mail: orders@abundant-health4u.com
Web Site: www.abundant-health4u.com

SHIPPING CHARGES

Total Weight	Ground	2nd Day Air	3 Day Express	Total Weight	Ground	2nd Day Air	3 Day Express
0-16 oz.	$5.48	$10.00	$4.95	401-416 oz.	$15..99	$53.80	$36.20
17-32 oz.	5.82	11.50	5.40	417-432 oz.	16.43	55.50	37.45
33-48 oz.	6.10	13.10	7.85	433-448 oz.	16.92	57.20	38.70
49-64 oz.	6.37	14.90	9.45	449-464 oz.	17.41	58.90	39.95
65-80 oz.	6.63	16.80	11.00	465-480 oz.	17.90	60.50	41.20
81-96 oz.	6.85	18.80	11.30	481-496 oz.	18.39	62.10	42.40
97-112 oz.	7.12	20.70	12.55	497-512 oz.	18.89	63.80	43.65
113-128 oz.	7.45	22.70	13.80	513-528 oz.	19.39	65.60	44.90
129-144 oz.	7.90	24.70	15.05	529-544 oz.	19.88	67.30	46.15
145-160 oz.	8.39	26.60	16.30	545-560 oz.	20.37	69.00	47.40
161-176 oz.	8.89	28.40	17.55	561-576 oz.	20.87	70.80	48.65
177-192 oz.	9.38	30.10	18.80	577-592 oz.	21.36	72.50	49.90
193-208 oz.	9.87	31.70	20.05	593-608 oz.	21.85	74.20	51.15
209-224 oz.	10.36	33.30	21.25	609-624 oz.	22.34	75.90	52.40
225-240 oz.	10.84	34.80	22.50	625-640 oz.	22.83	77.60	53.60
241-256 oz.	11.32	36.30	23.75	641-656 oz.	23.33	79.20	54.85
257-272 oz.	11.80	38.10	25.00	657-672 oz.	23.82	80.80	56.15
273-288 oz.	12.28	40.00	26.25	673-688 oz.	24.31	82.40	57.40
289-304 oz.	12.74	41.80	27.50	689-704 oz.	24.76	84.00	58.70
305-320 oz.	13.20	43.50	28.75	705-720 oz.	25.20	85.50	59.95
321-336 oz.	13.65	45.20	30.00	721-736 oz.	25.64	87.10	61.20
337-352 oz.	14.12	46.90	31.20	737-752 oz.	26.08	88.90	62.50
353-368 oz.	14.61	48.70	32.45	753-768 oz.	26.52	90.60	63.75
369-384 oz.	15.10	50.50	33.70	769-784 oz.	26.90	92.20	65.05
385-400 oz.	15.55	52.20	34.95	785-800 oz.	27.28	93.80	66.30
				801 oz. +	Call	Call	Call

International Shipping:
Global Priority Mail envelopes are $9.00 and hold one Reference Guide and one Quick Reference Guide.
Call for all other shipping costs.

BILLING INFORMATION (as it appears on the credit card statement)

Name:

Address:

City/State/Zip:

Phone #:

E-mail Address:

SHIP-TO INFORMATION (to which order will be sent)

Name:

Address:

City/State/Zip:

Phone #:

PAYMENT INFORMATION

☐ Visa   ☐ MC   Credit Card Number:
☐ Check/Money Order
   (Include with order form)   Exp. Date:

                          Signature:

Return Policy:
Any damaged or defective products must be reported within 10 days of receipt and will be replaced with an exact product replacement only. An RMA number must first be obtained from Abundant Health for all returns. Purchase price of returned items will be refunded less a 10% restocking fee. No refunds will be issued for any outdated, used, or damaged items.

Code	Wt. (oz)	Qty	Unit Price	Discount	Total
				-	=
				-	=
				-	=
				-	=
				-	=
				-	=
				-	=
				-	=
				-	=
				-	=
				-	=
				-	=
				-	=
				-	=
				-	=
				-	=
				-	=
				-	=
				-	=
SUBTOTAL:					=
Sales Tax (Utah residents only) x 0.0625:					+
(Add Ounces & See Chart on Products Page) **Shipping/Handling:**					+
TOTAL COST:					=

BILLING INFORMATION (as it appears on the credit card statement)

Name:_____

Address:_____

City/State/Zip:_____

Phone #:_____

E-mail Address:_____

SHIP-TO INFORMATION (to which order will be sent)

Name:_____

Address:_____

City/State/Zip:_____

Phone #:_____

PAYMENT INFORMATION

☐ Visa   ☐ MC   Credit Card Number:_____
☐ Check/Money Order
   (Include with order form)   Exp. Date:_____

                    Signature:_____

Return Policy:
Any damaged or defective products must be reported within 10 days of receipt and will be replaced with an exact product replacement only. An RMA number must first be obtained from Abundant Health for all returns. Purchase price of returned items will be refunded less a 10% restocking fee. No refunds will be issued for any outdated, used, or damaged items.

Code	Wt. (oz)	Qty	Unit Price	Discount	Total
				-	=
				-	=
				-	=
				-	=
				-	=
				-	=
				-	=
				-	=
				-	=
				-	=
				-	=
				-	=
				-	=
				-	=
				-	=
				-	=
				-	=
				-	=
				-	=
				-	=
			SUBTOTAL:		=
		Sales Tax (Utah residents only) x 0.0625:			+
(Add Ounces & See Chart on Products Page)		**Shipping/Handling:**			+
			TOTAL COST:		=